Q1
2005

Legal and Ethical Perspectives in Health Care: An Integrated Approach

2950664879

DEDICATION

This book is dedicated to our families. The family is that place where most of us first learn that ethical and legal conduct are worthy of our attention.

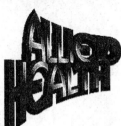

Legal and Ethical Perspectives in Health Care: An Integrated Approach

Raymond S. Edge, EdD, RRT
Dean, School of Health Professions
Maryville University-Saint Louis
Saint Louis, Missouri

John L. Krieger, Esq.
Member of American Bar Association
Member of Nevada State Bar
Member of Nevada American Inn of Court

Delmar Publishers

an International Thomson Publishing company I(T)P®

Albany • Bonn • Boston • Cincinnati • Detroit • London • Madrid
Melbourne • Mexico City • New York • Pacific Grove • Paris • San Francisco
Singapore • Tokyo • Toronto • Washington

Notice to the Reader

Publisher does not warrant or guarantee any of the products described herein or perform any independent analysis in connection with any of the product information contained herein. Publisher does not assume, and expressly disclaims, any obligation to obtain and include information other than that provided to it by the manufacturer.

The reader is expressly warned to consider and adopt all safety precautions that might be indicated by the activities herein and to avoid all potential hazards. By following the instructions contained herein, the reader willingly assumes all risks in connection with such instructions.

The publisher makes no representation or warranties of any kind, including but not limited to, the warranties of fitness for particular purpose or merchantability, nor are any such representations implied with respect to the material set forth herein, and the publisher takes no responsibility with respect to such material. The publisher shall not be liable for any special, consequential, or exemplary damages resulting, in whole or part, from the readers' use of, or reliance upon, this material.

Cover Design: Lost Acre Design, Douglas J. Hyldelund

Delmar Staff

Publisher: Susan Simpfenderfer
Acquisitions Editor: Dawn Gerrain
Developmental Editor: Debra Flis
Project Editor: Cori Filson
Production Coordinator: John Mickelbank
Art and Design Coordinator: Vincent S. Berger
Editorial Assistant: Donna L. Leto

COPYRIGHT © 1998
By Delmar Publishers
a division of International Thomson Publishing Inc.

The ITP logo is a trademark under license.

Printed in the United States of America

For more information, contact:

Delmar Publishers
3 Columbia Circle, Box 15015
Albany, New York 12212-5015

International Thomson Publishing Europe
Berkshire House
168-173 High Holborn
London, WC1V 7AA
England

Thomas Nelson Australia
102 Dodds Street
South Melbourne, 3205
Victoria, Australia

Nelson Canada
1120 Birchmount Road
Scarborough, Ontario
Canada, M1K 5G4

International Thomson Editores
Campos Eliseos 385, Piso 7
Col Polanco
11560 Mexico D F Mexico

International Thomson Publishing GmbH
Konigswinterer Strasse 418
53227 Bonn
Germany

International Thomson Publishing Asia
221 Henderson Road
#05-10 Henderson Building
Singapore 0315

International Thomson Publishing—Japan
Hirakawacho Kyowa Building, 3F
2-2-1 Hirakawacho
Chiyoda-ku, Tokyo 02
Japan

7 8 9 10 XXX 04

Library of Congress Cataloging-in-Publication Data

Edge, Raymond S.
   Legal and ethical perspectives in health care : an integrated
approach / Raymond S. Edge, John Krieger.
     p. cm.
   Includes bibliographical references and index.
   ISBN 0-8273-7684-7 (alk. paper)
   1. Medical ethics. 2. Medical laws and legislation. I. Krieger,
John, 1967-   .   II. Title.
R724.E274   1998
174'.2—dc21

          97-6627
          CIP

Table of Contents

1, 2, 4, 5, 6

Lesson 6

Lesson 6

CHAPTER 5 CONFIDENTIALITY AND VERACITY 79

Lesson 8 !

CHAPTER 6 ROLE FIDELITY 99

Preface

This text owes its birth to the students and practitioners who struggle with the legal and ethical principles of health care provision. Although often taught as separate disciplines, legal and moral aspects are always blended in practice. Although it is nice if the most ethical solution to a problem is also the most legal and vice versa, this is not always the case. One simply cannot attend to the one and ignore the other.

As an instructor of biomedical ethics and a practitioner of law, it seemed that an integration should be accomplished. This would be most useful for allied health and nursing specialists who must balance the demands of risk management and professional values on a daily basis. *Many of the programs that educate health care students often must choose between health care law and ethics, because the time allotted for non-science materials within the curriculum does not allow for two separate courses.* This is especially true in rapidly growing specialties, where the body of knowledge that must be mastered grows each year, and yet the time allotted for education remains the same. Often, the end result is a wink and a nod to the teaching of both legal and ethical aspects of practice, which serves to satisfy accreditation requirements, but leaves the students woefully unprepared for the issues they must face in practice. Whether the practitioner works at bedside, the laboratory table, or in the office, the services provided involve the lives and well-being of those served. In any such enterprise the practitioner often will find that it is not the science that brings them to frustration, but rather the complex legal, and ethical issues that must be resolved.

An important aspect of what this text is designed to promote is active participation within the classroom. The instructional objectives, case studies, review exercises, and appendices are important tools to facilitate the study. This is not an answer book, for in the disciplines of health law and ethics, there are no easy answers but rather broad fundamentals and challenging questions. The best use of this book in the classroom will require group processes, an active exchange of ideas, and the processes of critical reasoning. The review exercises found at the end of each chapter are designed to promote these activities in the class. Often to formulate an answer to the exercises, the students will be required to explore materials well beyond the text. An example of this can be found at the end of Chapter 3, where the student is asked to make a judgment based on an understanding of what was occurring in history during two separate periods. No answers are provided to any of these exercises, as the authors feel that the process of active engagement with ideas is more important than any particular answer. In fact, for most exercises there are many answers that could suffice. In these cases, the organization of the search is as important as the solution. This is also not the end all text for either subject, but rather the beginning place which, hopefully, will stimulate in the reader the desire to continue the exploration for a professional lifetime.

The chapters attempt to provide a seamless integration of materials between the legal and ethical disciplines. In many areas we were able to find complementary sub-

jects and cover them together, such as the legal requirements of privacy and the ethical duty of confidentiality. This was not always possible and certain areas are covered separately. To assist the reader in the study of health care law and ethics we
added five appendices to the text. Appendix A contains a list of the cases referenced
in the text, providing the citation for the case and the page number within the text
where a discussion may be found. Appendix B includes a discussion of normal
processes found within a lawsuit. Appendix C is an introduction to law library
research. Appendix D contains a listing of regional centers for the study of health
care ethics. Appendix E contains a representative sample of specialty codes of ethics.
A glossary is also included at the end of the text to assist the reader with unfamiliar terms. It is hoped that the reader will find the glossary and appendices useful
tools to assist in the organization of the material.

Acknowledgments

It is important to acknowledge the assistance we have had with this project, without which it would have remained only a good idea. Many of the ideas and exercises came from late night discussions with students who came to learn and stayed to be the best of teachers. Others came from class notes borrowed from a thousand sources over time, and unfortunately whose origins are lost. Where we could be sure of the source, it is provided credit; however, many of the ideas came from others, whose articles, conference talks, and private discussions are lost in the midst of time. To these we must proclaim with Blanche Dubois,"Who ever you are—I have always depended upon the kindness of strangers."

For others, the obligations are not lost in the midst of time, but are as fresh as today's conversation. Anyone who has attempted to do projects of this nature knows that they are accomplished by stealing time away from other obligations. Now that I am finished, I am appreciative that my family is still here.

I owe a special debt of obligation to Robert Francoeur who, although I have not told him personally before, has been a kind and generous mentor over the years. I owe a great debt of gratitude to Randy Groves, whose contrary, albeit at times valid, opinions regarding matters of health care ethics have helped bring mine into line with reason. I owe a sincere debt to my secretary, Ellen Harken, who was kind enough to edit the materials and to add a whole series of commas that somehow I had not thought needed. Without her, the readers would have had to contend with incredibly long sentences with sparse punctuation, which are hallmarks of what I fancy to be my style. The cartoon elements of Jeff Ek add to the understanding of the book and are deeply appreciated—it is nice to be around people with talent. And finally, I am indebted to Debra Flis, the Delmar editor who guided this book. Debra has the patience of Job and the task orientation of Simon Legree. These are not bad attributes when working with an author who seems to model his life after Scarlet O'Hara:"I'll think about that tomorrow."

I would also like to acknowledge the reviewers who provided valuable comments and suggestions. They include:

Theresa Perry, M.S.,CMA
Program Coordinator
Medical Assisting Program
Husson College
Bangor, Maine

Fatemeh Zakery, MHA, Ph.D.
Saint Louis College of Health Career
Saint Louis, Missouri

Elaine D. Schultz, RN, Med, MSN
Gerontologic Specialist
Professor of Nursing
Montgomery County Community
College
Blue Bell, Pennsylvania

Joseph Gordon
Instructor
Business Law, Business Ethics, Medical
Law, Medical Ethics
Davis Applied Technology Center
Kaysville, Utah

Paul J. Mathews, Eds, RRT, FCCM
Associate Professor-Respiratory Care
Education and Physical Therapy
Education
School of Allied Health
University of Kansas Medical Center
Kansas City, Kansas

Introduction

Our view of reality is like a map with which to negotiate the terrain of life. If the map is true and accurate, we will generally know where we are, and if we have decided on where we want to go, we will generally know how to get there. If the map is false and inaccurate, we generally will get lost.

M. Scott Peck in the *Road Less Traveled*

Key Terms

ethical	liability insurance	moral
legal	litigious	risk management

Regardless of the level of practice, the ability and opportunity to participate in the provision of health care is an awesome and wonderfully engaging enterprise. Perhaps no other industry is so exciting, meaningful, challenging, rewarding, frustrating, and just about any other adjective one wishes to add. These are meaningful professional careers. To enter the practice of health care is to enter into a social contract with other practitioners, your patients, and the community in general. This social contract calls for not only a particular set of clinical skills but also appropriate **legal, moral, ethical,** and social behaviors. For those who meet these obligations the practice of health care is personally and fiscally rewarding. At one level this book is designed to assist the practitioner in understanding the ethical and legal aspects of the health care social contract.

Like any other professional endeavor, the common area of practice belongs to each of us. It is unthinkable and unwise to believe that the health care arena will be maintained by some other group of specialists such as physicians, nurses, therapists, or whomever. The obligations of ethical and legal conduct, community service, and the refinement of knowledge are not the obligations of the few, but of many. Health care is a team effort, and all on the team are responsible for the outcomes. It is a common field where we labor, and like any other field, it requires that all those involved in the harvest maintain the space so that we can come again, and when we finally finish, leave it to others who will replace us in the labor.

Most of us see professional competence in terms of our clinical skills. Most often it is these skills that are judged as we prepare ourselves for entry into the profession. Our educational systems make reference to other professional attributes beyond clinical skills such as professional and ethical behavior, but in general unless students stray far from the path, their grades are based on being clinically quick. Yet, when we enter practice, the clinical questions are often those that seem most straightforward and it is the other attributes of being an ethical, legal, and professional practitioner that cause many to stumble.

We are in a time of great change for American health care. This is a **litigious** age. Our patient populations have come to expect miracles that cannot always be delivered. Practitioners at times find themselves seemingly between two forces, that of unhappy patients, aggrieved relatives, and their lawyers versus the **risk management** departments, other health care providers, clinical institutions, and insurance companies. Practitioners are expected to conduct themselves in such a manner as to protect their patients and at the same time avoid lawsuits against themselves and the institutions they serve. To make matters more complicated, this is also a time of legislative reform to the health care system where at times it seems the only thing that is truly stable is change.

It is hard to imagine that one can avoid the legal pitfalls of health care without some understanding of the basic structure of law. Part of the design of this text is to provide an introduction to law so that you can recognize situations that would take you beyond appropriate action. Understanding the legal ramifications of health care practice will allow for the avoidance of problems, and when that is not possible at least to indicate the need for an attorney or a conversation with the risk management department. For most of us, information regarding how to avoid legal problems will be at least as important as **liability insurance.**

Another aspect of professional practice is an attendance to ethical considerations. These are changing times for health care and in uncertain times, opportunities for ethical errors are compounded. The text will discuss basic principles such as confidentiality, patient autonomy, and justice in the context of modern health care practice. More importantly, the exercises within the text will offer several models in which to reason right answers when confronted with ethical problems with which you are unfamiliar. The moral practice of health care is an important responsibility for you as a practitioner.

This is also an age of rapid technological and social change that has pushed the frontiers of health care into uncharted territory. Many of the legal and ethical issues that are being faced are new. As examples, what is the legal status of frozen embryos if the donors have died? Are they heirs? What should we do with the information if we find a gene directly associated with violent criminal behavior? We currently have the ability to split cells and create two identical copies of a single individual. Should we? Is it ethical to use Third World nations as factories for scarce organs that are needed in the United States? Is it ethical and/or legal for a health maintenance organization to pay your primary care physicians an incentive if they order fewer tests and use fewer specialists? What place should an insurance company have in determining protocols that establish the length of stay for a particular patient group? What will be the meaning of the principle of confidentiality once we have a national data bank for health records? How will we protect individual privacy? How will we as a nation resolve the euthanasia question? Health care ethics and law are in an exciting stage of transformation as we enter the twenty-first century.

Most often health care law and health ethics are discussed in separate classes, yet the practitioner must attend to them both at the same time within the clinical setting. This text integrates both the discipline of health care law and health care ethics within a single narrative similar to how you will find it in the clinic. Being ethical and legal is not an either-or matter. As clinicians we must continually attend to both. To fail is to place your good name at risk, threatens the reputation of your specialty, may risk your personal fortune, and places your earning power in doubt. None of these are small matters.

In a clinical situation we most often base our decisions on a combination of pure technical knowledge, the facts of the particular case, and our prior clinical experience. These are somehow massaged into something which we call "clinical judgment." In ethical and legal considerations, factual knowledge contributes but rarely provides the final answer. The final decision is made by the weighing of personal values. Ethics in a sense is a generic term that describes the processes that one uses to come to decisions regarding issues of values. The ability to reason to a right answer in regard to ethical and legal questions is a real strength. One can have Nobel Prize winning clinical skills and yet come up empty if these are not combined with the ability to sort through ethical and legal considerations. The ethical and legal decisions that we make as practitioners have real consequences for ourselves and our patients. The purpose of this text is threefold, to assist the practitioner in (1) understanding the ethical and legal environment of health care, (2) making appropriate ethical and legal choices in practice, and (3) promoting ethical and legal leadership at the clinical site.

Beyond clinical, legal, ethical, and professional abilities is a set of generic overarching skills that must be mastered by all practitioners. Graduates of programs will enter a rapidly changing health care environment where nimble professionals will prosper and those unable to adapt to change will fall by the way. Graduates must be able to communicate orally and in writing, they must be able to collaborate in groups, they must be able to think critically. The narrow, uncritical thinker has only one opinion to assist in decision making. Individuals who can communicate, collaborate, think well and fairmindedly not only regarding their own viewpoints but also about beliefs and viewpoints that are diametrically opposed to their own, will be much in demand.

The context of health care law and ethics provides an excellent arena for the practice of communication, collaboration, and critical thinking. Although the text is filled with information, the authors of the text have attempted to avoid telling the reader what to think, believing that the true value of the information provided will be found when individuals are engaged in the process of thinking through and defending positions that they have organized for themselves. Throughout the text you will find exercises that will give you practice in refining generalizations, comparing and contrasting situations, transferring insights into new contexts, evaluating the credibility of sources, raising and pursuing significant questions, and generating your own perspective on the issues. These are all important abilities for practitioners who find themselves practicing in a rapidly changing health care environment. As you proceed through the text, the objectives at the beginning of each chapter will assist you in maintaining your focus of study. Finally, look up the key terms in the glossary as it will assist you in understanding the terms as they are being used by the authors.

When it comes to the legal and ethical aspects of health care we are rarely faced with decisions that call for simple right or wrong choices. However, while there may not be a clear right answer, there are many choices that must not be made. In these areas although there is room for much disagreement, that should not be taken to mean that all opinions have equal validity. Most practitioners would rather be ethical than unethical, legal than illegal. This text is designed to assist you in the process of making ethical and legal choices. The choices that we as practitioners make in these areas will speak volumes about ourselves and our professions.

CHAPTER 1

Human Value Development and the Foundation of Law

Goal

To understand the nature of human value development and the development of the American legal system.

Objectives

At the conclusion of this chapter, the reader should understand and be able to:

1. Differentiate between needs and values.
2. List the three value development stages of Lawrence Kohlberg.
3. Differentiate between moral systems and legal systems.
4. Explain why relativism is an inadequate basis for ethical decision making.
5. List three intentional torts that are often found in health care practice.
6. List four criteria that must be satisfied to sustain a claim of negligence.
7. Differentiate between public and private law.
8. Identify the basic principles involved in moral reasoning regarding health care and show their application to the code of ethics of your particular specialty.
9. Define the basic principles involved in health care.
10. Explain how informed consent and autonomy are related.
11. Outline the theoretical position of Carol Gilligan.
12. Explain the nature of the disagreement between Carol Gilligan and Lawrence Kohlberg found in their writings.
13. Define value cohort, within the context of the writings of Morris Massey.

14. Identify three basic principles and three basic misconceptions found in the study of law.

Key Terms

alegal	criminal law	nonmaleficence
altruism	defendant	plantiff
amoral	distributive justice	procedural justice
assault	ethics	relativism
autonomy	false imprisonment	res ipsa loquitur
battery	felony	respect for persons
beneficence	informed consent	role fidelity
civil law	invasion of privacy	stare decisis
common law	justice	statutory law
compensatory justice	liability	tort
confidentiality	misdemeanor	veracity
contract law	negligence	world view

NEEDS AND VALUES

> *When the words of a law are clear and free from all ambiguity, the letter of it is not to be disregarded under the pretext of pursuing its spirit.*

Pennsylvania Statutory Construction Act

> *The values by which we are to survive are not rules for just and unjust conduct, but are those deeper illuminations in whose light justice and injustice, good and evil, means and ends are seen in fearful sharpness of outline.*

Jacob Bronowski (1908–74), British scientist, author

The *why* of human behavior is the study of several academic specialties and a major preoccupation of sages, prophets, and philosophers throughout all ages. How is it that man has such a wide range of potential behaviors? How is it that, at one moment we seem to emulate the very angels themselves, and in the next, act as if we are still in the imagined state of nature described by Thomas Hobbes (1651), where life is nasty, brutish, and short? Although it is easy to see that behavior is nonrandom and designed to produce some end, it is not always easy to determine the cause and effect of our actions. One way to look at human behavior is to divide our actions as attempts to satisfy either our needs or our values.

Perhaps the best known work regarding the interaction of needs and behaviors is the hierarchy of needs by the humanist psychologist Abraham Maslow (1987). This seminal work provided an easily understood model of needs based on human motivation.

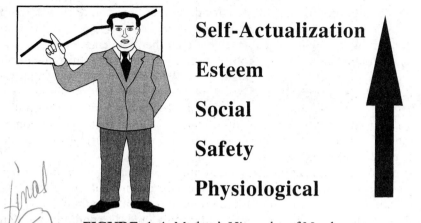

FIGURE 1–1 Maslow's Hierarchy of Needs

According to the theory, feelings of isolation result in need-based activities such as joining a bowling team, whereas food-gathering activities would be explained by motivation at the physiological level. Figure 1–1 lists the levels of Maslow's hierarchy of needs.

Although we might disagree with Maslow's explanation regarding a particular situation, under most circumstances the model is a persuasive explanation of observable cause-and-effect behaviors. Most observable human behavior does seem to be explainable as attempts to satisfy a given set of needs. If the question is asked, what a normal person would do in a given context, you are probably dealing with needs-based motivation. According to Maslow, as each need level is satisfied, the needs of the next level on the hierarchy become the dominant motivators for our actions. For example, once the physiological needs such as hunger are met, the individual no longer responds to that portion of the hierarchy and consequently moves to the next step. If the hierarchy of needs is correct, and the observer astute enough to determine which level of need was operational in a given context, then potentially they could predict the nature of the next action. However, we are rarely so astute in our observations that we can predict with any certainty what our fellow humans are likely to do.

Another problem with a needs-based theory is that at times human actions do not appear to be related to needs. In these circumstances, the individual seems to move away from needs-based considerations and appears to consult an inner subjective set of feelings, attitudes, beliefs, and opinions which comprise their personal value system. In these instances, individuals seem to ask themselves not what they would do, but rather what they should do.

To see how different the value system is from that of a needs system, one need only look at the conduct of the male passengers during the sinking of the *Titanic*. Obviously their need for survival was preeminent and could have explained a host of actions, including forcing their way onto the lifeboats. However, the predominate value of the era that men should protect women and children prevailed. Therefore, as the ship went down, the bands played and the men stood aside even at the peril of their lives. Similarly, the healthcare providers that sacrifice some level of personal safety to work with contagious patients, or the mother who takes on the park bully to protect her children, are acting from a position of value and are making decisions based on a belief about what one ought to do. An interesting aspect of value decisions is that they seem directly tied to specific cultural and historical contexts. One might wonder, given events similar to the *Titanic* tale, if we would see similar behaviors displayed in our modern age of gender equity. In a recent accident on board a ship the captain and crew were the first off, leaving the passengers to be rescued later. Times do change.

Our system of law is another set of determinants which is in place to shape the behaviors of people. We can think of law as a set of principles and processes by which people within a society seek to settle disputes and problems without resorting to force and violence. In some sense, law can be considered the minimum standard of expected performance between individuals in a society. Laws can be thought of as general rules of conduct whose compliance is enforced by governmentally imposed penalties. Laws govern the relationships among private individuals, organizations, government, and the private sector.

One can consider that the law establishes the lowest level of expected performance in the health care setting. To ensure that we as practitioners abide by this lowest standard, many of our codes of professional ethics contain rules that require us to stay within the law in our professional conduct. An interesting example of this can be seen in the American Medical Association's *1992 Code of Medical Ethics Current Opinions,* which states:

> *Ethical standards of professional conduct and responsibility may exceed but are never less than, nor contrary to, those required by law. . . . Ethical pronouncements of the Council on Ethical and Judicial Affairs and the House of Delegates should not be so interpreted, construed or applied as to encourage conduct which violates a valid law.*

On the surface this AMA standard seems reasonable and appropriate; however, consider that the physicians in National Socialist Germany performed horrendous experiments on individuals who they considered less than human. These physicians were well within the law of that nation but their acts have been judged immoral and reprehensible by the world.

Moral and ethical decisions can be seen as a less prescriptive and perhaps a higher standard of conduct than just obeying the law. Fortunately, under the circumstances of our practice, moral acts are generally legal acts. It is clearly possible, however, for an act to be medically correct, legally correct, and morally reprehensible to the individual practitioner. If you were to find yourself in such a situation, you must be prepared to remove yourself from the process or be prepared to take action based upon your own personal compass, knowing that there can be unfortunate consequences, regardless of the decision. Again, a quote from the American Medical Association (1992) guidelines is illustrative:

> *Violation of governmental laws may subject the physician to civil or criminal liability. Expulsion from membership is the maximal penalty that may be imposed by a medical society upon a physician who violates the ethical standards involving a breach in moral duty or principles.*

Lesson 4
pp 5 - 17

TABLE 1–1
Sanction comparisons between inappropriate legal, ethical, and professional etiquette

Area	Judgment	Sanctions
Ethics	Right or Wrong	Loss of professional reputation, loss of professional consortium, personal remorse
Legal	Legal or Illegal	Loss of professional reputation, loss of professional consortium, punishments determined under law
Professional etiquette	Proper or Improper	Professional disapprobation

As an example, if you choose to obey the law, you might place yourself in a situation in which you are going against your own personal values, diminishing your credibility in your own eyes. If, on the other hand, you obey your personal values and break the law, you must be prepared to face the social and legal consequences associated with your criminal activity and perhaps expulsion from the health provider community. The authors of this book will never recommend that you as an individual break any law; yet, we think that most see great value in the efforts of Martin Luther King Jr., Henry David Thoreau, and Mahatma Gandhi—all of whom would be less memorable if they had stayed within the laws of their time.

The practice of health care goes well beyond technical competence, and all practitioners must attend to the legal, ethical, and social etiquette requirements of their roles. Practitioners who fail to master these attendant duties will be a continual frustration to those who must work with them and will find themselves being sanctioned for their activities. Table 1–1 differentiates the types of sanctions commonly associated with lapses in appropriate legal, ethical, and professional etiquette. It should be pointed out that a single act could have consequences that involve our ethical, legal, and professional standing.

VALUE DEVELOPMENT

Human babies are born with a series of undifferentiated potentials. A good example of this undifferentiated potential is our ability to learn a language, yet the particular language is not proscribed by our genetic heritage. In this same sense, man has the innate capacity to acquire moral beliefs, but the value system that we develop is dependent upon the cultural framework in which we live. This capacity to become ethical beings and to conform to universal principles of mutual cooperation and **altruism** seems as old as the species itself. One of the earliest found skeletal remains of Neanderthal man was that of an individual, approximately 50 years of age, whose bones indicate that he suffered from a severe debilitating form of arthritis. His impediment made it unlikely that he could hunt or engage in strenuous activity, and therefore was dependent upon the caring of his group for his survival. The fact that he survived separated these early men from all other creatures. No other creatures in

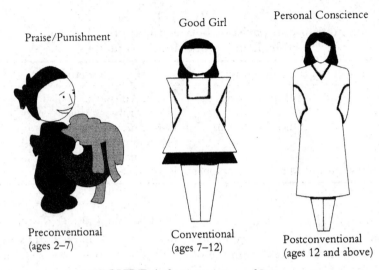

Praise/Punishment   Good Girl   Personal Conscience

Preconventional   Conventional   Postconventional
(ages 2–7)   (ages 7–12)   (ages 12 and above)

FIGURE 1–2 Orientation of Stages

the animal kingdom are willing or able to sustain a fallen individual. Although Neanderthal man may not have had words to express concepts such as love, altruism, and individual respect, individuals within the culture seemingly exhibited behaviors by which these terms are defined.

We are born into this world without a prescribed set of rules for what we should do in any given situation. Value development is a product of our interactions with our cultural environment. The foremost theorists in value development are Jean Piaget (1896–1980) and Lawrence Kohlberg (1981). Piaget's groundbreaking work, *The Moral Development of the Child* (1962), established much of the current thinking regarding value and moral development. Both Kohlberg and Piaget stressed that value development is intimately tied to the individual's cognitive and psychomotor development. Figure 1–2 identifies orientation stages that an individual passes through in value development according to Kohlberg's theory (Edge & Groves, 1994). In the first phase of the preconventional stage the child responds to the prevailing cultural values of right and wrong, good and evil. The child has little understanding of the values themselves and a reliance upon the authority of others. In the conventional stage the child conforms to societal expectations of family, group, or nation. This stage includes a form of good boy/good girl orientation as the child seeks to conform to expected social conventions. In the latter portion of this level, the focus becomes fixed on the rules, social order, and respect for authority. The focus of the postconventional stage is the development of a social contract and the making of autonomous decisions apart from outside authorities. In the final portion of this stage the individual develops an understanding of abstract qualities such as justice and respect for the rights and dignity of others. At this point the individual is in essence morally autonomous and capable of deciding what is right through the use of personal conscience.

According to the model the individual can be seen as growing through several stages of value orientation. For Kohlberg, the highest personal value for humans was equality, where the individual decided the issues based on an internal set of personal principles or rules. In recent years, Carol Gilligan (1982) has criticized the Kohlberg theory as being male centered, stating that perhaps the highest value for men was equality, but that women followed a different value development path that led them to value responsibility as the highest value. This gender difference, described by Gilligan, is somewhat borne out of studies using the typological profile created by Isabel Myers and Katherine Briggs (1980), known commonly as the MBTI. The MBTI examines an individual's placement within a set of normal human variables such as introversion and extroversion, intuition and sensing, thinking and feeling, and judging and perceiving.

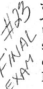

✷Men and women score equally on all the major dimensions of the instrument with the exception of thinking and feeling—the dimension most closely related to decision making. In this one dimension, a majority of the men tested prefer to make decisions based on analysis, rules, and principles which would be in keeping with Kohlberg's theory. The majority of women, however, preferred a decision-making process that includes the considerations of relationships, harmony, and responsibilities. These findings would indicate that men and women do tend to use different value criteria when making decisions and the findings seem to verify Gilligan's view that men and women follow different value development paths. In his writings after 1985, Kohlberg revised his scoring methodology to account for a possible gender bias.✷

Individually, we possess an organized system of thoughts, feelings, opinions, and beliefs **(world view)** with which we screen the events occurring around us. It is with this subjective screen, based on our culture and life experiences, that we judge the rightness or wrongness of actions as they pertain to what a person should do in a given situation. Whether an individual feels comfortable taking pens from work, pushing to the front of a line, buying goods beyond personal needs, obeying the law, or listening quietly as elders speak is a reflection of the individual's particular world view and value programming. Even when we feel that we have rejected or grown beyond the value programming of our childhood, we are often surprised that our decisions resonate with the events of the past.

> *Although a system may cease to exist in the legal sense or as a structure of power, its values (or anti-values), its philosophy, its teachings remain in us. They rule our thinking, our conduct, our attitude to others. The situation is a demonic paradox: we have toppled the system but we still carry its genes.*

> Ryszard Kapuscinski (1991), Polish journalist

The concept of being affected by the cultural programming of our past forms the basis of the work by Morris Massey (1980). He described four value groupings within American society seemingly related to the historical events of people's childhoods. Certain events that happen to us as a group (e.g., Great Depression, World War II, death of President Kennedy, Vietnam War) shape us as a generational value cohort. An excellent example of this cohort programming can be seen in the population that was young during the Great Depression era of the 1930s. As a group, this is a very security-conscious portion of our population. Whether real or imagined, the ideas of doing without, or "walking five miles to school through the snow," or "a penny saved is a penny earned" resonate through this whole population. Yet, these notions seem almost mythic to that portion of the population programmed in the mid '50s and '60s. Although some individuals may escape the impact of certain eras (for example, a hermit may escape the impact of urbanization and the idle rich may escape economic downturns), it is clear that certain events such as the assassination of President Kennedy have a profound effect upon the world view of those affected by the event. For a certain cohort of Americans, the events in Dallas in 1963 are seared into the collective memories in vivid detail, and as a group, some important element of optimism was forever lost.

BASIC PRINCIPLES OF HEALTH CARE

Over the course of our lives, each of us as humans develops a coherent set of beliefs, attitudes, feelings, and opinions, with which we judge the events of the world around us—good and bad, right and wrong, positive and negative. Table 1–2 is a listing of a group of value propositions that culturally we have come to recognize as universal principles of positive values.

Professional **ethics,** such as those found in health care and health-related law, are applied ethics. They are designed to promote ethical and legal practice within a profession. These are generally thought to promote the major purpose of the professional group. In health care, this is usually expressed as the pursuit of good health, with the prevention of death and the alleviation of suffering as secondary goals. The basic operative ethical principles that have been developed to assist health care professionals in determining right from wrong in value decisions regarding health care practice are **respect for persons, beneficence,** ✻ **nonmaleficence, justice,** and **role fidelity.** In practice, the principle of respect for persons has come to include the behaviors attendant with respect for personal **autonomy, confidentiality,** and **veracity.** It is from these basic principles that we derive the rules found in our codes of professional ethics. Table 1–3 lists some basic principles of health care. Although the principles are listed in a set order, it is not intended that they should be considered in any hierarchy of importance. ✻ THE ETHICAL PrinCiPLE OF DoinG No HArM.

Respect for Persons

The earliest traditions from which our health care principles stem are from the Cult of Aesculapius. According to these traditions the health care practice is strictly

TABLE 1–2
Universal Principles—Positive Values

• Honesty	• Benevolence
• Tolerance	• Charity
• Lawfulness	• Equality
• Veracity	• Personal Inviolability
• Love	• Justice
• Responsible Behavior	• Personal Privacy

a patient-practitioner interaction aimed at getting the particular individual well. In this light, care is to be aggressively patient centered, and the practitioner should not mix social, political, or economic considerations with the care of the individual patient. Important among these traditions are autonomy, confidentiality, and veracity, which speak to a special attitude of respect toward the individual.

Autonomy. Autonomy is synonymous with self-determination. Autonomy comes from the Greek terms *autos* (self) and *nomos* (governance). In health it has come to mean a special form of personal liberty, where individuals are free to choose and implement their own decisions, free from deceit, duress, constraint, and coercion. It is from this general principle that the secondary principle of **informed consent** flows. It is obvious that without adequate information regarding the nature of the condition, the available options, and the associated risks, a patient is not truly in a position where self-determination has validity.

Confidentiality. Confidentiality is perhaps the easiest to understand and the hardest to practice of all the basic principles of health care ethics. It is clear that if the patient felt that information regarding the patient's body or condition was the subject of public conversation, a wide gulf of distrust would exist between that patient and the provider. This fear of personal disclosure has, in the past, led minors with sexually transmitted diseases to suffer without care, afraid that the health care system was required to notify their parents. In modern health care, the use of computer terminals, which allow access to patient information in a variety of sites throughout the hospital, has made the control of this information difficult. Yet difficult or not, this is an important principle of practice whose abuse threatens to harm patients, the professions, and society in general who depend upon the services provided.

It is clear that providers need to communicate with patients the limitations of confidentiality in the modern setting. Beyond the patient-provider relationship are the legal obligations of the health care system to the rest of society. The patient should be told of any legal requirements that mandate the breaking of confidentiality and the nature of the disclosure.

Veracity. Veracity deals with the need for truth-telling in the patient-provider relationship. It is clear that if the patient does not disclose, or lies in regard to the nature of the illness, that this would inhibit the provider's ability to treat the patient. Equally

TABLE 1–3
Basic Principles of Health Care

• Respect for Persons	• Justice
confidentiality	• Role Fidelity
autonomy	• Beneficence
veracity	• Nonmaleficence

HIPPOCRATIC OATH

I swear by Apollo Physician and Asclepius and Hygieia and Panaceia and all the gods and goddesses, making them my witnesses, that I will fulfill according to my ability and judgment this oath and this covenant:

I will apply dietetic measures for the benefit of the sick according to my ability and judgment; I will keep them from harm and injustice.

I will neither give a deadly drug to anybody if asked for it, nor will I make a suggestion to this effect. Similarly I will not give a woman an abortive remedy. In purity and holiness I will guard my life and my art.

I will not use the knife, not even on sufferers from stone, but will withdraw in favor of such men as are engaged in this work.

Whatever houses I may visit, I will come for the benefit of the sick, remaining free of all intentional injustices, of all mischief and in particular of sexual relations with both female and male persons, be they free or slaves.

What I may see or hear in the course of the treatment or even outside of the treatment in regard to the life of men, which on no account one must noise abroad, I will keep to myself holding such things shameful to be spoken about.

If I fulfill this oath and do not violate it, may it be granted to me to enjoy life and art, being honored with fame among all men for all time to come; if I transgress it and swear falsely, may the opposite of all this be my lot.

FIGURE 1–3 Hippocratic Oath

---

clear is that lying to the patient, in regard to the illness impedes the patient's ability to make autonomous decisions. Health care is best provided in a relationship of trust where practitioner and provider are bound in an agreement of mutual truth.

Beneficence

In common English, beneficence has come to mean acts of charity and mercy. In regard to health care, however, it expresses a duty on the part of the practitioner to promote the health and welfare of the patient above other considerations, while attending to and honoring patient autonomy. Figure 1–3 is the Hippocratic Oath, which has several admonitions that commit the health care provider to the principle of beneficence. Like many of the fundamental principles of health care, beneficence seems to run counter to other important elements in the current health care arena, such as cost containment. There appears to be a real question as to whether a practitioner who is seeking to reduce costs by eliminating tests, treatments, and time in the hospital can at the same time be promoting the health and welfare of the individual patient above other considerations. *Good point is where the balance?*

Nonmaleficence

Most health care professional pledges, or codes of care, echo the principle paraphrased from the Hippocratic Oath statement, "I will never use treatment to injure or harm the sick." Although these seem quite similar to the duty of beneficence, some philosophers distinguish the two in the following manner:

Nonmaleficence—One ought not to inflict evil or harm.

Beneficence—   One ought to prevent evil or harm.

One ought to remove evil or harm.

One ought to do or promote good.

With beneficence, the obligation is toward positive action, toward preventing harm, and promoting good. With nonmaleficence, the obligation is stated in negative terms. We are to refrain from inflicting harm. In some sense, it is hard to imagine why we would need to be admonished to not harm our patients. Yet many of our modern therapies and practices make it necessary to do cost-benefit ratio analysis to determine when beneficence ends and maleficence begins. Both beneficence and nonmaleficence are important value principles for health care. The patient's assumption that health care providers are struggling incessantly to do them good and to keep them from harm is of great importance to morale. This is especially true for the patient who is garnering all available strength to fight an illness.

Justice

The principle of justice deals with the concepts of fairness, just desserts, and entitlements. What is due the individual? Like confidentiality, the maintenance of this principle seems simple in the abstract and complex in application. What does a just society provide in the way of **procedural justice,** or due process? What does a just society provide regarding **distributive justice,** when it must allocate scarce resources such as health care? When one is harmed, how does a just society respond in regard to **compensatory justice?** The recent cases when cigarette smokers and state governments have attempted to receive compensation from tobacco companies for the harm caused by use of their products suggest how important an issue compensatory justice could become in the future. If the courts were to allow the connection to be made and grant compensation to state governments, allowing them to recover their health care costs associated with tobacco usage, it is unclear how these companies could remain in business.

It is clear that as we reform our health care system, the principle of justice, in regard to equity and access to health care services, will become the major issue. What is fair? Must the system provide everything for everyone or will a decent minimum be acceptable for some elements of our society?

Role Fidelity

Modern health care is the practice of a team. It is no longer possible for a single individual to maintain the internal data bank of information, or the set of skills needed to provide rational care. The allied health specialties alone contain over 100 distinct areas of practice. When these specialists are added to that of nursing, they provide well over 80 percent of the care provided. Whatever the assigned role, the ethics of health care require that the practitioner practice faithfully within the constraints of the prescribed role. In most cases, the areas of acceptable practice are delineated within the scope of the practice section of the state legislation that enables that profession's practice.

THE FOUNDATIONS OF LAW

In his writings, the Greek philosopher Plato proposed an ideal state ruled by a wise philosopher king. In this state, disputes between individuals would be settled by the king applying unwritten laws guided by reason. Even in his own time, Plato came to understand that this was an unworkable ideal and agreed upon disputes being settled by authorities using written laws that were to be applied without regard to the circumstances of the individuals involved. It is from this neutral application of law that we take the tradition of a rule of law and not of people.

The basic sources for modern law are **common law** which emanates from judicial decisions, **statutory law** which arises from legislative bodies, and administrative law which flows from the rules, regulations, and decisions of administrative agencies. Common law is a set of principles that have evolved from the practices of the past and continue to evolve and expand from the judicial decisions that arise from court cases. Our system of law was derived from that of Great Britain; many of the legal principles and rules applied today had their origin in English common law. Cases arise out of disputes between individuals and, in deciding these cases, the judge examines earlier cases involving similar problems and circumstances to discover general principles that can be applied to the case at hand. This has given rise to the principle of **stare decisis,** which translated means "let the decision stand." The use of the principle stare decisis has provided the system with needed stability and yet has allowed for the creation of new principles as new or changing patterns of facts have emerged.

THE SYSTEM OF LAW

Our system of law can be divided into two basic elements—public and private law. The law that deals with the relationships between citizen and citizen, or that is concerned with the definition, regulation, and enforcement of rights in cases when both the parties involved are private citizens, is known as private law. Private law is concerned with the recognition and enforcement of the rights and duties of private citizens and organizations. **Torts** and **contract law** are two basic types of private law.

A tort is a private or civil wrong or injury, other than breach of contract, for which the court will provide a remedy in the form of an action for damages. The legal wrong committed upon the person may be a direct invasion of some legal right of the individual; the infraction of some public duty by which special damages accrue to the individual; or the violation of some private obligation by which the damages accrue to the individual. Every tort action has three elements: the existence of a legal duty owing from **defendant** to **plaintiff**, a breach of that duty, and damages which are a proximate result. Torts are usually classified into three broad categories: negligent torts, intentional torts, and torts in which the **liability** is assessed irrespective of fault (strict liability), such as claims against the manufacturers of defective medical products. Judges have long recognized that tort law can be used to influence behavior. As an example, if an individual is harmed by a medical product and the manufacturer can be sued by the customer, the company is more likely to provide additional instructions and warning labels on the devices (Anderson & Anderson, 1987). Some common forms of intentional torts that have implications within the health care setting are (Pozgar, 1993):

1. **Assault** and **Battery**
2. Defamation of Character
3. **False Imprisonment**
4. **Invasion of Privacy**

A basic difference between intentional torts and **negligence** is intent, which is present in intentional torts and absent in negligence. A second important difference is that intentional torts involve a willful act that violates another's interest, whereas in negligence, the problem is as likely to be an omission of an act that is deemed reasonable. Negligence also takes several forms, of which the most common are (Pozgar, 1993):

1. Malpractice—carelessness or negligence on the part of a professional.
2. Malfeasance—the execution of an unlawful or improper act.
3. Misfeasance—the improper performance of an act that leads to injury.
4. Nonfeasance—the failure to perform an act, when there is a duty to act.
5. Criminal negligence—the reckless disregard for the safety of another.

To sustain a claim of negligence, evidence of the following must be in place (these are often called the four Ds of a negligence claim):

Duty—A provider-patient relationship must be established. A duty to care must exist.

Dereliction of Duty—A breach of duty; when the provider fails to act as an ordinary competent provider would have acted in a similar situation.

Direct Cause—The breach of duty was the direct cause of the injury, damage, or loss.

Damages—An injury or loss actually took place.

Within the text, subjects such as defamation of character, malpractice, and assault and battery will be amplified within the sections that deal with our moral duties that are most closely related to our legal obligations. As an example, the subject of privacy will be examined within the context of our moral obligation to maintain patient confidentiality.

In breach of contract, there is a failure, without legal excuse, to perform any promise that comprises the whole or part of the contract. The formal contract is established when both parties have promised to be bound within the agreement. Thus, when one party offers to do something in exchange for the other party's agreement to do something, the contract is formed by the acceptance of the offer.

Contractual duty can occur as the result of signing formal documents or can arise out of implication. For example, in a case when the patient shows up in the emergency room and is met by the receiving nurse, fills out the paperwork, and tells the nurse the main problem, it implies that the patient is willing to pay for the services. Conversely, having the patient fill out the paperwork and getting the medical history on the case implies a promise to provide treatment.

Public law deals with the relationships between private parties and the government, and is that branch of law that is concerned with the state in its political or sovereign capacity. It consists generally of constitutional, administrative, criminal, and international law. Constitutional law is that branch of national and state law that deals with the organization, invested powers, and framework of government. Under our national constitution and the various state constitutions, legislative bodies are given the power to enact laws to govern the people. Examples of statutory law, at the national level, might be the creation of such agencies as the Social Security Administration and the Internal Revenue System. Important state statutes that impact the provision of health care include those related to:

- health providers practice acts
- informed consent
- peer review
- Good Samaritan Act
- living will statute
- child abuse laws
- competency determination
- emergency medical services

Practice acts for health care providers are examples of statutory law at the state level. Administrative law is that body of rules and regulations, orders and decisions, that is created by administrative agencies to implement their powers and duties. OSHA rules and regulations are examples of administrative law. **Criminal law** is an important aspect of public law which prohibits conduct deemed injurious to public order and provides for punishment of those found to have engaged in prohibited practices. It should be noted that many times an act can have both private **(civil law)** and criminal (public law) ramifications. An example of this can be seen in the now notorious O.J. Simpson cases. Mr. Simpson was first acquitted of the death of his wife and Ronald Goldman under criminal law and then was convicted in a civil case filed for wrongful death. The important differences between criminal and civil law can be seen in the level of proof required between the two case types and the reparations required. The level of proof in civil cases is less rigorous and the reparations called for is monetary rather than punitory.

Crimes are divided, by their seriousness and levels of punishment, into felonies and misdemeanors. The **felony** is the far more serious breach of law and is punishable by death or imprisonment in a state or federal penitentiary. A **misdemeanor** is a crime punishable by less than a year incarceration in a jail or house of correction. Examples of common misdemeanors are the theft of small amounts of money, disorderly conduct, or breaking into an automobile. Legislators enact laws that determine whether an act is a crime and whether it will be considered a felony or misdemeanor. Some activities such as murder, rape, sodomy, larceny, manslaughter, burglary, robbery, and arson have been determined by common law to be felonies. The general thrust of public law, in all of its forms, is to assist the society in attaining its valid public goals.

FUNDAMENTAL PRINCIPLES OF LAW AND LEGAL MISPERCEPTIONS

Like ethics, law is guided by fundamental principles. The first of these is a concern for justice and fairness. The second is plasticity and change. Although the law from the outside is seemingly complete and solid, it is a shifting process that reacts to its environment. The third principle is that acts are judged on the universal standard of the reasonable person. What would a similarly trained, reasonable and prudent person have done in that particular situation? The fourth fundamental principle is that of individual rights and responsibilities. Failure to meet one's responsibilities affects one's rights. The doctrine of personal responsibility is fundamental to the rule of law. It holds that every person is liable for his own actions (Hubbard, 1982).

Because law seems clearer and less subjective than questions regarding ethics, several misperceptions about the nature of law have developed. First, there is a feeling that law is somehow all inclusive and that if you needed a legal determination, all you would need to do is apply the correct legal precedent. The law, in fact, is incomplete and always growing. This is especially true in areas such as health care and technology, where new environments are being created that have yet to be explored by law. It is possible in these areas for something to be neither legal nor illegal. A possible example of this pertains to the legal rights of human clones. For instance, although it is scientifically possible to split a single egg and create two identical human beings, we have not developed the legal body of doctrines to deal with the complex issues that might come should we begin this practice.

Clones yes, but what of Embryos & frozen sperm?

✳ A second misperception arises out of the view that law is prescribed and certain. That is, if one does this, the law will do that, with the act determining a fixed consequence. Yet, given that there are areas for which we have no legal rulings, there cannot be a certainty how these gaps will be filled. Even in areas where we have legal precedence, growth and change occur. One need only consider the current debate regarding civil rights to see how the law, at one time, sanctioned preferential treatment based on considerations of race and gender, and now seems to be moving to condemn such considerations.

✳ A third misperception is that the law tells us what to do. In this thinking, legal acts are those things we should do and illegal acts are to be avoided. In most cases it is prudent to view the law as a guide to proper behavior, yet it would be a mistake to confuse legal and ethical behavior. For periods of time, the use of contraceptives was illegal in certain jurisdictions, and yet the decision to control one's own reproduction seems a very appropriate human right. Were the citizens using contraceptives and controlling their reproductive lives wrong? Illegal? Perhaps. Maybe or maybe not.

CONCLUSION

This chapter prepared the foundation for the integrated study of the legal and ethical aspects of health care. Health care law and ethics are two different disciplines to which every health care provider must attend as they practice their specialty. Unlike many clinical questions, answers to ethical and legal problems are often not well defined. Within the specialty educational programs, often the time allotted to the study of these subjects is not sufficient to the needs of the graduate as these are rapidly changing times. Yet, changing or no, our ability to handle the legal and ethical questions with which we are faced in our practice setting will make all the difference in regard to our professional lives.

Unfortunately many Americans are like the students described in *The Closing of the American Mind* by Allan Bloom (1987). The one value with which these individuals feel comfortable is that truth is relative. This proposition is based on an accommodation to a pluralistic culture. History is viewed as a past when men thought that they had the truth, and in the name of this truth, justified outrageous persecutions, wars, slavery, xenophobic racism, and even witch burning. The point that these students take from this reading of history is that the "true believer" is a dangerous person, and that only in the avoidance of thinking that your way is the right way, can we survive. Openness and tolerance have become, for these students, the only plausible stance in the face of various claims to truth and an appropriate lifestyle. With this belief in **relativism,** the rational person then would not be concerned with correcting the mistakes from the past, but would rather decide that all truth is relative and consider one view equal to all other views.

Few health care practitioners would be comfortable in taking a relativistic view of values or law. In our common practice, we must constantly attend to the dictates of law, professional conduct, and personal values. The decisions that we must make are of such an important nature that the flip of a coin will not do.

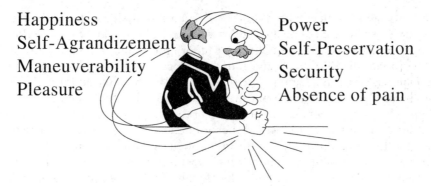

Happiness
Self-Agrandizement
Maneuverability
Pleasure

Power
Self-Preservation
Security
Absence of pain

FIGURE 1–4 Hedonistic World View

Others in our society have advocated a hedonistic value system where *is* and *ought* are the same and the individual becomes devoid of other-regarding impulses. For such an individual, the major guideposts for decisions are desire and aversion, and nothing can be right or wrong apart from them. This attitude of self-absorption was captured in the popular slogan, "He who dies with the most toys wins." Figure 1–4 lists the values associated with this world view. However, individual self-interest is inadequate as a base for legal and moral decision making in health care. Some answers truly are better than others—some decisions must not be made. To take an **amoral** or **alegal** position that somehow all answers to moral or legal questions are equal and that individuals are a law unto themselves, would be unacceptable in health care practice.

The philosopher Nietzsche was correct in his declaration that we are valuing animals. In the practice of health care, each of us must come to understand the nature of the legal and professional environment. Unlike the beasts of the forest whose decisions are governed by a prescribed set of instincts, we are condemned to lives of freedom and choice. In the practice of health care, a position of "anything goes" is unacceptable.

Legal Case Study: *Ybarra v. Spangard*, 154 P.2d 687 (Cal. 1944)

In this case the patient entered the hospital with abdominal pain and was diagnosed as having acute appendicitis. An appendectomy was arranged, with the surgery to be performed by Drs. S and Dr. T. Dr. R was the anesthetist in charge. Dr. R adjusted the patient for the operation by pulling his body to the head of the operating table. The patient remembers Dr. R laying him back against two hard objects at the top of his shoulders, about two inches below his neck. When he awoke from the operation he felt a sharp pain about halfway between the neck and the point of the right shoulder.

Dr. T ordered diathermy treatments for the patient while he remained in the hospital to combat the pain. However, the pain did not cease but spread down to the lower part of his arm, and after his release from the hospital the condition grew worse. The patient eventually was unable to rotate or lift his arm, and developed paralysis and atrophy of the muscles around the shoulder. Later, the patient consulted with Drs. G and F, both of whom concluded that his paralysis was the result of trauma or injury by pressure or strain applied between his right shoulder and neck. Prior to the operation, the patient never had any pain or injury to his right arm or shoulder.

The patient sued Drs. R, S, and T under a doctrine of negligence known as ***res ipsa loquitur,*** which is a Latin phrase that means "the thing speaks for itself." In this case, the paralysis was not an event that would normally occur in an operation for an appendectomy except for negligence. Prior to the operation, the patient's arm and shoulder were perfectly healthy and therefore could not have been a contributory cause. Furthermore, due to the fact that the patient was unconscious throughout the operation, he was unable to identify which doctor was responsible for the trauma to his shoulder and neck area. The court therefore held that when a patient receives unusual injuries while unconscious and in the course of medical treatment, all health care providers who had control over the patient's body or the instrumentalities which may have caused the injuries may be liable for negligence.

The court also noted that "assisting physicians and nurses may be employed by the hospital, or engaged by the patient, [consequently] they normally become the temporary servants or agents of the surgeon in charge while the operation is in progress, and liability may be imposed upon him for their negligent acts." Hence, Drs. S and T could be held to be negligent, even if Dr. R was solely responsible for the paralyzing injury to the patient.

1. Which form of negligence best fits this case?   *8 OR 1*

2. Are all the elements for a claim of negligence found in the case? Identify each of the four Ds. *Yes. There was a patient provider relationship Dr. R should have been more aware of the patient's position, because of Dr. R's placement of the patient, the patient sustained an injury. There has obviously been a loss since the patient suffered paralysis of the right arm.*

REVIEW EXERCISES

1. The following quote is from Maya Angelou, author of *I Know Why the Caged Bird Sings.*

    All of childhood's unanswered questions must finally be passed back to the town and answered there. Heroes and bogey men, values and dislikes, are first encountered and labeled in that early environment. In later years they change faces, places and maybe races, tactics, intensities and goals, but beneath those penetrable masks they wear forever the stocking-capped faces of childhood.

    a. The concept expressed that somehow our values find their roots in the experiences of our childhood is most in keeping with which value theorist? *Kohlberg*

    b. List three personal values that you hold that can be directly attached to an experience or teaching you heard in childhood. *Respect for parents + grandparents*

2. Morris Massey uses the phrase, "You are what you are because of where you were when." In this chapter, we described a group shaped by the Great Depression and World War II. Write a value statement for them, in regard to the following topics. Start each statement with "A person should . . ."
    a. patriotism
    b. value of work
    c. family member roles
    d. cooperative action

3. Now visualize an imaginary time and place in which children are brought up in a situation where these circumstances are common: single-parent families, poverty, street gangs, nonmeaningful work, violent streets where people drive by and kill strangers, inadequate schools, and

popular media that pander to a nightmarish mixture of sexuality, violence, and consumerism. Write a value statement for this imaginary group in regard to patriotism, value of work, family member roles, and cooperative action. Start each statement with "A person should . . ."

4. Write a value statement that corresponds to your views regarding the following topics. Again, begin each statement with "A person should . . ."
   a. abortion
   b. divorce
   c. family
   d. finding a wallet with $1000

5. Write a paragraph regarding the gender difference in value development noted in the works of Gilligan and Kohlberg. Is this a natural difference, or one caused by the roles that women have been assigned by our culture? Do you feel that the ideals of the current feminist movement will eliminate this difference in the decision-making process?

6. List two examples of the following:
   a. Statutory Law
   b. Administrative Law
   c. Constitutional Law
   d. Criminal Law
   e. Private Law

7. A competent elderly patient tells you, "I want to go home." You respond with, "We won't let you go home, you're not capable of taking care of yourself." You may have just created the elements of what tort?

8. The patient tells you, "I don't want the treatment." You respond with, "Your doctor has ordered the treatment and told me to make you take it, even if I have to hold you down." You may have just created the elements of what tort?

9. Describe the beneficial effect to our system of law gained from the principle of stare decisis.

10. Would the following scenario produce a viable negligence action? If so, which type is the best fit? If not, what element is missing? Defend your answer.

    Following his return home from the hospital the patient became aware that the respiratory therapist had given him a treatment that was meant for the patient in the next bed. The therapist did not check the wristband on the patient. This was a deep breathing treatment designed to make the patient cough and clear his lungs.

11. The Hippocratic Oath found in the chapter is one of the oldest codes of health care ethics. Identify the sections that deal with the principles of confidentiality, beneficence, nonmaleficence, justice, and role fidelity. Patient autonomy and veracity do not seem to be principles addressed in the code. If it is true that they are omitted, why do you suppose this occurred? What does this tell you about codes of ethics?

REFERENCES

American Medical Association. (1992). *1992 code of medical ethics current opinions.* Chicago: Council on Ethical and Judicial Affairs.

Anderson, G. & Anderson, V. (1987). *Health care ethics.* Rockville, MD: Aspen Publication.

Angelou, M. (1996). *I know why the caged bird sings.* Westminster, MD: Random House.

Bloom, A. (1987). *The closing of the American mind.* New York: Simon and Schuster.

Edge, R. & Groves, R. (1994). *The ethics of health care.* Albany, NY: Delmar Publishers.

Gilligan, C. (1982). *In a different voice.* Cambridge, MA: Harvard University Press.

Hobbes, T. (1651). *Leviathan parts I and II.* New York: The Bob Merrill Company. (1958).

Hubbard, F.P. (1982). *Law and ethics.* In N. Bell (Ed.), *Who decides.* Clifton, NJ: Humana Press.

Kapuscinski, R. (1991). *Independent on Sunday.* Quoted in *Columbia Dictionary of Quotations.* Columbia University Press.

Kohlberg, L. (1981). *Philosophy of moral development.* San Francisco: Harper and Row.

Maslow, A. (1987). *Motivation and personality* (rev. ed.). New York: Harper and Row.

Massey, M. (1980). *People puzzle: Understanding yourself and others.* Englewood Cliffs, NJ: Prentice Hall Co.

Myers, I. (1980). *Gifts differing.* Palo Alto, CA: Consulting Psychological Press.

Piaget, J. (1962). *The moral judgment of the child.* (M. Gabain, Trans.). New York: Collier Books.

Pozgar, G. (1993). *Legal aspects of health care administration.* Gaithersburg, MD: Aspen Publication.

Tbarra V. Spangard, 154 p. 2d 687 (Cal. 1944).

CHAPTER 2

Reasoning in the World of Values

Goal

The major instructional goal is to examine the common theories and methods used in making value decisions.

Objectives

At the conclusion of this chapter, the reader should understand and be able to:

1. List the theorists who are considered the fathers of contemporary duty-oriented, consequence-oriented, and virtue-ethics reasoning.

2. Outline the theoretical position known as utilitarianism, and analyze a clinical problem following its framework.

3. Outline the theoretical position of Kant, and analyze a clinical problem following his duty-oriented reasoning.

4. Explain how rule utilitarianism is similar to duty-oriented reasoning.

5. List the major criticisms of duty-oriented, consequence-oriented, and virtue-ethics reasoning.

6. Outline the theoretical position known as virtue ethics and analyze a clinical problem following its framework.

7. List several sources from which basic principles have been derived by duty-oriented theorists.

Key Terms

agape

biographical Life

categorical
  imperative

consequence-
  oriented reasoning

duty-oriented
  reasoning

equal consideration
  of interest

ethics

euthanasia

| hedonic calculus | mean | principle of utility |
| hedonism | morality | utilitarianism |

VALUE CONFRONTATIONS

All sciences are under the obligation to prepare the ground for the future task of the philosopher, which is to solve the problem of value, to determine the true hierarchy of values.

Friedrich Nietzsche (1844–1900), German philosopher

Every man should expend his chief thought and attention on his first principles; Are they or are they not rightly laid down? And when he has duly sifted them, all the rest will follow.

Socrates (496–399 B.C.), Greek philosopher

As health care providers, we are often surrounded with the comfortable world of the science of health care practice. It is a splendid arena, grounded in reason, scientific method, and human experience. Questions in regard to drug preparations, pathologic entities, and appropriate therapeutics often seem to have straightforward and comfortable answers. We know that if we apply the right set of equations or follow the correct procedures, that a best answer comes forward. In some situations, not only the best answer, but the only answer. It is a safe world where answers are reproducible and consistently verifiable. One need only to present the facts and everyone comes into agreement.

And yet, one does not finish the earliest of the clinical internships before the discovery is made— that this arena of comfortable agreement is only the smallest, and perhaps, not even the more interesting aspect of our practice. In the real arena of health care, where patients, families, and practitioners meet, rarely is there only one answer, rarely is it comfortable, and knowing what is medically correct, is rarely enough. This is the arena where values play a commanding role in determining what is right and good for the patient.

It is our values that tell us what is right and wrong, good and evil, and imply a preference in regard to correct human behavior. Roughly speaking, our values go beyond telling us what is, to what ought to be. This rather subjective screen with which we surround ourselves often countenances strong feelings or intense attitudes, which are backed by rational justifications.

Although we tend to think of value problems in the big ethics sense, that is, those problems that are involved in choices dealing with life and death, we are also bedeviled by everyday questions that call for judgment, based on a perception of right and wrong. The following list of problems is similar to those that practitioners face on a day-to-day basis.

- Is it right or wrong for a nurse to take a gratuity from a patient if the nurse has provided excellent service?

- Is it okay for a physician to own a portion of a diagnostic clinic, and refer patients to that clinic?

- Should the pharmacist criticize a physician who will not change a drug order even though the order is clearly not in the best interest of the patient?

- What is the medical technologist's duty when another technologist makes an error?

- Should the discharge planner tell a patient who asks about the quality of the medical care, that in the planner's opinion, the physician is a jerk?

- If the radiographer X-rayed the wrong patient, but did not harm the patient in the process, would the radiographer need to confess the error?

- As a physical therapist, if the patient could not afford the care, but needed it, would it be okay to falsify insurance papers to get the appropriate care for your patient?

- As a respiratory care practitioner, would it be okay to accept a finder's fee from a home health equipment company to which you referred your hospital patients?

Although none of these questions involves life or death decisions, they call for value judgments and are subject to very different answers, depending upon the value structure and general world view of the individual. In health care practice, however, although value questions are by nature subjective, some answers are better and more appropriate than others.

Some practitioners feel that these are not matters of **morality** at all, but questions of institutional policy and/or legal dictates. For instance, it is not only unethical, but also against the law, for a respiratory therapist working in a hospital to accept a finder's fee from a home care company for recommending that company to patients. In many instances, law serves the same functions as ethics, promoting well-being and social harmony and resolving conflicts of interest. Yet, crucial differences exist between law and morality. It is quite possible for someone to determine that an act was legal and yet, unethical. This does not invalidate the law. Antiabortion advocates would hold that health care providers who perform abortions are unethical, yet few would deny that it is a legal practice. The Tuskeegee research case, when black men with syphilis were left untreated even after the advent of antibiotics so that researchers could continue to study the terminal effects of the disease, was reprehensible, unethical, mean spirited, and all of the other value-laden words you might use, but at the time, was it illegal? Even if it were legal, would you not have wanted the nurse involved to have blown the whistle on the research on the basis of how unethical it was, even at the risk of her professional position? (Ad Hoc Advisory Panel, 1973)

As a citizen who is also a health care provider, if I arrive on the scene of an automobile accident, I am not legally obliged in most jurisdictions to attempt rescue. Yet, what about my ethical obligations as a health care provider? Am I not ethically obliged to provide assistance? Many aspects of our personal and professional lives are not covered by law.

Another difference between law and ethics is the manner in which sanctions are imposed. With law, the sanctions for inappropriate actions are usually physical or financial, (e.g., fines, imprisonment). With moral infractions, the sanctions are more likely to take the form of expulsion from the community of practitioners, loss of reputation, and personal remorse.

ETHICAL ASSESSMENT

One of the most frustrating aspects of practice is that in questions of values, you will often find yourself in disagreement with other individuals whom you respect and know to be honorable. In that we reason from our own personal world view, it is clear that even the best intentioned individuals can come to very different solutions. In that values are not subject to scientific analysis or deal with items that are easily quantifiable, value arguments are often deeply felt and rarely won. Because of the intense feelings associated with our values, we often come to believe that those with opposing views are not only wrong, but somehow evil in their wrongness. It is in the arena of values where we often see the individual taking a stand and acting as a majority of one. As professionals, it is necessary, even in our opposition, to attempt to be constructive not destructive in the methods we use when we come to disagreements over issues involving personal values. Accommodation in regard to the issue of abortion might be more easily attained, if each side had not cast the other as "baby killers" or "anti-women terrorists."

To acknowledge that individuals can come to different opinions in regard to value issues, is not to say that all opinions have the same credibility, and that no particular answer is better than another. Often we will find ourselves with no "right" answer or several "right" answers that seem to fit the situation. To make better value decisions, we must often get beyond our first initial thoughts and feelings in regard to these basic issues and build a framework for examining these problems. Several theoretical positions have been proposed that allow us to examine issues that are value laden.

Some will base their opinions on formal philosophical or religious beliefs, while others will try to weigh the potential outcomes seeking to choose that which provides the greatest good for the greatest number. Still others really do not use a formal system at all to determine the right answer, but will rely upon current practice or past experiences as their guide. Table 2–1 differentiates what is assessed, with evaluative terms in regard to outcomes.

When attempting to solve these problems, often individuals will either appeal to some previously established principle or rule or will attempt to calculate the consequences of the various options. When we examine statements often associated with the abortion issue, we can see these two separate decision-making methods coming into play:

- I should not because life is sacred! (appeal to a rule or principle)

- I should because I have the right to my body! (appeal to a rule or principle)

- I should because this is an unwanted pregnancy which interferes with my life plan! (appeal to consequences of the choice)

- I should not because abortion trivializes life and if we allow this, they will come for the elderly and infirm next! (appeal to consequences of the choice)

- I should because the pregnancy endangers my life. (appeal to consequences of the choice)

TABLE 2–1

Ethical Systems	Evaluation Criteria	Outcomes
Ethical System	Evaluation	Judgment
Duty Oriented	The Act Itself	Right – Wrong, Obligatory – Optional
Consequence Oriented	Consequences	Good – Bad – Neutral
Virtue Ethics	Good Practice	Virtuous – Lacking in Virtue

Notice that in each of the rationales the individual is either appealing to a principle or rule or to the consequences of the pregnancy. In the first two statements, the person is appealing to a rule or principle to justify her decision. The consequences of the decision are not in question. "I shall not because life is sacred" or "I shall because I have a right to do with my body whatever I choose" are both **duty-oriented** forms of reasoning in that they appeal to a rule or principle in justifying the decision. When we examine the next three rationales, the individual involved appears not to be appealing to a principle or rule, but rather to the consequences of this particular pregnancy. The consequences of having or not having an unwanted baby are defended in terms of interference with a life plan, or endangering the life of the mother or creating an insensitive society where all life is trivialized. An appeal to consequences is the major element of **consequence-oriented** reasoning.

As value problem solvers, we generally rationalize our decisions by an appeal to an established authority, rule, or principle, or by avoiding particularly odious consequences. The following scenario finds a practitioner evaluating both systems—that of deciding by principles or by examining the consequences—before finally selecting a choice with which he can be comfortable.

Let us suppose that you have been providing home care for Mr. Jones, a COPD patient, and he has come to trust you and respects you for the care provided. Mr. Jones has no family, and is very wealthy. During your conversations, he has told you of his great admiration for the auto racer Mario Andretti. On your last visit, he appears very agitated and you are thinking of calling 911 to summon an ambulance. Before that transpires, he calls you to him and indicates a large box which appears to contain a great deal of money (five million dollars in small unmarked bills), and presses a note into your hand, that makes you his agent in regard to the money. He pleads with you that if he dies, you are to take the money to Mario, and ask him to add Mr. Jones's name to the advertisements on his racing car as a symbol of his sponsorship. In that he is very agitated and given that the situation is unlikely to occur, and you wish to humor him, you agree. He then thanks you, obviously relieved, sighs, and dies.

You do call 911, but of course, it is too late. You then pick up the box to carry out your promise. After all, "a promise is a promise!" As you proceed to your car and drive away, you begin to think about all the rules that you were brought up with; "Thou shalt not steal," enters your mind. "Do unto others as you would have them do unto you" seems somewhat appropriate for the occasion. You finally decide that in good conscience you cannot keep the money yourself, but do you really have to give it to a very wealthy racecar driver, just so that the late Mr. Jones can have his name painted on the car? You then decide to give the money to the American Lung Association, after all Mr. Jones died of a pulmonary disease, and you base your decision on two other sayings you grew up with: "The ends justify the means" and "The greatest good for the greatest number."

What has happened in this particular (albeit unlikely) scenario is that the health care provider first looked at the problem using a duty-oriented process to determine whether he should keep his promise. In this, the focus was on the act itself. Is it necessary to keep one's promises? The Golden Rule and "a promise is a promise" are rules that look only at the act itself to judge the right or correct response. When he switched his thinking to the "greatest good for the greatest number," he was not evaluating the act, but rather using a consequence-oriented rationale to examine his options.

TELEOLOGICAL (CONSEQUENCE-ORIENTED) THEORIES

Teleological theory is taken from the Greek word *telos* which means "end." The basic concept is that the right act is that which brings about the best outcome. Often individuals will attempt to use consequence theories when they seek to divide scarce resources such as health care. In doing this they may deny an individual access to a heart transplant, if the money could be spent on providing vaccine for thousands. This would be done on the basis of the good of the many outweighing the good for an individual.

With consequence-oriented reasoning, the rightness or wrongness of decisions is based upon outcomes, or predicted outcomes. Those following a consequence-based theory would decide that what is right is that which maximizes some good, such as pleasure and happiness, or ameliorates suffering. The right thing to do then results in being the good thing to do as measured by outcomes. These theorists may argue about what constitutes the good, but once decided they would have no problem theoretically deciding upon a right course of action. In their works focused on the health care setting, T. L. Beaucamp and L. B. McCullough (1984) offer health (prevention, elimination, or control of disease), relief from unnecessary pain and suffering, amelioration of handicapping conditions, and the prolongation of life as intrinsic goods. Table 2–2 provides a listing of a variety of consequences that have been claimed as intrinsic goods (Frankena, 1973).

Utilitarianism

Utilitarianism (Mill, 1863) is the most common form of consequence-oriented reasoning. Jeremy Bentham (1748–1832) and John Stuart Mill (1806–1873) are considered the fathers of the theory which holds that the good resides in the promotion of happiness, or the greatest net increase of pleasure over pain. To elevate the theory beyond a "pig philosophy," John Stuart Mill defined happiness as a set of higher order pleasures such as intellectual, aesthetic, and social enjoyments rather than mere sensual pleasure. However one defines happiness or pleasure, for utilitarians, it is the ends—not the means—that count. The purest form of this line of reasoning is act utilitarianism, when the decision is based on listing the possible alternatives for action, weighing each in regard to the amount of happiness or utility it provides, and selecting the course of action that maximizes happiness and minimizes suffering. Bentham (1789) invented a system of calculating the amounts of pleasure gained and pain avoided which he called **hedonic calculus** (Pojam, 1995).

TABLE 2–2
Proposed Intrinsic Goods

- life, consciousness, and activity
- health and strength
- pleasure and satisfaction of all or certain kinds
- happiness, beatitude, contentment
- truth
- knowledge and true opinion of various kinds, wisdom
- beauty, harmony, proportion in objects contemplated
- aesthetic experience
- morally good dispositions or virtues
- mutual affection, love, friendship, cooperation
- just distribution of goods and evils
- harmony and proportion in one's own life
- power and experiences of achievement
- self-expression
- freedom
- peace, security
- adventure and novelty
- good reputation, honor, esteem

There is some criticism that this form of reasoning may lead to **hedonism** in which one group derives pleasure from the pain of others, justifying the actions on the basis of utility. You can see this in the New Testament story where Caiphas, the High Priest, advises the Council to turn Jesus over to the Romans for crucifixion. He advises, "You know nothing at all; you do not understand that it is expedient that one man should die . . . that the whole nation should not perish" (John 11:50 KJV). To overcome this objection, some newer consequentialist formulations have required the principle of **equal consideration of interest** be shown, where the individual is not allowed to increase her share of happiness at the expense of another. Each person's happiness must be considered equally. Figure 2-1 is a flow chart model of how decisions are made using a utilitarian orientation (Edge & Groves, 1994).

One real problem of act utilitarianism (hedonic calculus or no) is that the individual must somehow predict and calculate the various levels of happiness promoted by each choice. This is made doubly hard by the fact that you are dealing with two superlatives—greatest good for greatest number. In your measurements, do you focus on doing good to large numbers, or should your focus be on the greatest good? A second problem is the seeming loss of self and personal congruence. A person who shifts from one position to another, basing each decision on the perceived levels of happiness and pain avoidance, would seem very inconsistent and confusing to others. The following is a list of criticisms that have been brought against utilitarian reasoning:

1. The calculation of all the possible consequences of our actions, or worse yet, our inactions, appears impossible.

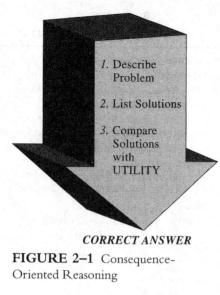

CORRECT ANSWER

FIGURE 2–1 Consequence-Oriented Reasoning

2. Utilitarianism may be used to sanction unfairness and the violation of rights. To maximize one person's or one group's happiness, it may be necessary to infringe on the happiness of another individual or group.

3. Utilitarianism is not sensitive to the agent-relativity of duty. We are inclined to think that parents are obligated to care for their children, and physicians are wrong to harm patients. Both of these examples could be allowed under utilitarianism if doing so maximized overall utility.

4. Utilitarianism does not seem to give enough respect to persons. Under this theory, the ends justify the means, so it may be moral to use a person merely as a means to our ends.

5. Under utilitarianism it is justifiable to prevent others from doing what we believe to be harmful acts to themselves. Such a paternalistic view could justify unacceptable governmental intervention into the private lives of individuals.

6. Utilitarianism alone does not provide a basis for our own moral attitudes and presuppositions. If followed, utilitarianism may recommend behaviors that are in conflict with personal fundamental moral beliefs and give rise to a sense of loss of self (Edge & Groves, 1994).

A formulation of utilitarianism that seems to avoid the problem of exact quantification required in act utilitarianism, is rule utilitarianism. Rule utilitarians prospectively examine an act to see if it would meet the requirements of the **principle of utility.** They then determine whether a rule can be created that could be applied in similar cases. Rule utilitarianism requires that the rule bring about positive results when generalized to a wide variety of situations. Rules forbidding the abridgment of free speech or the "promise is a promise" rule might qualify as acceptable under rule utilitarianism, even if under certain rare situations they may bring about a decrease in happiness or pleasure.

Situation Ethics

On the surface, these theories seem quite straightforward. Utilitarianism relies on a single principle that potentially answers every question. Consequence ethics are often persuasive in that they give comfort to our modern cynicism in regard to absolute truths, and speak to our better selves in respect to tolerating the views and cultures of others. This is especially true in such recent formulations of consequence-oriented reasoning as Joseph Fletcher's *Situation Ethics* (1966), where the good is **agape,** which can be defined as general goodwill or love for humanity. He holds that human need determines, in the final analysis, what is or is not ethical. Under the principles of this theory, if an act helps people, it is a good act; if it hurts, it is a bad act.

In his writings, Fletcher provides six guidelines for making ethical choices:

1. Compassion for people as human beings
2. Consideration of consequences
3. Proportionate good
4. Priority of actual needs over ideal or potential needs
5. Desire to enlarge choice and reduce chance
6. Courageous acceptance of the need to make decisions and the equally courageous acceptance of the consequences of our decisions

As can be seen, the six guidelines provide for no appeal to an absolute principle, no authority upon which one can rely. The only possible test of rival views lies in the consequences. This proposal is similar to the clinical model of medicine, where the best therapeutic regime choice is the one that is most likely to result in an improvement in patient well-being.

DEONTOLOGICAL (DUTY-ORIENTED) THEORIES

Deontological ethicists feel that the basic rightness or wrongness of an act depends upon its intrinsic nature rather than upon the situation or the consequences. This position is often described as a deontological theory, taken from the Greek word for "duty." An act in itself would either be right or wrong; it could not be both. To the duty-oriented theorist, utilitarianism is anathema as it seeks to determine moral rightness by nonmoral values (e.g., happiness and pain avoidance). These theorists hold that it is not consequences that should be examined, but rather the rightness or wrongness of the act itself.

This particular world view is codified in several major ethical systems and religions. Most duty-oriented systems depend upon a set of rules or principles that are

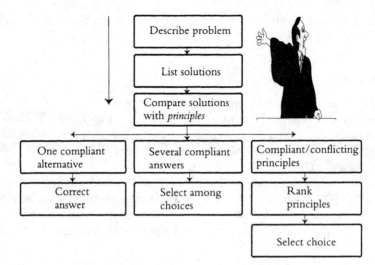

FIGURE 2–2 Duty-Oriented Reasoning

accepted as being universal. When judgments are to be made, the individual finds a corresponding universal principle or rule that fits. Yet, some duty-oriented theorists do not depend upon rules, but rather feel that individuals must consult their own personal moral perceptions to make determinations as to the rightness or wrongness of an act. The admonition of "Let your conscience be your guide" is consistent with these views. Figure 2-2 provides a flow chart model of how decisions are made in a duty-oriented system (Edge & Groves, 1994).

Kantian Ethics

In the classic work, *Foundation of the Metaphysics of Morals* (Kant, 1785), the greatest philosopher of the German Enlightenment, Immanuel Kant (1724–1804), held that the consequences of an action were essentially irrelevant. Kant based his moral philosophy on the crucial concept that humans are rational beings and that a central feature of this rationality was that we could reason to moral principles. Once found and understood these rational moral principles would be consistent and nonoverridable truths. These truths would not be based on contingency or potential consequences, but would rather be universal, necessary, and absolute. Kant held that morality is derived from rationality, not from experience, and that obligation is not grounded in the nature of man or in the circumstances of the situation, but in pure reason. These universal truths are applied to all people, for all times, in all situations. The human mind works the same way, regardless of who you are, where you are, or when you are. An action could be known to be right when it was in accordance with a rule that satisfied a principle he called a **"categorical imperative."** By *categorical* he meant they do not admit exceptions. An *imperative* is a command derived from a principle. These imperatives were formulated by finding a maxim that could be understood as universal law. The imperatives seem to have three elements: (1) universal application, that is, binding upon every individual, (2) unconditionality, and (3) demanding an action. An example of this might be the unconditional duty of a lifeguard to enter the water to save a drowning person. The mental process for the lifeguard would be a series of questions, "Should all paid lifeguards attempt to rescue drowning individuals?" "Is this duty to rescue unconditional?" and finally, "Does this particular incident require the actions of a lifeguard?" If the lifeguard answered "yes" to all three questions, then the lifeguard would, according to Kant, have a binding moral duty to act.

One such maxim relevant to health care ethics is, "We must always treat others as ends and not as means only." Kant saw people as having an absolute value, based upon their ability to make rational choices. Accordingly, our dignity derived from this capacity and this was violated whenever a person was treated merely as a means to an end (a thing) and not a person. From this one maxim you could derive the other principles used in the ethics of health care. An action then could be judged right or wrong by determining its relationship to a categorical imperative, even without knowledge of the particular circumstances.

Recently, the papers told of a family who could not find an acceptable bone marrow transplant donor for their daughter who suffered from a rare form of cancer. In order to gain acceptable bone marrow, they decided to have an additional child, hoping that the child would provide the match. Kantian theorists would find this action unacceptable, as the baby was being used as a means, rather than as an end of its own. The following are a list of criticisms that have been brought against Kantian ethics:

1. The exceptionless character of Kant's moral philosophy makes it too rigid for real life. Real-life situations are so varied that it is impossible to create rules that can guide us in all circumstances.

2. Morality cannot be derived from pure reason. The fact that we can feel pain and pleasure is central to morality. It is unlikely that we would care about morality if we did not feel pain or pleasure.

3. The disregard of the consequences of our actions can lead to disastrous results. We all have been hurt by well-meaning people who were overly concerned to "obey the law." It is often the spirit of the law, rather than the letter, that provides the arena for rational decisions. The Robert Bland proverb, "We may grasp virtue so hard that it becomes vicious," captures the essence of not considering the consequences of our decisions.

4. Even though nonhuman animals feel pain and pleasure, for Kant they do not have any independent moral standing because they are not rational beings.

5. It is possible to be faced with a conflict between two duties equally supported by an imperative. (The nurse who promises not to reveal that a patient has asked questions about euthanasia is asked by the family if the matter was discussed.) (Edge & Groves, 1994)

Duty-oriented theorists obviously wish to promote a good result; however, they feel that merely serving the good is not an adequate foundation for ethics. For these theorists the right action is one based upon a correct principle regardless of the results.

For instance, if life is sacred, then taking a life is wrong, regardless of the circumstances leading to the act. Duty-oriented theorists argue among themselves as to how principles are derived; some claim the basis to be natural law, whereas others look to religious dictate, intuition, social contract, pure reason, or common sense.

John Rawls and the Social Contract

One influential formulation of duty-oriented reasoning is the contract theory of John Rawls (1971). He envisions that the social contract begins at a time when the participants are shielded from knowledge of the end status of those making the decision. Thus if two individuals were making decisions in regard to slavery, and if neither knew who in the end were to be assigned the role of owner and slave, each would decide against slavery as an institution unless that institution somehow served both individuals' advantage. In this theory, Rawls proposes that if a reasoning individual were placed in a social situation requiring a value choice without knowing the role in the situation (Rawls calls this the original position), that the individual would choose the alternative that supported or favored the most disadvantaged person. This then becomes a restatement of the Golden Rule. According to Rawls, actions are morally defensible only if each of the participants would choose to be the recipient of an identical action by someone else under identical circumstances. The first principle of the social contract is justice which secures basic liberties for all individuals within the covenant:

> *Each person possesses an inviolability founded on justice that even the welfare of the society as a whole cannot override. For this reason justice denies that the loss of freedom for some is made right by a greater good shared by others . . . the rights secured by justice are not subject to political bargaining or to the calculus of social interest.*

Following this line of reasoning, the concern of an ethical society would be toward the care and support of its most disadvantaged citizenry as they are the ones who are least able to speak for themselves. This is a decidedly duty-oriented position in that it establishes the duty of moral equality, which could not be bargained away regardless of social interest or the welfare of the society as a whole.

The pro-choice advocate who bases her view on the constitutional guarantee to privacy, the pro-life advocate who believes life is sacred and therefore abortion is wrong under all circumstances, and the priest who maintains the confidentiality of the confessional even in the case of unreported incest, are all following the dictates of a duty-oriented or absolutist system. As health care providers, it is the exceptionless character of the duty-oriented position that gives most practitioners pause, as we always seem to be in situations of gray rather than black or white.

Mixed Duty-Oriented Systems

In an attempt to expand the deontological system, William Frankena (1973) created a two-principled position known as "mixed deontological ethics." In place of the principle of utility focused on the measurement of happiness and pain avoidance, Frankena substitutes first the principle of beneficence, and secondly justice.

TABLE 2–3
Subprinciples of Beneficence

* One ought to prevent evil or harm
* One ought to remove evil
* One ought to do or promote good

Beneficence requires that we strive to do good, yet does not require that we quantify the amount of good derived or evil avoided. Table 2–3 lists the hierarchical arrangement of the subprinciples included in the principle of beneficence.

These subprinciples would be considered in hierarchical order in making decisions, but may be overridden by the second major principle in the theory, the principle of justice. There is always a presumption of equality of treatment. Yet, what happens when the two principles themselves (beneficence and justice) conflict? In these instances, Frankena calls for the use of personal intuition as a guide to resolution of conflicts between the two principles.

It is clear that neither consequence nor duty-oriented systems have produced a theory that can be accepted under all circumstances. Both duty and consequence ethics pose grave problems in modern decision making. As an example, if we take the question of the sanctity of life and an absolutist view prevailed, modern medicine and technology might be placed on the side of saving every living individual from death, regardless of intolerable costs, suffering of the family, or inability to restore life in a meaningful sense. Conversely, if a utilitarian view prevailed, we might see arguments that would allow certain categories of handicapped individuals to be subjected to **euthanasia** on the basis that their removal served the best interest of society. Today, health care decision making is often based on an uneasy truce between the absolutist and consequentialist views, as practitioners seek a viable middle ground. In practice, rarely do you meet the individual who fails to consider the consequences of the situation, or one who is comfortable with decision making without reference to principles.

VIRTUE ETHICS

The moral virtues, then, are produced in us neither by nature nor against nature. Nature, indeed, prepares in us the ground for their reception, but their complete formation is the product of habit.

Aristotle (384–322 B.C.), Greek philosopher

The failure of duty-based or consequence-based ethical systems to produce a theoretical position able to overcome the major criticisms of each, has led some theorists to return to the teachings of Aristotle and explore ethics, not understood in measurements of outcomes or the establishment of rules and principles, but as an attribute of character. "How should I carry out my life if I am to live well?" replaces the current "How do I know which action is correct?" The emphasis is taken off individual actions and the quandaries in which we find ourselves and put instead on what we can do to produce the sort of character that instinctively does the right thing. This adaptation of the philosophy of Aristotle has become known as **virtue ethics** (MacIntyre, 1981).

In his teachings, Aristotle distinguishes two kinds of virtue, intellectual and that of the character. Goodness of character was considered neither natural nor unnatural, and was thought to be produced by the practice of virtue. This practice created the habit of taking pleasure in virtuous acts, which then acted as a sign of a good life. In a sense, Shakespeare's advice in *Hamlet* was correct, "If one were to have virtue, one must first assume it." Aristotle's traits of a virtuous character are listed here.

1. Virtuous acts must be chosen for their own sake.

2. Choice must proceed from a firm and unchangeable character.

3. Virtue is a disposition to choose the mean.

Virtuous acts that flow from a force of habit create a disposition of moderation toward the **mean** and away from extremes. We all have experienced times when we needed to swing hard against the directions in which our passions were leading us. (Not every passion has a mean. For instance, there is no mean of murder; as murder is itself an extreme in interpersonal conduct.) Better examples can be found in courage, liberality, pride, ambition, good temper, truthfulness, shame, and justice.

Beyond character virtue, Aristotle also believed in intellectual virtues such as practical wisdom. This he defined as the power of deliberation about things good for oneself. Neither practical wisdom nor character virtue could exist independently from each other.

A modern formulation of these concepts is found in the works of Alasdair MacIntyre (1981). MacIntyre holds that many different conceptions of virtue revolve around ideal characters associated with a variety of traditions. He isolates and describes several idealized characters such as Homeric (strength and warrior), New Testament (humility and slave), and Early American (industry and capitalist). Beyond these ideals, he believes in a core idea of virtue, of which courage, justice, and honesty are essential components.

The practice of health care specialties creates an arena where specialty-specific virtues are defined and exhibited. These social roles, specific to health care and the specialty that one chooses, provide the standards of excellence which MacIntyre relates to virtue. It is through obedience to these rules, and the adoption of common achievement goals, that lead us to some perceived good. To enter into the role of the nurse, technologist, physician, priest, or teacher is to enter into a set of correct practices, and to accept the authority of these as standards of that role. In the example of the nurse, once the individual accepts and enters that practice, duty is determined by the nursing role, and the traditions of that specialty. Figure 2-3 displays how decisions are made reasoning from a position of virtue ethics (Edge & Groves, 1994).

Today's view of good practice is grounded in the history of our particular specialty. When one enters into a specialty, you not only enter into a relationship with all your contemporaries, but also with those who preceeded you in the role. This is especially true of those who have preceeded us and have made major contributions to the profession. Every new nurse is, in some way, entering a field with specialty

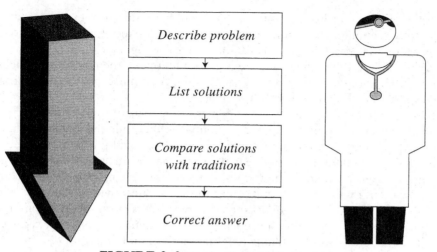

FIGURE 2–3 Virtue-Oriented Reasoning

practices shaped by Florence Nightingale. In this way, we learn from tradition, but tradition also learns from us.

A major problem with using virtue ethics in the health care situation is the changing nature of our specialties. What may be considered a virtue at one period may be inappropriate in the next. Perhaps the best example is nursing. Good practice in the '50s and '60s contained ample portions of virtues such as submissiveness and respectfulness that today are being replaced with such virtues as patient advocate and patient teacher. Health care specialties are in a period of rapid transition, with seemingly daily changes. It is quite possible that on the same shift one could have several groups of nurses with differing views of what the "good nurse" is all about.

Like duty-oriented and consequence-oriented systems, virtue ethics has been subject to criticism. The following is a list of problems associated with virtue ethics:

1. Virtue ethics generally do not provide specific directions in regard to decision making.

2. In that virtue ethics relies on traditional practices, it does not quickly respond to changes in the practice that require new sorts of moral responses.

3. The derivation of duty from one's social role is liable to lead to or perpetuate classism, sexism, etc.

4. A traditional emphasis makes morality depend on past experience rather than on reason. This environment provides little respect for creative solutions or personal autonomy.

5. Practitioners often find themselves attempting to address more than one set of idealized roles, which may come into conflict (e.g., the need to be a team player or the need to be a whistle-blower, as in a case of negligent care by co-workers) (Edge & Groves, 1994).

Yet, even given its limitations there is something persuasive about virtue ethics. If we truly examined our actions as practitioners and looked at what went into our decision-making processes, in calculations of what is right or wrong in regard to -professional duties, we would find we often are following the dictates of an idealized role. We are asking ourselves, "What does the good nurse, physical therapist, or radiographer do when faced with this situation?"

In virtue ethics we are not calculating increases in pleasure and amounts of pain avoided, or seeking to find an appropriate duty-oriented rule or principle to apply, but are being guided by the duties imposed by our role and position in the health care team and society. Yet, what is one to do when confronted by situations for which role practices are yet to be created, practice duties that have no traditional counterpart? A current example of this new arena of health care, for which the past offers little guidance, is the nurse or respiratory therapist who is put in the position of not only being asked to disconnect a ventilator from a patient in a persistent vegetative state, but also to remove the feeding tube and intravenous lines.

CONCLUSION

As humans, each of us develops a more or less consistent and coherent set of attitudes, feelings, and opinions, with which we judge the world of actions around us, making determinations of what is good or bad, right or wrong, positive or negative. Our personal value system or world view appears to be culturally derived by the events of our lives, and the traditions of our people.

Several ethical systems have been proposed to assist us in bringing order to value-laden decision making. Clearly, the settling of these issues by the flipping of a coin is unacceptable, as it would lead to an ethical pluralism, where any choice is as good as another. To allow a moral, neutral society is not in keeping with social order and progress. Currently, the most common ethical systems derived to assist us in making these value judgments are duty orientation, consequence orientation, and virtue ethics. Table 2–4 examines each of these ethical systems. Each of these general systems, with which we look at ethical problems, have contemporary advocates and detractors.

None of the common ethical systems examined in this chapter have been found to overcome all of the legitimate criticisms and none, at this point, have universal acceptance. When we examine our personal decision-making systems, we may often use a duty-oriented system in some decisions, and be consequentialistic or virtue-ethics oriented in others. An individual could be very duty oriented and absolutist in regard to an issue such as abortion, and yet approach the withdrawal or removal of life support from an outcomes or virtue-ethics orientation. It has been noted that just as in the fox hole there are no atheists, in the practice of health care there is little comfort in decision making without a situational framework or the reliance on principle. Van Rensselaer Potter (1973), who is credited with coining the word *bioethics*, explained that this new discipline had as its focus the traditional task of health care ethics, that of aiding the individual practitioner to make decisions and to live with oneself. **Ethics,** then, is a generic title that we give to systems that seek to bring sensitivity and method to the human task of decision making in the arena of moral values.

TABLE 2–4 Ethical Systems

General Category	Examples	Definition
Duty Oriented	Kantian Ethics Hebrew–Christian Ethics Oxford Intuitionists Contractarians	The rightness or wrongness of an act is determined by principles or rules.
Consequence Oriented	Utiliarianism Situation Ethics Egoist Ethics	The rightness or wrongness of an act is determined by considering the potential effects of the act.
Virtue Orientation	Virtue Ethics	The rightness or wrongness of an act is determined by an examination of correct practices.

Legal Case Study: National Commission on Gay and Lesbian Youth Suicide Prevention

On December 5, 1995, Senator Kerry presented a bill before the Senate to establish the National Commission on Gay and Lesbian Youth Suicide Prevention. The bill sought to establish a commission who could "identify the root causes and report on possible methods to prevent suicide among gay and lesbian adolescents." Senator Kerry emphasized that this is a national problem because one-third of all teen suicides occurred among gay and lesbian youth. Senator Kerry stated, "We cannot ignore the obvious fact that gay and lesbian youth are subject to enormous societal pressure" (Referenced to the 141 Cong. Rec. S 18028 December 5, 1995).

1. What type of law is being created by Senator Kerry? common law? civil law? public law? private law? statutory law? regulatory law? criminal law?

2. Defend this law from a duty, consequence, and virtue-ethics perspective.

REVIEW EXERCISES

1. For this case, first justify your decision using duty-oriented reasoning and then follow using consequence-oriented and virtue-ethics reasoning.

> Let us suppose that you are a paramedic and arrive at an emergency scene. The situation is that a group of scouts have entered a cave that is now filling with water. They were led into the cave by a rather large scoutmaster. Unfortunately while leading them out of the cave, the scoutmaster somehow managed to get stuck in a narrow opening

with only his head and shoulders protruding out. With his upper torso stuck outside the cave, it appears that the scoutmaster will survive, but all the boys below will drown if they cannot escape.

After you have checked all possible escape routes and have attempted to extricate the scoutmaster, it becomes clear that the only way to save the boys is to cut up the scoutmaster into pieces so that he can be removed. This is, unfortunately, not the Winnie the Pooh story where Rabbit could wait until poor Pooh lost weight.

What is the correct action for this case? Justify your answer with either a legal or ethical principle.

2. Kant requires that his imperatives be universalized. Consider the following as a rule:

Whenever I cannot get my homework done for a course, I shall pay another student to do the work, and claim it as my own.

Universalized, the rule would state: Whenever anyone needs homework done, and cannot get it done, they should pay someone else to do it and claim it as original work.

Would you accept that as a reasonable proposition? What happens to the grading process if you accepted this? If it were understood by the instructors that this was a universal proposition, why would they give homework?

3. List two basic value principles that you could see yourself accepting without any consideration of consequences. You might consider the imperative that we must always treat others as ends in and of themselves rather than as a means to an end.

4. List four "good practices" that are inherent in your health care specialty.

REFERENCES

Ad Hoc Advisory Panel. (1973). *Final Report of the Tuskeegee Syphilis Study,* 5–15. Washington, DC: United States Public Health Service.

Aristotle. *Niocomachean ethics.* (T. Irwin, Trans.) (1985). Indianapolis, IN: Hackett Publishing Company.

Beaucamp, T., & McCullough, L. (1984). *Medical ethics: The moral responsibilities of physicians, 37.* Englewood Cliffs, NJ: Prentice Hall.

Bentham, J. (1989). *An introduction to the principles of morals and legislation.* In Louis Pojman (Ed.), *Ethical theory.* Belmont: Wadsworth Press. (Reprinted from original work published 1789.)

Edge, R., & Groves, R. (1994). *The ethics of health care.* Albany, NY: Delmar Publishers Inc.

Fletcher, J. (1966). *Situation ethics.* Philadelphia, PA: Westminster Press.

Frankena, W. (1973). *Ethics,* 87–88. Englewood Cliffs, NJ: Prentice Hall.

Hitt, W. (1990). *Ethics and leadership.* Columbus, OH: Batelle Press. John 11:50 KJV.

Kant, I. (1785). *Foundation of the metaphysics of morals.* (L. S. Beck, Trans.). Indianapolis, IN: The Bobbs Merrill Co. Inc. 1959.

MacIntyre, A. (1981). *After virtue.* Notre Dame, IN: University of Indiana Press.

Mill, J.S. Ed. (1863). *Utilitarianism.* Buffalo, New York: Prometheus Books. (reprinted 1897) New Testament. King James version. John 11:50.

Pojam, L.P. (1995). *Ethics: Discovering the right and wrong.* Belmont, CA.: Wadsworth Publishing Company.

Potter, V.R. (1973). *Bioethics: Bridge to the future.* Englewood Cliffs, NJ: Prentice Hall.

Purtillo, R. (1993). *Ethical dimensions in the health professions.* Philadelphia: W.B. Saunders Company.

Rawls, J. (1971). *A theory of justice.* Cambridge, MA: Harvard University Press.

Shakespeare, W. *Hamlet.* (In *Hamlet,* act 3, section 4, to Gertrude).

Winslow, G. (June 1984). *From loyalty to advocacy: A new metaphor for nursing,* 32–39. Hastings Center Report.

CHAPTER 3

The Nature of Rights in Ethical and Legal Discourse

Goal

The major instructional goal is to explore the language of rights and the nature of the obligations that are attendant to these rights.

Objectives

At the conclusion of this chapter the reader should understand and be able to:

1. Define what is meant by a claim to a moral right.
2. Explain how rights and their attendant correlative obligations are grounded in the same overarching principles and rules.
3. Define and differentiate between the following types of rights:

   Moral rights

   Legal rights

   Positive rights

   Negative rights

   Perfect obligations

   Imperfect obligations

4. List three examples of positive and negative rights.
5. Explain how operating from the *original position* would naturally lead to choices that are founded on the principle of justice and collective choice.

6. Contrast the development of rights from a natural rights, consequential, and contractarian position.

7. Explain why the modern tendency to justify all claims on the basis of rights has a negative effect upon the value of rights as a concept used in ethical discussion.

8. List four correlative obligations that may be rightfully claimed from us by our patients as a result of our being health professionals.

9. List four examples of natural rights that have found their way into our society as legal rights.

10. Outline the rights problem associated with the Supreme Court's creation of a negative right in regard to abortion.

11. Differentiate between rule and act utilitarianism. Explain why rule utilitarianism seems a better base for the claims to a right than act utilitarianism.

Key Terms

action	**Golden Rule**	**perfect obligation**
act utilitarianism	**imperfect obligation**	**rights**
correlative obligations	**original position**	**rule utilitarianism**

THE PROBLEM OF RIGHTS

We hold these truths to be self evident, that all men are created equal; that they are endowed by their Creator with certain unalienable rights; that among these are life, liberty and the pursuit of happiness.

Thomas Jefferson

The assertion of such rights (natural rights), is absurd in logic and pernicious in morals.

Jeremy Bentham

One interesting, but perhaps peculiar aspect of humanity and of our society in particular is the multiplication of claims to personal **rights.** People advocate a right to die, a right to health care, a right to smoke hemp products, nonsmokers' rights, smokers' rights, animals' rights, women's rights, abortion rights, and a right to a guaranteed annual income with periodic paid holidays. In Fuji, a group of miners claimed a personal right to a sex break during work hours (Bassom, 1981). It is almost as if we have lost the ability to provide arguments for something without appealing in the language of rights. One might wonder why the nonsmoker could not have framed the statement as "I would rather not be required to breathe in foul air" rather than "I have a right to breathe clean air." We are either living in an age of sudden awareness where we have evolved and are now aware of a whole new set of rights, or we are confusing what we want with what is somehow our due.

Although it is not the author's intent to judge the merit of any of the previously mentioned claims for rights, it would seem that until we can come to some agreed upon definitions, these claims become almost meaningless. It is clear that human imagination and creativity can create more claims to rights than we could possibly honor. Rights have been described variously as entitlements, interests, powers, claims, and needs (Bandman & Bandman, 1995). Regardless of how rights are defined, they appear to be desirable and beneficial. If one is a possessor of a right, one apparently need not feel gratitude to others for its possession. Somehow the right is ours, something that one owns, or is one's due and not dependent upon the good will of others. Rights are not claims to a privilege which is dependent upon the free will, kindness, or pleasure of another person. When we say that someone has a right to something, we are not indicating that it would be nice or charitable if they received it, but rather that they must be provided the object or service in question. To quote Maurice Cranston (1967), "A right is something of which no one may be deprived without a grave affront to justice." Rights can be thought of as "trumps which take precedence over mere expediency or social benefit" (Dworkin, 1978).

If a right is something that is ours, something that we need not feel gratitude to others for its possession, then what are we to make of statements such as the American Hospital Association's *A Patient's Bill of Rights* (Figure 3–1)? It is clear that if it is a listing of legitimate rights, then the listing cannot be considered to be a gift given by the health care providers, or in this case the American Hospital Association. If the patient already had these rights, then the statement is only a reaffirmation of what is already owned. The source of the patient's claim is beyond the listing, and found either in sanctions of law, good practice, or moral duty.

The language of rights will permeate health care discussions for the foreseeable future. Perhaps the most important of these discussions will be centered on the ongoing current debate as to whether a right to health care exists for all citizens. Along with this issue, we will argue out the rights for the unborn, a right to die, animal rights, and a host of others. Although it is comforting to base our legal rights to goods and services upon natural rights, it is not a necessary condition; many legal rights will be based on an assessment of available resources and the need to guarantee a certain quality of life for all citizens. It is necessary to recognize in all of this that not all human wants should be turned into moral or legal rights.

One use of rights language that must be separated from the establishment of obligations and justified claims is that which is found in such declarations as the United Nations Universal Declaration of Human Rights (1948). The authors of these documents were laying out an expression of hope for the future of mankind rather than an expression of realities that would be grounded in law or legitimate claims. These expressions of hope have great symbolic value, but it is difficult to explicate the status of the rights claimed in the sense of **correlative obligations.**

AHA Policy   A Patient's Bill of Rights

This policy document presents the official position of the American Hospital Association as approved by the Board of trustees and House of Delegates.

Management
Advisory

Patient and
Community Relations

Introduction

Effective health care requires collaboration between patients and physicians and other health care professionals. Open and honest communication, respect for personal and professional values, and sensitivity to differences are integral to optimal patient care. As the setting for the provision of health services, hospitals must provide a foundation for understanding and respecting the rights and responsibilities of patients, their families, physicians, and other caregivers. Hospitals must ensure a health care ethic that respects the role of patients in decision making about treatment choices and other aspects of their care. Hospitals must be sensitive to cultural, racial, linguistic, religious, age, gender, and other differences as well as the needs of persons with disabilities.

The American Hospital Association presents *A Patient's Bill of Rights* with the expectation that it will contribute to more effective patient care and be supported by the hospital on behalf of the institution, its medical staff, employees, and patients. The American Hospital Association encourages health care institutions to tailor this bill of rights to their patient community by translating and/or simplifying the language of this bill of rights as may be necessary to ensure that patients and their families understand their rights and responsibilities.

Bill of Rights*

1. The patient has the right to considerate and respectful care.

2. The patient has the right to and is encouraged to obtain from physicians and other direct caregivers relevant, current, and understandable information concerning diagnosis, treatment, and prognosis.

   Except in emergencies when the patient lacks decision-making capacity and the need for treatment is urgent, the patient is entitled to the opportunity to discuss and request information related to the specific procedures and/or treatments, the risks involved, the possible length of recuperation, and the medically reasonable alternatives and their accompanying risks and benefits.

   Patients have the right to know the identity of physicians, nurses, and others involved in their care, as well as when those involved are students, residents, or other trainees. The patient also has the right to know the immediate and long-term financial implications of treatment choices, insofar as they are known.

3. The patient has the right to make decisions about the plan of care prior to and during the course of treatment and to refuse a recommended treatment or plan of care to the extent permitted by law and hospital policy and to be informed of the medical consequences of this action. In case of such refusal, the patient is entitled to other appropriate care and services that the hospital provides or transfer to another hospital. The hospital should notify patients of any policy that might affect patient choice within the institution.

4. The patient has the right to have an advance directive (such as a living will, health care proxy, or durable power of attorney for health care) concerning treatment or designating a surrogate decision maker with the expectation that the hospital will honor the intent of that directive to the extent permitted by law and hospital policy.

   Health care institutions must advise patients of their rights under state law and hospital policy to make informed medical choices, ask if the patient has an advance directive, and include that information in patient records. The patient has the right to timely information about hospital policy that may limit its ability to implement fully a legally valid advance directive.

5. The patient has the right to every consideration of privacy. Case discussion, consultation, examination, and treatment should be conducted so as to protect each patient's privacy.

6. The patient has the right to expect that all communications and records pertaining to his/her care will be treated as confidential by the hospital, except in cases such as suspected abuse and public health hazards when reporting is permitted or required by law. The patient has the right to expect that the hospital will emphasize the confidentiality of this information when it releases it to any other parties entitled to review information in these records.

7. The patient has the right to review the records pertaining to his/her medical care and to have the information explained or interpreted as necessary, except when restricted by law.

8. The patient has the right to expect that within its capacity and policies, a hospital will make reasonable response to the request of a patient for appropriate and medically indicated care and services. The hospital must provide evaluation, service, and/or referral as indicated by the urgency of the case. When medically appropriate and legally permissible, or when a patient has so requested, a patient may be transferred to another facility. The institution to which the patient is to be transferred must first have accepted the patient for transfer. The patient must also have the benefit of complete information and explanation concerning the need for, risks, benefits, and alternatives to such a transfer.

*These rights can be exercised on the patient's behalf by a designated surrogate or proxy decision maker if the patient lacks decision-making capacity, is legally incompetent, or is a minor.

FIGURE 3–1 A Patient's Bill of Rights. Reprinted with permission of The American Hospital Association, copyright 1992.

9. The patient has the right to ask and be informed of the existence of business relationships among the hospital, educational institutions, other health care providers, or payers that may influence the patient's treatment and care.

10. The patient has the right to consent or to decline to participate in proposed research studies or human experimentation affecting care and treatment or requiring direct patient involvement, and to have those studies fully explained prior to consent. A patient who declines to participate in research or experimentation is entitled to the most effective care that the hospital can otherwise provide.

11. The patient has the right to expect reasonable continuity of care when appropriate and to be informed by physicians and other caregivers of available and realistic patient care options when hospital care is no longer appropriate.

12. The patient has the right to be informed of hospital policies and practices that relate to patient care, treatment, and responsibilities. The patient has the right to be informed of available resources for resolving disputes, grievances, and conflicts, such as ethics committees, patient representatives, or other mechanisms available in the institution. The patient has the right to be informed of the hospital's charges for services and available payment methods.

The collaborative nature of health care requires that patients, or their families/surrogates, participate in their care. The effectiveness of care and patient satisfaction with the course of treatment depend, in part, on the patient fulfilling certain responsibilities. Patients are responsible for providing information about past illnesses, hospitalizations, medications, and other matters related to health status. To participate effectively in decision making, patients must be encouraged to take responsibility for requesting additional information or clarification about their health status or treatment when they do not fully understand information and instructions. Patients are also responsible for ensuring that the health care institution has a copy of their written advance directive if they have one. Patients are responsible for informing their physicians and other caregivers if they anticipate problems in following prescribed treatment.

Patients should also be aware of the hospital's obligation to be reasonably efficient and equitable in providing care to other patients and the community. The hospital's rules and regulations are designed to help the hospital meet this obligation. Patients and their families are responsible for making reasonable accommodations to the needs of the hospital, other patients, medical staff, and hospital employees. Patients are responsible for providing necessary information for insurance claims and for working with the hospital to make payment arrangements, when necessary.

A person's health depends on much more than health care services. Patients are responsible for recognizing the impact of their lifestyle on their personal health.

Conclusion

Hospitals have many functions to perform, including the enhancement of health status, health promotion, and the prevention and treatment of injury and disease; the immediate and ongoing care and rehabilitation of patients; the education of health professionals, patients, and the community; and research. All these activities must be conducted with an overriding concern for the values and dignity of patients.

A *Patient's Bill of Rights* was first adopted by the American Hospital Association of 1973. The revision was approved by the AHA Board of Trustees on October 21, 1992.

©1992 by the American Hospital Association, 840 North Lake Shore Drive, Chicago, Illinois 50611. Printed in the U.S.A. All rights reserved. Catalog no. 157750.

THE NATURE OF RIGHTS

A right can be thought of as a justified claim. In this sense, if you have a moral right to personal property, then others have an obligation to respect your claim to that property. Rights can be justified by moral or legal principles and rules, or in some cases a claim to both moral and legal justification. An interesting aspect of rights theory is that built within the concept of rights is a correlative thesis of right and obligation. In this sense a right creates an obligation in others to behave in a certain way, to either provide goods or services or refrain from interference. As an example, the patient's right to informed consent obligates the health care provider to supply appropriate information. If it is possible to examine the obligation of the health care provider, we could ascertain the patient's right to informed consent, or vice versa. If we could examine the patient's right to informed consent, then we could reason ourselves to the obligation of the health care provider. The correlative thesis implies that both the obligation and the right are being justified by the same overarching principles or rules (Beauchamp & Childress, 1989).

We often think of rights as being absolutes, yet, they must compete in the social context with other competing claims. Even the right to life, which seems rather foundational, must compete with the right to life of others who have an equal claim to their lives, and with social considerations and moral judgment in regard to self-defense and killing in time of war. In health care, we have all seen cases when generally accepted rights, such as a right to informed consent and personal autonomy in regard to health care choice, are overridden when they came into competition with other rights in a social context. In the language of rights, we often find the following formulation to explain the obligations and limits of rights.

If John has a right to X, then others have no justification in interfering with John's pursuit or possession of X, so long as John's exercise of his right to X does not infringe upon the rights of others. In deathbed situations, often the family will wish for the health care providers to do everything for their loved one. In a sense, they have a right to expect that everything will indeed be done and the providers have an obligation within a reasonable context to see that everything is provided. Yet, one's death is uniquely one's own, and if the patient chooses to exercise the autonomy of choice and asks that all heroics be avoided, then the family's rights to calling for heroics can be interfered with and infringed upon.

HISTORICAL BACKGROUND OF RIGHTS REASONING

Historically, the language of rights and their concepts came into general political and moral discourse in the middle ages. **Natural rights** were generally equated to the law of God and found their most succinct expressions in forms such as the **Golden Rule.** With the age of reformation, both local jurisprudence and international law came to be discussed in the light of natural rights. In the writings of such men as Grotius, Pufendorf, and Locke, the legitimacy of nation states could be determined by the respect they paid to the inherent natural rights of citizens (Golding, 1978). We saw some reflections of this in the world's attitude toward the apartheid state of South Africa and the shifting American policy of attaching favored nation status to human rights improvement in states such as the People's Republic of China.

Natural liberties are universal moral rights and are thought to exist prior to and independent from the guarantees of a social contract or institutionalized government. The concept writ large into our culture that all men are "endowed by their Creator with certain unalienable rights; that among these are life, liberty, and the pursuit of happiness" (Jefferson, 1776) is an expression of the universality of natural liberties and moral rights. These are often called *negative rights*, in that they obligate others from interference. The right to liberty is actually a statement of a personal right to be free from interference of the exercise of that right, such as enslavement. The expression, "human rights," seems to have been used first by the American firebrand patriot, Thomas Paine, in his translation of the revolutionary French *Declaration of the Rights of Man and Citizens* (1789). In his writings, Paine seems to use human rights and natural rights as synonymous terms.

Human rights, when differentiated from natural rights, seem to flow from a recognition that all humans (Homo sapiens) are equally separated from the beasts of the field and are unique unto themselves. As we grow and mature, we come to recognize our common human origins and the needs that are required for our development. If I am without food, I hunger, and if this continues long enough, I die. Not only do I know this of myself, I know this for all human beings. There are basic needs that we all share and have come to recognize and respect as a person's just due, if he is to remain human. There are some in the animal rights groups that find this form of reasoning to establish human rights speciesists, much in the same vein as racists, sexists, etc. These common needs are not the province of humans alone and yet most do not grant these rights to animals based on a recognition of their shared needs.

These claims to goods or services are often termed *positive rights*. These fundamental shared needs form the basis for our concepts of universal human rights. This agreement, in regard to universal human rights, is a recognition that as humans we are interdependent, and the welfare of one is the responsibility of all.

Not every human right can be satisfied in all situations. If, for instance, I thirst for water and no water is available, I continue to thirst. Having a right without a means to exercise it does not negate the right—it continues to exist. Other humans know that as they need water, so do I if I am to remain alive and human. I can justly demand water from them if it is available beyond their needs. If they have only enough for themselves, my right to their water becomes inoperative, in effect canceled out by their needs. I still have a human right to have my needs fulfilled, yet I may not demand what others require to remain alive without violating their fundamental human rights.

It is believed that natural rights and human rights are so basic and universal that individuals may know of their existence and truth by reason alone. Thomas Aquinas (1225–1274) stated in the *Treatise on Law* (1988):

> To the natural law belong those things to which a man is inclined naturally; and among these it is proper to man to be inclined to act according to reason. . . . Hence this is the first precept of law, that good is to be done and promoted; and evil is to be avoided. All other precepts of the natural law is based upon this; so that all the things which the practical reason naturally apprehends as man's good belong to the precepts of the natural law under the form of things to be done or avoided.

The point that Aquinas made is that some moral principles do not depend upon feeling, observation, or demonstration, but are stable, eternal, irresistible, and certain—at least to those who are wise enough to understand their terms. If understood, they would be as unarguable as the statement, "All calico cats are cats." Natural rights then are basic truths which can be understood and known by human reason alone and are not dependent upon outside dictates.

The Old Testament story of Cain and Abel is illustrative of the nature of natural rights. In the story, God questions Cain about the whereabouts of his brother. In his answer, Cain indicates an understanding that indeed he has done wrong. In that Cain and Abel were reported to be the third and fourth humans to walk the earth, and given that the story takes place in a time prior to the Ten Commandments, how did Cain know that he had erred? It appears that Cain knew the admonition against killing from reason alone, and God was therefore justified in punishing him for breaking this natural law.

The ideas of Thomas Aquinas are somewhat echoed in the works of John Locke (1959) who wrote of self-evident principles whose veracity the "mind can not

TABLE 3–1
Suggested Criteria for Personhood

- One who could be said to have interests, a person for whom something can be said to be good for personal sake.
- One who has cognitive awareness, a being of memories, expectations, and beliefs.
- One who is capable of relationships. Interpersonal relationships seem to be at the very essence of what we idealize in truly being a person.
- One who has a sense of futurity. How truly human is someone who cannot realize there is a time yet to come as well as a present? The words "What do you want to become?" only makes sense in relation to a person.
- One who is capable of self-motivated activity.

doubt, as soon as it understands the words." According to Locke, the law of nature ". . . . teaches all mankind that, being all equal and independent, no one ought to harm another in his life, health, liberty or possessions." To Locke, these were not matters of truths that one could accept without demonstration or experiment but rather became known and self-evident by these processes.

The concepts of natural and human rights seem based on humankind being the measure of all things. In that these rights are restricted to persons, several criteria have been established to examine the nature of personhood. Table 3–1 provides a list of common criteria found in discussions of personhood (Edge & Groves, 1994).

Common within these criteria is the species requirement, which states that only members of our species (Homo sapiens) have the status of persons. A second criteria often used is rationality. Only rational beings capable of autonomous action can be thought to have human rights. This criteria has figured prominently in discussions on whether humans can cease to be persons if they fall into a permanent state of unawareness. Other criteria commonly discussed are the capability to use language, being self-aware, and having a sense of time and the ability to form relationships.

Currently the criteria for personhood is more argued than agreed upon. Some in society desire to establish criteria that would extend the meaning of personhood to other entities such as aliens and animals. Others wish to move the criteria to such a basic level that helpless infants and those in vegetative states are included. Others refuse to be drawn into the discussion at all, fearing that any agreed upon criteria today might provide the basis for the labeling of some minority group in the future as being essentially nonpersons. Table 3–2 lists key concepts drawn from the historical traditions of natural law.

TABLE 3–2
Key Concepts from the Natural Law Tradition

- Humans possess a rational nature, provided as a gift from God.
- Even without a knowledge of God, one can discover natural laws.
- Natural laws are unchangeable and universal.
- Natural law exists independently from social contract.
- Inability to effect natural rights does not extinguish them.

CONTRACTARIAN AND CONSEQUENTIALIST RIGHTS THEORY

Some philosophers believe the whole concept of natural or human rights is patent nonsense. Jeremy Bentham was an implacable foe to the concept of natural rights, holding that they were "absurd in logic and pernicious to morals" (Hart, 1982). Therefore, if the concept of rights could not be thought of as stemming from basic human reason or as a preexistent endowment of a kind creator, on what other rational foundation may rights be justified? In his work, *Utilitarianism* (1863), John Stuart Mill set out the following in regard to right and wrong which might lead us to a source for rights from a utilitarian view.

> We do not call anything wrong unless we mean to imply that a person ought to be punished in some way or another for doing it; if not by law, by the opinion of his fellow creatures, if not by opinion then by the reproaches of his own conscience. This seems to be the real turning point in the distinction between morality and simple expediency. It is part of the notion of Duty in every one of its forms, that a person might rightfully be compelled to fulfill it. Duty is a thing that may be exacted from a person as one exacts a debt. Unless we think that it can be extracted from him we do not call it his duty. Reasons of prudence, or the interest of other people, may militate against actually extracting it; but the person himself, it is clearly understood, would not be entitled to complain. There are other things, on the contrary which we wish that people should do, which we like or admire them for doing, perhaps dislike or despise them for not doing, but yet admit that they are not bound to do, it is not a case of moral obligation; we do not blame them, that is we do not think that they are proper objects of punishment.

What Mill described as being the distinction between morality and simple expediency is better stated as the distinction between that which is morally required and morally valuable. For Mill, duties were subdivided into two sets: duties of **perfect obligation,** which have inherent within them assigned correlative rights, and duties of **imperfect obligation,** which do not give birth to any right. The basis of perfect obligations was the realm of required duty, whereas imperfect obligations were those in which the act was obligatory, but the particular occasions of performing them are left to our choice. Examples of imperfect obligations can be found in areas of charity and beneficence which we are called upon to practice but not toward any particular person or any prescribed time (Sumner, 1989). The difference, then, is the specified requirement of a duty as opposed to what one might expect on the basis of generosity or beneficence.

Rights then are claims that can be justified on the principle of collective agreement. For Mill, what others were calling moral rights, were claims that were morally justified, that were also backed by the force of law or public opinion. "To have a right, then, is, I conceive, to have something which society ought to defend me in the possession of. If the objector goes on to ask why it ought? I can give him not other reason than general utility" (Mill, 1863). Yet, general utility in the sense of **act utilitarianism,** when the merit of each act is judged only on the pleasure it brings or on the pain it avoids, would be a crude tool upon which to base a system of rights, in that they would be seen to shift in the changing circumstances of each and every situation. A better model would be that of **rule utilitarianism,** when an act may be prejudged as right or wrong presuming that it conforms to a rule previously validated by the principle of utility. For example, a rule that forbids the abridgment of free speech could be selected under rule utilitarianism, because under most circumstances it promotes utility; that is, in most instances such a rule increases pleasure and avoids pain.

We would then adopt the rule against the abridgment of free speech and apply it to all similar situations, even though in rare circumstances it brings about a decrease in pleasure or happiness. One could imagine a society accepting and enforcing a great number of claims to rights, validated by the principle of utility, if by doing so they tended to promote general happiness and their omission produced the reverse of happiness.

This still begs the question as to whether there are distinct moral rights that are separate from rights supported by social sanction. It seems that what Mill is saying is that if a moral justification is worthy of social protection, that is, an enforceable sanction, then it is a moral right. Yet for some, the fact that there is an antecedent moral right is what has led us to create the social sanction that protects it.

According to Thomas Hobbes (1651), life in the state of nature prior to the formation of government was "solitary, poor, nasty, brutish and short." Rather than an era of peace and tranquility populated with noble savages, Hobbes envisioned a nightmare of violence, where each individual decided only for himself and against all others. In this version of a state of nature, there could be no industry, no crops grown, and no security or peace found, and certainly no rights whose claims were equally understood and honored.

> *To this war of every man against every man, this also is consequent; that nothing can be unjust. The notion of right and wrong, justice and injustice, have there no place. Where there is no common power; there is no law, no injustice. Force and fraud are in war the two cardinal virtues. Justice or injustice are faculties neither of the body nor the mind. If they were they might be in a man alone in the world, as well as in his senses and passions. They are qualities that relate to men in society, not in solitude.*

(Hobbes, 1651)

For Hobbes, nature did not teach lessons of innate human rights, but rather that human nature itself created the need for a Leviathan, something so large that it could crush individual will and bring about acceptable behavior from the chaos. In this era, only the law of self-preservation existed. For Hobbes, the Leviathan, which needed to be larger than the individual, was a justification for the monarchy, but would later be reduced by others to ideas including a social contract or government.

The Hobbesian model does not solve the question of human rights, as it posits a world where the strong and the ruthless, armed with force and fraud, are the only ones who are allowed to come to the bargaining table. It is difficult to see how the principle of justice that would allow equal protection for all could come from such a gathering. Perhaps a more useful model is that of John Rawls (1971), who offers a kinder and gentler arrangement as the context for the social contract. Rawls imagines an **original position** that is designed to promote rational choice and fairness. In the original position all individuals are free and equal. There is a veil of ignorance, which denies each of the agents knowledge of who is to receive the rights to goods and services. When the decision is made, it would need to be made so that the most disadvantaged individual would be willing to accept that position. This formulation of social justice can be seen in the fair opportunity rule (Beauchamp & Childress, 1989) (Figure 3–2).

In this light, let us consider two agents attempting to determine whether slavery would be a good thing. Neither knows of the other's natural assets or social position. Neither knows who is to be the slave, if that is the choice. It is clear that in

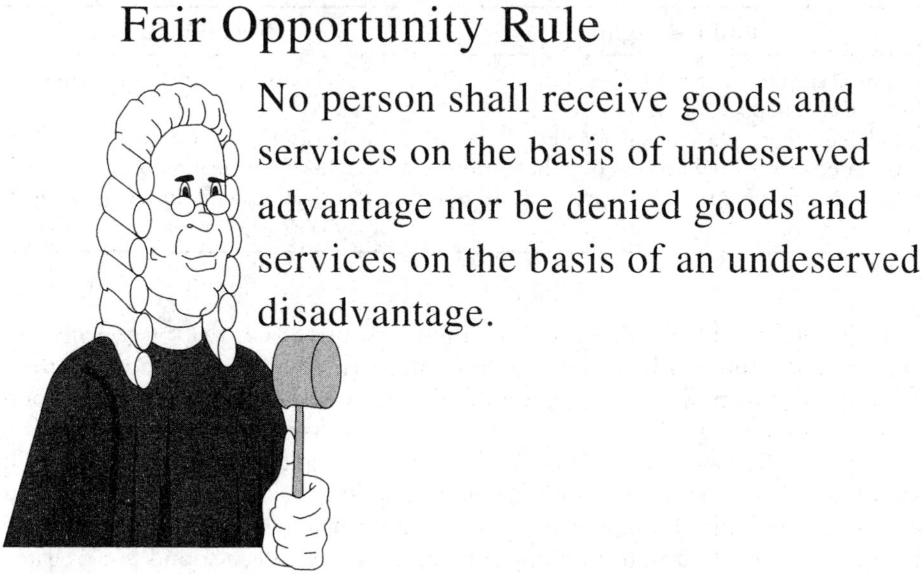

Fair Opportunity Rule

No person shall receive goods and services on the basis of undeserved advantage nor be denied goods and services on the basis of an undeserved disadvantage.

FIGURE 3–2 Fair Opportunity Rule

this original position, neither would choose to have slaves. If the choices were made from this original position, the principle of justice would prevail, as Rawls (1971) has removed the opportunity for either of the individuals to exploit the determination to their advantage.

Contractarians are those that believe that individual rights are grounded in the principle of justice and collective choice, and it is this collective choice that forms the basis of morality. Yet, there are those who state that Rawls, in his setting up of the original position, has already posited the concept of a moral right to equal concern and respect. If this is true, then it would seem that these rights would need to have existed prior to the collective choice procedure (Sumner, 1989).

LEGAL RIGHTS

Whatever individuals feel to be the original source of rights, whether from the laws of nature, a generous creator, or social contract, it is more likely that they will be accorded their just due if backed by the sanction of law. Some rights have been seen as being of such importance that they have become legal rights. These are rights not only asserted as moral prerogatives, but afforded governmental guarantees. Legal rights are created through constitutional guarantees, legislative statutes, judicial review, and governmental agencies. They are ubiquitous, and each of us lives in a literal sea of legal claims that shape our behaviors. These claims can be as comprehensive as a constitutional guarantee, or as small as whether you must separate your garbage into recyclables and nonrecyclables. The following are examples of a few common positive and negative rights that have been afforded the sanction of law:

Positive Rights	Negative Rights
American Veterans' right to health care	Equal opportunity in employment
Right to a public education	Freedom of religion
Indigent right to health care (Medicaid)	Right to bear arms
Licensed drivers' right to use of public roads	Right to personal property
Citizens of Ballwin, MO, to garbage collection	No taxation without representation
	Right to an abortion

In general, we have found it easier to put into place laws that protect negative rights, which require others to refrain from interfering with our just claims, than in framing laws that provide positive or welfare rights, which call for provision of goods and services. This can be seen in the current controversy regarding a right to abortion. In the 1973 case of *Roe v. Wade,* the Court ruled that the woman's negative right to privacy, that is, a right to noninterference, provided a right to abort her fetus, within certain limits. This negative right is justified by considerations of the principle of autonomy. This right to noninterference has even been found to abrogate a husband's veto of his wife's and her physician's decision to terminate the pregnancy (*Danforth* case, 1976).

What is not included in the negative right to noninterference in the decision to have an abortion is the positive right to a claim to the resources and services required for an abortion. The current controversy, in regard to denying poor women public funding for legal abortions, is based on this difference between negative and positive rights. In wanting to argue that poverty ought not to exclude some women from exercising the negative right to noninterference in regard to abortions, individuals are seeking to create a positive right justified under the principle of distributive justice.

Notice that positive rights are recipient rights, which are rights to receive goods and services from another person, organization, or government. Only legal persons can receive legal rights. Although there are laws regarding the safe and humane treatment of animals, these are not based on animals having special rights which must be protected. In that animals do not hold the status of legal persons under the law, it is hard to imagine for them legal rights. The characteristics that are commonly attributed to a legal person are found in Table 3–3 (*Cochran's Law Lexicon*, 1973).

In that the law has granted the status of "persons" under the law to include ships and corporations, animals could perhaps in the future also be granted this status. When you examine the attributes of legal persons, it would not seem a far stretch that animals might fit into this category. Animals in truth can be injured, they can be benefited, and certainly could be thought of as having an interest in avoiding pain. At this moment, however, animals share the same legal category as buildings, pieces of art, or furniture; they are considered property.

We should also note that legal rights may or may not be based on established moral claims. The fact that citizens of Ballwin, MO, have a claim to garbage collection is, perhaps, a matter of consensus in regard to quality of life issues rather than basic moral convictions. Legal rights obviously differ between jurisdictions, vary from nation to nation, and in that they are products of human action, can be made

TABLE 3–3
Attributes of Legal Persons

- Persons that can be injured.
- Persons that can be thought to have interests.
- Persons that can be benefited.

and unmade. An excellent example of this shifting with time can be seen in the civil rights legislation of our nation. In our earliest time, humans with black skins were considered property that could be bought and sold. At a later time they could not be legally enslaved, but could be denied the rights of other citizens to the vote under the Jim Crow laws. Currently, under the law, African-Americans must be treated equal to all, and if past discrimination can be proved, must be given recompense by affirmative action policy. One would hope that as time passes and past inequalities are remedied, the legal status of African-Americans will again change.

While it is clear that legal rights are often used to reaffirm moral rights, they do not necessarily coincide. Many legal rights such as the right to drive and the right to garbage collection in your neighborhood are not born in deep moral principle. Likewise, there are many moral rights not sanctioned by law.

The enforcement of legal rights is a rather clear process, with a designated set of factors (fines, punishments, constraints) that tend to coerce others to honor an individual's claims. On the other hand, moral rights depend upon a more informal set of processes which include contempt, blame, and social ostracism, that are designed to induce appropriate behavior.

MORAL AND LEGAL RIGHTS

Moral or natural rights have several different aspects not necessarily shared by legal rights. First, they are universal, and if an individual has this right, then all relevantly alike individuals also have the same rights regardless of historical time or laws of the nation. Second, moral rights provide equality among humans. If a single individual has a moral right, then all individuals of that class have the same right and possess it equally. Men cannot have more moral rights than women, whites over blacks, Christians over Moslems, etc. When it comes to moral rights, we are all born equal. Third, moral rights are believed not to be the product of human creativity, but are inherent to our species. They cannot be brought into existence by democratic vote or taken away by despotic action. These rights continue to exist, even if the means of effecting them are denied.

Some would question the value of a moral right if in fact it was ignored under law. One might argue that each individual has the moral right to personal autonomy in the area of reproduction, and that the government has no right to tell individuals how many or how few children they should have. Yet in the People's Republic of China there is a stringently enforced one child per family policy. What is the value of the moral right if it can be ignored by those in power?

To provide greater protection of moral rights, many people believe that moral rights should be converted to legal rights and provided the sanction of law. In the case of the recent efforts to create an equal rights amendment for women, proponents would argue that this should come into the law based on the moral claims for equality. Obviously, those who claim a right for the unborn, special rights for children, animal rights, and others are seeking to base these in our foundational claims to universal moral rights.

CONCLUSION

Just as inflation erodes the value of currency by decreasing its purchasing power, so too, does the inflation of rights language erode the value of these concepts as justified claims. Regardless of whether you have come to believe that rights are innate, or formed as a result of a social contract, they remain an important and vital aspect of the legal and ethical practice of health. In the foreseeable future, all patient care providers will be discussing the issue of rights as they relate to the patients we serve. The parents who wish to decline lifesaving care for their children, the child who wishes a prescription for contraceptives without parental consent, and the physical therapist who is forced to charge less than what the market will bear for his services due to a governmentally imposed cap are all involved in aspects of the rights controversy.

The concept of human rights with their attendant creation of obligations must be limited only to fundamental human needs. Table 3–4 lists three basic considerations that should be examined prior to declaring new human rights. The most important of these is dilution, when our creativity as humans causes us to claim rights well beyond limits that can be honored and thereby reduces the meaning of rights as a concept. Soren Kierkegaard (1946), the father of Christian existentialism, was correct in asserting that ethics should not become merely a statistical exercise. Human rights cannot be created or lost by opinion polls. The daily will of the people is a fickle foundation. It must be remembered that in early Nazi Germany, well before the atrocities of the holocaust death camps, the popular will of the people first reduced the rights of the mentally ill. It is clear that in this beginning, they came to forget that the most basic of our human rights is the right to be recognized and respected as equal human beings.

In our daily practice as health care providers, more good will be done by honoring the basic human rights that we already have come to know by experience and reason than in imagining a whole host of new ones. Our professions place upon us

TABLE 3–4
Considerations in Declaring New Human Rights

- Not all human wants can or should be converted to justified human rights.
- The human ability to declare rights is greater than our ability to fulfill them.
- The dilution of human rights by adding new ones, threatens established claims.

special obligations and additional duties to protect the rights of those we serve. These rights form part of the condition of practice and bind us not only to our patients, with whom we have entered into a voluntary contractual agreement, but also to society as a whole. For society and our patients' rights to be operative, we must as practitioners assume the correlative obligations that give them meaning.

Each of us needs to develop a framework for thinking about these issues and the claims they represent. Obviously, when rights claims are deployed on all sides of a single issue, they become diluted and their meaning, in regard to understandable obligations, is lost. Our failure to form a certain base for the development of human rights does not negate their importance. They are in some way fundamentally important, as they are the essence that we share with all humanity. The respect of human rights is the independent standard by which we judge the merit of nations and the actions of individuals. Most practitioners would feel quite uncomfortable in a world where the rights we have intuitively come to accept, regardless of their source, were to be removed from our moral scales.

LEGAL CASE STUDY 1: A Question of Rights (*Danforth v. Planned Parenthood of Central Missouri*, 428 U.S. 52.(1979)).

In 1974, the Missouri legislature, in response to *Roe v. Wade*, passed an act which, among other things, required a married woman to obtain the written consent of her husband before she could seek an abortion from a doctor. The act was challenged by several Missouri doctors acting as a class for all doctors who perform abortions and all those patients within the state of Missouri desiring a termination of their pregnancies. The Supreme Court was once again faced with the rights of the pregnant mother. Missouri was attempting to give a right of consent to the husband. The Court reasoned, however, that *Roe v. Wade* specifically excluded the state from any rights in the first trimester of pregnancy; hence, the state could not grant the husband a right of consent because the state did not have any rights to convey to the husband. The Court held the Missouri law unconstitutional and stated:

> When a woman, with the approval of her physician but without approval of her husband, decides to terminate her pregnancy, it could be said that she is acting unilaterally. The obvious fact is that when the wife and the husband disagree on this decision, the view of only one of the two marriage partners can prevail. Inasmuch as it is the woman who physically bears the child and who is the more directly and immediately affected by the pregnancy, as between the two, the balance weighs in her favor.

LEGAL CASE STUDY 2: (Referenced from *Elliot v. Board of Weld County Commissioners*, 796 P.2d 71 Colo. Ct. App.(1990)).

In Colorado, members of a county commission passed an ordinance that prohibited smoking in all county buildings. Inmates incarcerated in a jail located in that county brought an action against the county stating that they had a liberty and a property right to smoke. The inmates reasoned that because Colorado law required public facilities to include an area for smokers, the inmates also should be afforded such a facility in jail. However, the court disagreed with the inmates' interpretation of Colorado law, and stated that there was no constitutional right to smoke in jail or prison.

1. What was the difference, if any, between the two claims for rights as illustrated by the two cases?

2. What would be the basis for a right to smoke?

3. Examine the conflict of rights found in the *Danforth* case. On what basis was the decision made? Was the court saying that the husband had no rights in the matter?

REVIEW EXERCISES

1. In our culture we often talk of special rights for those whom we consider innocent, such as babies and children. How might such rights have evolved and become justified?

2. In considering positive rights and negative rights, where would you place the right to silence, as found in the Fifth Amendment to the Constitution?

3. We often talk of recipient rights, such as the rights that American veterans have to health care. Could one create recipient obligations in regard to this right? As an example, could we predicate this right to health care on the obligation that the veteran would refrain from smoking, drinking to excess, etc.? Would this be a good idea? If a right is something for which one need not feel grateful to others, how could others create legitimate obligations in regard to the right?

4. In the chapter discussion regarding abortion, we found that the negative right to abortion only created an obligation to noninterference. In this light, do we currently have a negative right to health care?

5. In theory, once one understood the right, one should be able to reason out the correlative obligations.
   a. List at least two obligations to each of the items found in *A Patient's Bill of Rights* provided in the chapter.
   b. Which of the included patient's rights are currently provided the sanction of law?

6. It is clear that not all wants can or should be converted into rights. Yet, it seems as if we are being inundated by demands from various groups expressed in the language of rights. If a right can be defined as a justified claim, provide the justification under some ethically acceptable principle for the following claims to rights.
   a. Nonsmokers' rights
   b. Smokers' rights
   c. Gay rights
   d. Marijuana smokers' rights
   e. Animal rights
   f. Women's rights

7. The philosopher John Rawls states that the basic social arrangement is an agreed upon contract to advance the good will of all who are in the society. In this communal effort, all would work toward equal distribution of goods and services unless an unequal distribution would serve to everyone's advantage. Others have argued that when this view of an enlightened collective social protection is added to the fair opportunity rule (Figure 3–2), you can begin to see an actual right to health care. What is your opinion in regard to a right to health care?

8. In some rights discussions, individuals speak of "option rights." These are loosely defined as your sphere of autonomy, where you have the right to freedom of action without interference from others. Which of the rights found in *A Patient's Bill of Rights* could be considered option rights (where one is free to do or not do what one has a right to do)?

9. It appears that philosophers who hold a contracterian view feel that rights stem from a collective social decision and that these rights gain their power by the fact that they are important enough to be protected by law or at least social sanction. Theorists like Thomas Aquinas and Locke on the other hand feel that rights exist presociety and come from sources such as a consequence of God's creation.

   These are two very different orientations to rights. Which do you feel provides the strongest protection for the weakest among us, e.g., the elderly, the handicapped, the premature infant? Explain your answer.

10. In the chapter, the examination of the writings of Hobbes made it seem as if he were justifying the institution of a monarchy, while the doctrines proposed by Aquinas were in keeping, or at least acceptable, to the Catholic Church. If indeed these writers were in some real sense responding to certain institutions or changes taking place in their time, what historical factors would explain Locke and his declared rights to life, health, liberty, and possessions?

11. In an excellent essay, Joel Feinberg imagined a place called Nowhereville. This imaginary place is very much like our own except for the fact that there are no rights. In keeping with this idea, imagine a hospital setting in which no one had rights. How would it differ from the hospitals that we now know? Could it be made to function?

12. In William Golding's classic novel, *Lord of the Flies* (1962), a situation occurs when a small chubby child with the nickname Piggy loses his glasses to a bully. Piggy asserts his claim to the glasses in the language of rights, arguing that he has a right to them.

    In the story the bully rolls a rock down on Piggy, killing him and thus ending the discussion. Did Piggy have a right to his glasses? If not his glasses, did he surely have a right to his life? From where might such rights have come? Did Piggy's weakness in respect to enforcing his rights decrease his legitimate claims?

REFERENCES

Aquinas, T. (1966). Summa theologica. In *Social thought in America* (p. 265). Boston, MA: Beacon Press.

Aquinas, T. (1988). *Treatise on law.* Wash D.C. Regnery Publishing, Inc.

Bassom, M. D. (1981). Introduction to the fourth conference on rights, 3. In M. Bassom (Ed.), *Rights and responsibilities in modern medicine.* New York: Alan R. Liss, Inc.

Bandman, B., & Bandman, E. (1995). *Nursing ethics.* Norwalk CT: Appleton and Lange.

Beauchamp, T. L., & Childress, J. F. (1989). *Principles of biomedical ethics* (p. 57). New York: Oxford University Press.

Cochran's law lexicon. (1973). (W. Gilmer, Ed.). Cincinnati, OH: W.H. Anderson Company.

Cranston, M. (1967). Human rights, real and supposed. In D. D. Raphael (Ed.), *Political theory and rights of man* (p. 23). Bloomington, IN: Indiana University Press.

Danforth v. Planned Parenthood of Central Missouri. 428 U.S. 52 (1976).

Dworkin, R. (1978). *Taking rights seriously* (p. xi), Cambridge, MA: Harvard University Press.

Edge, R., & Groves, R. (1994). *The ethics of health care.* Albany, NY: Delmar Publications.

Golding, M. P. (1978). The concept of rights: A historical sketch. In B. Bandman & E. Bandman (Eds.), *Bioethics and human rights* (pp. 44–50). Boston: Little Brown.

Golding, W. (1962). *Lord of the flies.* (Intro. by E. M. Forster.) New York: Coward-McCann, Inc.

Hart, H. L. A. (1982). *Essays on Bentham: Studies in jurisprudence and political theory.* Oxford, England: Clarendon Press.

Hobbes, T. (1958). *Leviathan parts I and II.* New York: The Bob Merrill Company (Original work in 1651).

Jefferson, T. (1776). *The Declaration of Independence*.

Kierkegaard, S. (1946). Attack on Christendom. In R. Bretall (Ed.), *A Kierkegaard anthology* (p. 446). New York: The Modern Library.

Locke, J. (1959). *Essay on human understanding (1)*. New York: Dover Press.

Mill, J. S. (1952). Utilitarianism. In R. M. Hutchins (Ed.), *Great books of the western world*. Chicago: Encyclopedia Britannica, Inc.

Paine, Thomas. (1979). *The rights of man*. Westminster, MD: Everymans Library.

Rawls, J. (1971). *A theory of justice*. Cambridge, England: Clarendon Press.

Sumner, L. W. (1989). *The moral foundation of rights*. Oxford, England: Clarendon Press.

United Nations (1948). *United Nations Universal Declaration of Human Rights. In making sense of human rights: Philosophical reflections on the Universal Declaration of Human Rights*. Berkeley CA: University of California Press. (1987).

CHAPTER 4

Autonomy versus Paternalism: A Contest Between Virtues

Goal

The general goal of this chapter is to outline the nature of the conflict between autonomy and paternalism in health care, and to discuss the ethical and legal issues associated with patient autonomy. Secondary goals will be to emphasize the requirements of informed consent and competency determination.

Objectives

At the end of this chapter the reader should understand and be able to:

1. Define paternalism.
2. Describe how paternalism in its best sense is a result of provider beneficence.
3. List and describe the four models of provider-patient interaction as outlined by Ezekial and Linda Emanuel. Explain which of the models are best suited for today's practice.
4. Define and list the elements of informed consent.
5. Differentiate between the professional community standard and the reasonable patient standard, and explain how the latter best serves the needs of the autonomous patient.
6. Explain why a more subjective standard than the professional community standard or the reasonable patient standard may be needed to protect patient autonomy.

7. Define therapeutic privilege, list the situations where it is used, and explain the problems of benevolent deception.

8. List several groups in our society that would have limited autonomy.

9. Outline the major elements of competency determination.

10. Explain how the First Amendment protection of the Constitution protects the autonomy of religious individuals who have beliefs that conflict with current medical practice.

11. Explain the rationale used by the courts to allow adults with particular religious beliefs to refuse lifesaving therapies for themselves, but not allow them to refuse for their children.

12. Explain the standard of decision making that sets the legal requirement for informing the patient regarding material risks associated with a particular treatment.

13. List the common functions associated with institutional ethics committees.

Key Terms

abandoned

actionable

ad litem

amicus curiae

authentic

competency

false imprisonment

Joint Commission on Accreditation of Healthcare Organizations (JCAHO)

paternalism

patient-centered standard

professional autonomy

professional community standard

reasonable patient standard

VALUE PREFERENCE AS THE BASIS OF HEALTH CARE DECISIONS

Self-determination has to mean that the leader is your individual gut, and heart, and mind or we're talking about power, again, and its rather well-known impurities. Who is really going to care whether you live or die and who is going to know the most intimate motivation for your laughter and your tears is the only person to be trusted to speak for you and to decide what you will or will not do.

June Jordan, U.S. poet, civil rights activist.

Perform (your duties) calmly and adroitly, concealing most things from the patient while you are attending to him. Give necessary orders with cheerfulness and sincerity, turning away his attention from what is being done to him; sometimes reprove sharply and emphatically, and sometimes comfort with solicitude and attention, revealing nothing of the patient's future or present condition.

Hippocrates, Decorum, in 2 Hippocrates

If the health care practitioner is a professional to whom patients turn in times of need, and if health is a universal good, it would seem that patients, who are strangers to the specialized world of medicine, would lie quietly and allow the medical team to work on their behalf. The problem with this statement lies in the fact that, although health is a universal good, it is not the only one. The good life, like beauty, is a subjective matter and is in the eyes of the beholder. The good life, however, which is determined, contains many other factors beyond health. At times, these other desirable factors have a higher personal value.

A hypothetical case that looks at how a variety of factors interplay to shape decisions is that of a professional athlete who contracts a neurological disease, which is rapidly debilitating and then terminal. The athlete's physician knows of a drug that, if taken, will extend her life by ten years. Without the medicine, the prognosis is two to three years of normal activity followed by a rapid onset of debilitation and finally death. Following the physician's recommendation, the athlete takes the medication. Unfortunately, the medication affects her balance and she cannot continue to play at the professional level. She is faced with the problem of taking the medication and extending her life to ten rather noncompetitive years with the immediate ending of her career, or not taking the drug and shortening her life by seven or eight years. Without the drug, however, she would gain two to three years in which to fulfill her professional contract and earn millions.

In this hypothetical case, the athlete discontinues the treatment against her doctor's recommendations. The desire to compete and fulfill the multimillion dollar contract has a higher personal value than a life extension of seven or eight years of noncompetitive life. The example shows that health care decisions are not only matters of medical expertise, but also matters of individual value preferences.

AUTONOMY VERSUS BENEFICENCE

One irony of health care is that in an earlier age when practitioners had less to offer by way of scientific evidence for their cures and nostrums, society allowed them a greater role in medical decision making. Now, when every treatment is subjected to scientific method and scrutiny, patients are demanding and receiving a greater role in the decision-making process. The scope of the distance we have come in this process from physician **paternalism** to patient autonomy can be seen from two excerpts—one from the Code of Ethics of the American Medical Association (1848) and the other from the American Medical Association, Fundamental Elements of the Patient-Physician Relationship (1992).

> *The obedience of a patient to the prescriptions of his physician should be prompt and implicit. He should never permit his own crude opinions as to their fitness, to influence his attention to them. A failure in one particular may render an otherwise judicious treatment dangerous and even fatal.*

1848 Code of Ethics, Section 6

> *The patient has the right to make decisions regarding the health care that is recommended by his or her physician. Accordingly, patients may accept or refuse any recommended medical treatment.*

1992 Fundamental Elements of the Patient-Physician Relationship

It is clear that faith in the practitioner and in his or her judgment plays an important role in the healing process, yet the only one who can truly make an authentic decision for the patient is the patient. What is the health care provider to do when the patient appears to be making choices that are not in the patient's best interest? When, if ever, is paternalism justified, either legally or morally?

The most eloquent statement and defense for personal autonomy is found in the essay, "On Liberty" by John Stuart Mill (1859). In this work, the author holds that the only purpose for which power can be rightfully exercised over any other member of a civilized community against that member's will, is to prevent harm to others.

> His own good, either physical or moral, is not a sufficient warrant. He cannot be compelled to do or forebear because it will be better for him to do so, because it will make him happier, because, in the opinion, to do so would be wise or even right. These are good reasons for remonstrating with him, but not for compelling him or visiting him with any evil in case he does otherwise.

The issue is more complex than who is in charge or even who knows best. The real issue is which of the basic ethical principles holds supremacy in a given situation. Should it be the personal liberty of self-determination under the principle of autonomy even at the expense of forcing the health care provider to do less than could be done, or practitioner beneficence when care is provided, even in cases when the patient wishes to be left alone? Should alert, rational patients be allowed to refuse reasonable care if that decision sacrifices their lives or health? A secondary question is what duty do health care providers have in this choice? Can the practitioner assist after the patient has made a decision that is medically incorrect, and if followed, would lead to personal harm?

What of the practitioner's **professional autonomy?** Can a patient's desire to be treated in a particular way overcome the autonomy of the health care provider? For instance, if a patient demanded an abortion from a physician with a pro-life view, whose autonomy should prevail?

Professional autonomy allows the practitioner to withdraw from circumstances that are contrary to basic personal values and beliefs. It does not, however, overcome the personal autonomous choices regarding health care made by a competent adult. If the provider has entered into a patient-provider relationship, and the practitioner feels it necessary to withdraw services, care must be taken to ensure that the patient is not **abandoned.** When a treatment relationship exists between a physician and a patient, abandonment law requires that all necessary care be provided unless the relationship is terminated by the patient, or the provider after having given adequate notice and an opportunity to secure an alternative source of care.

The attitudes of some practitioners toward patient autonomy can be brought into focus by considering what is meant when we say, "Mr. Jones is a good patient," or "Physicians and nurses do not make good patients." Often, what is meant is that Mr. Jones follows orders and that physicians and nurses are assertive and noncompliant. In this light, "good" indicates an individual who allows the medical staff to make all the decisions.

Emphasis on patient autonomy is a relatively new phenomenon—the evolution of this body of study seems to be away from provider paternalism, even if the paternalism is guided by the best motives. In American society, it is the children and elderly who most often have their autonomy limited under the guise of paternalism.

These two groups and the mentally ill are the ones most often judged incapable of assessing risk to themselves.

Patient-Provider Relationship

Ezekial and Linda Emanuel (1992) proposed a series of hypothetical models used for the examination of the physician-patient relationship. In these models the relationships take four basic forms: paternalistic, informative, interpretive, and deliberative.

Paternalistic Model. In the paternalistic model, the interaction is designed to ensure that the patient makes the decision that best promotes the patient's well-being. The health care provider presents selected information in such a way as to encourage consent to the intervention that is most medically appropriate. The essential role of the health care provider is that of guardian.

Informative Model. The health care provider in the informative model provides the patient with the relevant information and allows the patient to select the desired intervention. The concept is rooted in the idea that patients know their value systems, and need to receive the facts to make their appropriate, authentic patient-centered decisions. The central role of the health care provider in this model is that of technical specialist.

Interpretive Model. The interaction in the interpretive model is designed to elucidate patients' values and what they really want. The provider then helps the patients select the interventions compatible with those values. The health care provider is functioning in the role of advisor.

Deliberative Model. Under the deliberative model, the health care provider seeks to help the patient determine and choose the best health care values related to the particular clinical situation. The health care provider helps the patient in value clarification and in understanding the aspects of the various potential interventions. The provider not only discusses what the patient could do, but also what the patient *should* do in a particular situation. The essential provider roles of these interactions are teacher and friend.

In the examination of these interaction models, the paternalistic model is clearly the most manipulative and perhaps illegal, if the end result is that the patient does not receive adequate information to provide an informed consent. For rational adults, a paternalistic model that predetermines the end result is demeaning at best, and if practiced, would do harm to the basic human rights of the autonomous individual.

In the informative model, the problem is if informed consent is addressed and the provider has perhaps complied with the legal necessities of information. The question here is not a legal one, but rather an ethical one. Has the provider satisfied the principles of beneficence or role duty? In truth, this rather limited scientific or technical role for the practitioner not only serves the patient poorly, it diminishes the health care provider's role to one that is least satisfying to both patients and practitioners. Health care providers are paid for this professional judgment.

In regard to legal and ethical requirements, the interpretive and deliberative models seem to have merit in both a legal and ethical sense. They provide the information required by law so that the patient can make an informed consent, and they honor the patient's personal autonomy. Between the two, the interpretive model is the least likely to truly serve the authentic choice of the patient in that it relies on the provider coming to the right conclusions in regard to what would be an authentic choice for another. In an advisor's role, one is usually telling someone what is the best choice, rather than allowing the choice to be **authentic**. The teaching function of the deliberative model would seem the best in assisting patients to formulate plans that are most authentic to themselves.

INFORMED CONSENT

It is from the struggle between paternalism and autonomy that the basis for the doctrine of informed consent is derived. The term came into common usage after appearing in the **amicus curiae** brief filed on behalf of the American College of Surgeons in the 1957 case of *Salgo v. Leland Stanford University* (Brody, 1992). Informed consent as both a moral and legal doctrine emerged as a product of the last half of the twentieth century, as judges sought to protect the patient's right to greater freedom of choice. Informed consent binds the physician to an adequate disclosure and explanation of the treatment, and the various options and consequences. It should be emphasized that it is a physician's prerogative and obligation, and whereas other health professionals may assist, it is the doctor who has the duty to fully explain procedures and treatment to patients. Simply stated, informed consent requires that before any risky or invasive procedures may be performed, the health care practitioner must inform the patient of pertinent details about the nature of the procedure, its purpose, potential risks involved, and any reasonable alternatives that may be available. It is important to recognize that informed consent does not require full understanding or full voluntariness to be in place. If these criteria were truly required, autonomous action would be a rare event. Table 4–1 lists the elements of informed consent found in most definitions (Anderson & Anderson, 1987).

TABLE 4–1
Elements of Informed Consent

1. Disclosure: The nature of the condition, the various options' material risks, the professional's recommendation, and the nature of consent as an act of authorization.
2. Understanding: Most states require that the physician provide information at a level that a hypothetical reasonable patient could understand.
3. Voluntariness: No efforts toward coercion, manipulation, or constraint are allowed. The patient must be in a position to practice self-determination.
4. Competence: Decisions in regard to competence usually take into account experience, maturity, responsibility, and independence of judgment.
5. Consent: An autonomous authorization of the medical intervention.

STANDARDS OF DISCLOSURE

It is informed consent that allows autonomous self-determination. The main struggle in the courts has been to determine what standards should govern the level of disclosure. Two standards have been proposed: the **professional community standard** and the **reasonable patient standard.**

Professional Community Standard

With the professional community standard, the health care provider is bound to provide the amount of information that would be expected from other reasonable practitioners within a community in similar situations. This formed the basis of the decision in the *Natanson v. Kline* (1960) case which involved what a physician must disclose in regard to the side effects of cobalt therapy. This standard was based on the concept that the practitioner and patient were bound by a special fiduciary relationship where the difference in levels of information and patient trust binds the professional to act in the patient's behalf without allowing any conflict of interest. The amount and nature of the information provided would be determined by the traditions of the particular practice and the professional community standard. Application of this standard, however, seems to have numerous problems, as the focus is not on patient understanding, but rather on the physician's standard of practice. Because there is often a wide gap between the social, economic, and educational levels of the physicians and their patients, even with the best of intentions, this standard does not necessarily lead to a level of communication that allows for true patient autonomy.

Reasonable Patient Standard

Reasonable patient standard holds that the amount and type of information needed is that which a hypothetical reasonably prudent person, in similar circumstances, would need to understand the nature of the condition and the various options. This standard was articulated in *Cantebury v. Spence* (1972) when the court ruled that "True consent to what happens to one's self is the informed exercise of a choice and that entails an opportunity to evaluate knowledgeably the options available and the risks attendant upon each." The rationale for this standard is that the type and amount of information needed must be at the patient's level, if the patient is truly to be autonomous as a decision maker. Yet, it must be understood that the traditional reasonable person as described in law cannot be equated to the ordinary person or the average person. This idealized person is one who is never subject to irrational fears or personal idiosyncrasies. One leading treatise on tort law provides the following characterization of the reasonable person:

> *He is not to be identified with an ordinary individual, who might occasionally do unreasonable things; he is a prudent and careful person, who is always up to standard.*

(Keeton, 1984)

One criticism of the reasonable patient standard is the nature of the highly idealized hypothetical person. Who is to say that this person is anything like a particular patient with regard to personal beliefs, cognitive abilities, and social background? What perhaps is needed is a **patient–centered standard** that relies on the unique nature and abilities of an individual patient to determine the amount of disclosure needed to satisfy the requirements of informed consent. This more subjective standard would allow a greater differentiation based on patient preference. A patient who values a pain-free life is very different from one who values an extended life regardless of pain, or as in the case of the professional athlete, a person who values a shorter life, but with full athletic prowess above all other considerations, is possibly quite different from some hypothetical reasonable person.

Another aspect of informed consent is the determination of how much information is necessary. At what level does a risk appear so unlikely that it can be left unsaid? The courts have not provided a bright line indicating the level of material risk that determines these decisions. As will be seen from the cases found in Chapter 7 related to AIDS, the courts have, at times, required disclosure when the risk of infection was infinitesimal. What the courts have provided as a guideline speaks not to the physician nor generally acceptable professional practice, but rather the determination is on the patient side of the equation. The disclosure of known risks and untoward results must be based on matters that are material to the individual patient's needs and decisional process (Southwick, 1978). A risk is material and therefore should be disclosed if it would be likely to affect the patient's decision.

Over time, the courts have been forceful proponents of informed consent and autonomy over paternalism. In several landmark cases, an absolute need for individual self-determination has been required. There is, however, a limited role for paternalism in the area of therapeutic privilege. Therapeutic privilege is the legal exception to the rule of informed consent that allows the caregiver to proceed with care without consent in cases of emergency, incompetence, information concerning dangers that patients of average sophistication would already know, and when the patient, due to depression or instability, could be harmed by the information. The latter case is a rather controversial form of therapeutic privilege, as the decision to withhold information is based on "sound medical judgment" and opens the door for professional determinism at the expense of patient autonomy.

An important case in the autonomy versus paternalism issue was that of *Schloendorff v. The Society of New York Hospital* (1914). In the *Schloendorff* case, the courts outlined a rigid respect for personal autonomy: "Under a free government at least, the free citizen's first and greatest right which underlies all others—the right to the inviolability of his person, in other words, his right to himself. . . ." This right to self was supreme, and guaranteed by the U.S. Constitution through the Fourteenth Amendment to the Bill of Rights. Unwanted touching is assault and threat of assault is battery. These violations of rights are torts for which American law provides a legal remedy. Unwanted medical treatment is in these cases **actionable,** even if the health care provider is attempting to do good. Doing good is not enough if the good performed is without the consent of the patient. In the *Schloendorff* case, a woman was admitted to the hospital, suffering from a stomach malady. The patient refused surgery but allowed the physician to examine her under ether. During the examination, the surgeon found fibroid tumors that needed to be removed and proceeded to remove them, feeling that the care was medically expedient. In his review, Justice Cardozo wrote:

> The wrong complained of is not merely negligence. It is trespass. Every human being of adult years and sound mind has a right to determine what shall be done with his own body; and a surgeon who performs an operation without his patient's consent, commits an assault for which he is liable in damages.

In the document *Current Opinions* of the Council on Ethical and Judicial Affairs, of the American Medical Association (1992), these limitations are outlined in Section 8.08 on informed consent.

Informed consent is a basic social policy for which the following exceptions are permitted:

1. In cases when the patient is unconscious or otherwise incapable of consenting and harm from failure to treat is imminent. Even when a genuine emergency exists, the physician should attempt to secure the consent of relatives.

2. When the risk of disclosure poses such a serious psychological threat of detriment to the patient as to be medically contraindicated.

3. The physician is not privileged to withhold information from the patient merely because divulgence might prompt the patient to forego needed therapy.

4. Even when the patient's reaction to risk information is reasonably menacing, disclosure to a close relative of the patient to secure consent for proposed treatment may be an avenue open to the physician.

In regard to consent and minors, it is difficult to state a position because situations and state statutes differ. In the emergency setting, when parents are unavailable, when there is an immediate threat to life or health, or when delay would cause permanent damage, there is no legal requirement for consent. The prudent health care provider, however, will have made a good faith effort to reach the parents or someone standing in a parental relationship, if the patient's health allows the extended time delay. It is also useful practice to document the emergency nature of the incident by professional consultation.

In nonemergency treatment situations involving minors, the providers must determine the age of majority for their area. Common law sets the age of majority at 21 years, but many jurisdictions differ across the nation. The fact that an individual is married and can vote or purchase alcohol does not provide adequate proof that a minor may provide legal consent for medical treatment. It is important that health care providers know the age of majority for their jurisdiction. Obviously, once this age is attained, the individual is considered an adult.

Yet, there are many cases in which a mature minor may seek health care without parental consent. This situation is common in cases of family planning, sexually transmitted diseases (STDs), or for medical conditions relating to pregnancy. In these cases, the test of the minor's ability to provide consent is often the level of maturity as measured in part by age, but more importantly, by the minor's ability to comprehend the nature of personal decisions. In these cases of age-discretion decisions, factors such as emancipation and marriage may play a major part in these determinations.

Critics such as Jay Katz (1982) have likened informed consent to a fairy tale. He argues that although the doctrine is enchantingly appealing in its simplicity, it does not live up to its promise of delivering decisional authority to the patients. The reality of current medical practice does not fulfill the promise and is often perfunctorily performed, not so much as to convey information and open dialogue between physicians and patients, as to comply with the legality of the law. One indication of this problem is a 1982 survey provided in President's Commission for the Study of Ethical Problems in Medicine and Biomedical and Behavioral Research, which reported that 75 percent of all physicians surveyed believed it to be their responsibility to try to persuade a patient to accept the medically indicated course of treatment. Katz argued that "once kissed by the doctrine, frog-patients" do not become "autonomous princes."

In some sense, however, the criticism by Katz is not a criticism of the principle of informed consent, but rather in how it is implemented. In an excellent article entitled "Enhancing Patient's Autonomy," Lorys (1994) calls on health care providers to go beyond fulfilling the letter of the law to capturing the spirit of true informed consent. This would require providers to allow time for patient reflection before the decision, especially in cases when pain, confusion, high technology, and teaching schedules threaten to coerce the patient and turn the process into little more than a perfunctory explanation of risks and benefits. According to Lorys, for patient decision making to be autonomous, the following four elements must be in place:

- Patient has decision-making capacity.
- Patient not impaired by factors that interfere with autonomous choice.
- Patient provided information regarding nature of illness, various options, and associated risks.
- Patient has opportunity to question and receive answers in relation to issues involved.

FALSE IMPRISONMENT

It is among debilitated patients that the intentional tort of **false imprisonment** is most likely to occur. This tort involves the unlawful restriction of another's freedom. Actual physical force is not necessary to prove this claim. A reasonable fear that force, which may be implied by words, threats, or gestures, will be used to detain a person is often sufficient. The health care provider that forces a patient to remain until the bill is paid or forms signed may be liable under the tort of false imprisonment. These cases often involve patients who have been involuntarily committed to a mental institution. In the case of *Stowers v. Wolodzko* (1971), the patient was committed by her husband and psychiatrist; however, following the commitment, the psychiatrist held the patient incommunicado, refusing to allow her to contact an attorney or a member of her family. The court found the psychiatrist's actions constituted false imprisonment arising out of unlawful restraint of the patient's freedom.

Certain state statutes have allowed the detention of mental patients who were considered a danger to themselves, to property, or to others. These statutes may also allow the hospital to detain a patient with a contagious disease. Those who are mentally ill or contagious may only be restrained to the degree necessary to protect themselves from harm, or to prevent them from harming others. In these cases, it is wise to document the situation carefully, noting the reasons for the detention, the harm that would arise from the patient leaving, and the patient's insistence on leaving.

COMPETENCY DETERMINATION

The presumption under common law is that competent adults are at liberty to consent to or refuse health care. The practitioner, as a general rule, must respect and abide by the decisions of an autonomous patient. This right to refuse treatment even when an individual's life is threatened is a test of our conviction regarding personal self-determination. This general rule, however, cannot apply when the patient's decision is based on incomplete information, lack of understanding, or external controlling influences that preclude independent judgment. Table 4–2 outlines the moral and relevant factors that often influence physicians' decisions in regard to honoring the wishes of the critically ill (Siegler, 1977).

If we examine an illustrative case of a young man injured shortly after returning home from the war, we can see the effects of the six factors from Table 4–2 in play. In this case, the individual was a hometown war hero, and while waiting for an opportunity to begin a career as a commercial pilot, he was involved in an oil field/natural gas accident that left him severely burned, disfigured, blind, and without the use of his hands. Although badly injured, it became apparent that he would survive the incident and that his claim against the petrochemical company was such that he would never, under reasonable circumstances, be in financial need.

Early in his care, however, it became apparent to the young man that he was facing an extended period of rehabilitation and treatment for his burns. At that time, he

TABLE 4–2
Common factors used in decisions regarding patient competence

1. The patient's ability to make choices about care. Does the patient have sufficient information and intellectual capacity to make a rational choice?
2. The patient's consistency with known values.
3. Age. It would seem that a more mature patient's refusal in life-threatening circumstances can often be more easily respected than the refusal of a much younger patient.
4. Nature of the illness. Whether the illness can be diagnosed and what the prognosis is can be significant, especially if complete recovery is possible with appropriate treatment.
5. The attitudes and values of the physician responsible for the decision. The physician's moral and religious background, as well as attitudes toward life and death have a role in the physician's recommendations.
6. The clinical setting. When authority is diffused among a health care team, decisions must be reached in a different way from those used in such private settings as the physician's office or in the patient's home.

decided that, in actual fact, he did not want to continue the painful treatment or to live the life of a blind, disfigured person.

At this early stage of care, it may be concluded that the pain and medications had prevented the young man from making a rational, authentic decision in regard to stopping treatment. If allowed, his decision to stop treatment would have meant an early death due to infection. Using criteria one from Table 4–2 (patient's ability to make choices about care), the medical staff may decide that the pain and medications were limiting his ability to make a rational choice, and therefore continue the care despite his protestations. Using the patient's blindness and physical handicap as a rationale, the physicians authorized the patient's mother to sign consent forms for the continuation of his care.

As time passed, the young man continued to protest the care, and the physicians had him undergo psychiatric evaluation to determine his competence. The results of this evaluation were that, indeed, the patient was competent and that the decision was authentic. The patient did not wish to continue care, based on his evaluation that the pain of the treatment was greater than the value of his future life. He simply did not value an extended life that left him disfigured, blind, and without the use of his hands.

At that time, if the physicians had attended to criteria two (authentic decision), three (age), or four (prognosis of condition), they may have allowed for his self-determination, because the decision appeared authentic, his maturity was not in question, and the nature of the prognosis was such that he would not be returned to a state of health that he valued. However, the physicians decided to continue the treatments, basing the decision on criteria five (attitude and values of the physicians) and six (clinical setting), which do not take into account the desires of the patient or the determination of **competency.** The decision rested more on the physician's personal values and those of the patient's mother, lawyer, and the institutional decision-making system. The treatment was continued although the patient was somewhat mollified by the idea that if he would put up with the treatment, he could later make his own decisions in regard to ending his life without constraint.

This case points out that the factors listed in Table 4–2 do indeed outline considerations used by physicians for decision making; however, they provide no clear mechanism for the decisions themselves. If we intend to honor the autonomy of our patients, then only criteria one (ability to make decision), two (authentic decision), and three (age) need be considered. What seems to be needed is a systematic method by which the focus of the decision-making process is patient based. The real questions that need to be addressed are: Is the patient in a position to make an authentic decision, and should we allow the patient to make this decision under these circumstances? With certain categories of individuals such as children, the mentally incompetent, and those coerced by pain or trauma to the point of incapacity for rational reasoning, the decision to limit personal autonomy is often an easy decision, and frequently made.

The Presidential Commission for the Study of Ethical Problems in Medicine and Biomedical and Behavioral Research (1982) identified three approaches to the determination of competency. These approaches could be categorized as outcomes, status, and functionality. Outcomes criteria would use community values as the standard by which competency is measured. Status criteria would measure indices such as age and mental and physical status. Functionality would examine the individual's actual functioning in decision-making situations. Most believe that the functioning category works best, as it is focused on the issue of whether the patient can make competent decisions.

The difference between an outcomes approach and a functional approach can be seen in the original case and appeal of *Lane v. Candura* (1979). Mrs. Candura, a 77-year-old widow and diabetic, contracted gangrene in her lower right leg. After a period of reflection, Mrs. Candura decided against her physician's recommendation of having her leg removed. The court held that she had closed her mind to the options, and that she was incompetent because her choice was irrational. This is an outcomes approach, for the court reasoned that, obviously by not choosing to have her leg removed, she was risking her life, therefore her choice was irrational, therefore she was incompetent. The appeals court took a different approach to her decision and concentrated upon her ability to appreciate her situation and the various alternative options. The appeals court held that, while Mrs. Candura's choice may have seemed unfortunate, it was "not the uninformed decision of a person incapable of appreciating the nature and consequences of her act." In these cases, it is important for health care providers to honor the competent determinations of the individual patient. As a matter of law, the patient is assumed competent. All testing to assess competency must begin with the premise that the patient is competent unless proven otherwise.

In general, a competent adult has the absolute right to refuse medical treatment, even if the refusal is life threatening. At question is patient autonomy, which is positively confirmed by being able to answer yes to two questions: Does the patient understand and appreciate the nature of the illness and the consequences of the various options that may be chosen? and Is the decision based on rational reasoning? The decision itself need not be rational, but the reasoning process should be.

COMPETENCY DETERMINATION AND RELIGIOUS FREEDOM

The First Amendment to the Constitution creates a problem for the requirement that patients prove their competency by rational reasoning. Given First Amendment protections for religious belief, the requirement regarding the need for rational processes should be modified to include the protection of decisions based on faith, that is, "a belief held to be true, in regard to things unseen." A corollary question needs to be added to the previous two questions in these cases: Is this seemingly irrational thinking, based on a religious belief, acceptable and entitled to First Amendment protections? To be protected, a belief must be held by a sufficient number of people for an extended time period, or be sufficiently like other beliefs that are held by other groups that are considered orthodox.

In regard to Jehovah Witness faith, the courts have provided a generally consistent picture concerned with honoring the decision to not accept transfusions. Orthodox Jehovah Witnesses believe that in the Old and New Testament scriptures, the Lord declares that his followers should not partake of blood:

> *For it is the life of all flesh; the blood of it is for the life thereof; therefore I said unto the children of Israel, Ye shall not eat the blood of no manner of flesh; for the life of all flesh is the blood thereof; whosoever eateth it shall be cut off.*

Leviticus 17:14 KJV

But that we write unto them, that they abstain from pollutions of idols, and from fornication, and from things strangled, and from blood.

Acts 15:20 KJV

To Jehovah Witnesses, the acceptance of a transfusion places them in a situation where they may indeed prolong their lives here on earth, but places them in jeopardy of being eternally cut off from their God.

The decision to honor a decision made as an act of faith is not based on whether an individual's faith is rational to the health care provider, but rather on whether the decision is being made by an autonomous adult. In a Chicago case when the woman repeatedly told her physician that she understood the consequences of her action, but as an act of faith could not take a transfusion, the courts held:

Even though we may consider the appellant's beliefs unwise, foolish or ridiculous, in the absence of an overriding danger to society we may not permit interference . . . in the waning hours of her life for the sole purpose of compelling her to accept medical treatment forbidden by her religious principles and previously refused by her with full knowledge of the probable consequence.

In re Estate of Brooks, (1965)

The decision by an autonomous Jehovah Witness patient to not accept a lifesaving blood transfusion could be honored. Health care providers would do so on the basis that the patient understands the nature of the condition and the consequences of the options, thereby satisfying question one. In regard to the requirement of rationality, the provider would need to take into consideration the First Amendment protection of the patient's rights, as the decision is not a matter of reason, but of faith. It is interesting to note, however, that if the patient appealed not to a protected orthodoxy, but rather to someone such as the Smedley the Powerful who dwells under Mount Hood, providers may consider the decision delusionary and limit the autonomy to protect the patient.

The autonomy of a member of the Jehovah Witness faith or other orthodox religions that restrict medical care, however, does not extend the refusing of medical care to their children. The courts have held that parents no longer exercise the power of life and death over a child.

Parents may be free to become martyrs themselves. But it does not follow that they are free. . . . to make martyrs of their children before the children reach the age of full and legal discretion when they can make that choice for themselves.

Prince v. Massachusetts, (1944)

In these cases, the courts will usually appoint a guardian **ad litem** for the specific and limited purpose of making treatment decisions on behalf of the child. The child is usually not removed from the home or control of the parents, except for the limited area of medical decision making.

In nursing homes across the United States, there are estimated to be 80,000 patients with some level of dementia. Most of them, following our guidelines, could be determined incompetent to make decisions in regard to their medical care. In the acute hospital setting, about 50 percent of the decisions to not resuscitate if the patients begin to fail, involve incompetent patients. The question of competency determination, and who makes the decisions when incompetence is determined, is a problem that will continue to bedevil modern medical care until systems are developed to handle these cases.

INFORMED DEMAND FOR FUTILE TREATMENT

The question of futility has become a major problem in some cases. What is to be done when health care providers make the decision that all further efforts with regard to treatment are futile? The American Thoracic Society (1991) provided the following statement in regard to the obligation of health care professionals in cases when all continuance of life-sustaining therapy appears futile:

> A physician has no ethical obligation to provide life sustaining intervention that is judged futile . . . . even if the intervention is requested by the patient or surrogate decision maker. To force physicians to provide medical interventions that are clearly futile would undermine the ethical integrity of the medical profession.

Although it may not be an ethical obligation to provide life-sustaining care that is determined futile, the courts have not always been willing to overcome patient autonomy in these decisions. In January 1990, an 85-year-old woman was taken from a nursing home to Hennipin County Medical Center for emergency treatment of dyspnea from chronic bronchiectasis. Ms. Helga Wangele required emergency intubation and was placed on a ventilator. During a weaning attempt, Mrs. Wangele had a cardiac arrest and was resuscitated. Following this event, the patient was in a persistent vegetative state as a result of severe anoxic encephalopathy. The attending physicians concluded that the continuation of life support was futile and that treatment could not reverse the underlying disease process or restore the woman to a state of acceptable function. Although continued treatment was determined to be futile, the patient was not brain dead (*Brody, 1992*).

The physicians approached the husband in regard to removing the ventilator. In this conversation, the husband informed them that although his wife had not given her opinion regarding the matter, he wanted everything done, and that the physicians should not play God. It was his opinion that his wife was not better off dead, and that removing the ventilator was just another sign of the decay within the culture.

It seemed to the health care staff that the request was entirely inconsistent with rational health care and the need for cost containment. Although the costs for the continued care would be paid by Medicare, the physicians felt that the case had already received a fair share of the resources that had been pooled for the benefit of the community. An editorial in the *Minneapolis Star Tribune* (1991) summed up the matter in the following manner:

> The Hospital's plea is born in realism, not hubris. They (the physicians) should be free to deliver, and act on, an honest and time-honored message: "Sorry, there is nothing more we can do."

Given the impasse between what appeared to be medically rational and the husband's clear authentic choice, the matter was decided in the courts. On July 1, 1991, the court appointed the husband to represent his wife's interests. Three days later the patient died of multisystem organ failure.

It is clear that these are difficult decisions that attempt to balance the moral integrity of the health care providers against our obligation to enable and allow the autonomous and authentic choices of patients and their families. On the surface we are again arguing autonomy versus beneficence.

How much do we limit autonomy if we begin by limiting the patient's right to demand futile treatment? Upon examination, a right to demand futile treatment in and of itself does not fit the health care environment. In health care, while we have obligations to help rather than hurt, and to work unceasingly on behalf of the patient, this is not an equivalent to "the customer is always right." A patient with chest pain may not demand that a cardiac bypass be done.

Yet these are also value-laden decisions and in value-laden cases, generally, the values of the patient rather than the practitioner should prevail. In one case a physician was counseling a patient in regard to a DNR order and indicated that providing CPR would only give the patient a 1 in a 1,000 chance of survival. The patient replied, by asking what her chances would be if the CPR was not provided? Who determines what chance of life is too high to consider?

The following is a set of suggestions that would allow for the development of a rational futility policy:

- Institutional policy should be developed to assist in conflict cases between health care providers and the patients who are demanding what is considered futile care. These policies, however, should be guided by several criteria. Where possible, the criteria should protect the patient's autonomy, decrease the opportunities for decisions based on the value-laden judgments of the provider rather than true futility, shield the patient from societal decisions in regard to cost containment, and maintain the communication links between patients and providers.

- The values of the patient must be understood and taken into consideration.

- The decision to override patient autonomy must be based on principles supporting the integrity of the profession, rather than individual provider conscience, and the decision must be articulated in this fashion.

- The decision should be shielded from the value decisions of the wider society that the providers may serve.

- These policies do not abrogate the requirement of the providers to provide full, honest, and supportive communication in regard to the plan of care.

- The policy must contain opportunities for patient and family negotiation regarding the decision and an invitation to accept the futility judgment.

- Decisions to remove life-supporting therapy on the basis of futility must be subject to peer review and take into consideration the health care goals of the participants, which may include nonbiomedical objectives (Tomlinson T. & Czlonka, D. 1995).

It is clear that we have not come to a resolution regarding futility. The frustration of the issue when health care practitioners are required to provide futile care has been likened to the daughters of Danaus described by Ovid (Alpers & Lo, 1995). These young women were condemned to draw water in leaky buckets from which the water inevitably spilled. It would seem that if the treatment was as futile as the mythical transporting of water in a leaky bucket, the professional integrity of the profession would require that the treatment be suspended with or without agreement of the patient or the surrogate.

INSTITUTIONAL ETHICS COMMITTEE

An institutional ethics committee (IEC) can be defined as an interdisciplinary body of health care providers, community representatives, and nonmedical professionals who address ethical questions within the health care institution, especially on the care of patients. The impetus for such a committee came from the high profile cases involving Karen Ann Quinlan and Baby Doe (Anderson & Anderson, 1987). The President's Commission for the Study of Ethical Problems in Medicine and Biomedical and Behavioral Research (1982) advocated research into ethics committees.

Often ethics committees are seen as an alternative to court litigation. Health care providers were struggling with new issues that came as the result of previously unimagined lifesaving medical technology, and team medicine where literally hundreds of practitioners were responsible for some aspect of the care. The committees were seen as a way to safeguard the patient's interests by serving on a consultative basis to analyze ethical dilemmas; to educate health care providers, patients, and families; and to guide hospital policy. Figure 4–1 lists the most common functions associated with ethics committees. Note that decision making is not one of the functions listed—these committees play an advisory role.

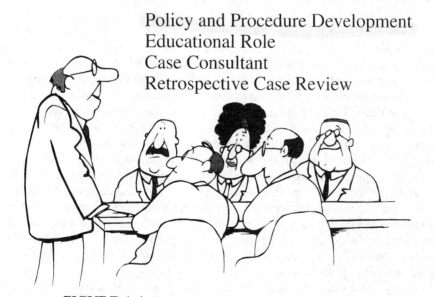

Policy and Procedure Development
Educational Role
Case Consultant
Retrospective Case Review

FIGURE 4–1 Common Functions of Ethics Committees

In 1992 the **Joint Commission on Accreditation of Healthcare Organizations (JCAHO),** the accrediting agency for hospitals and other health care organizations, required the establishment of organizational mechanisms for addressing conflicts with the health care setting. In most organizations covered by JCAHO this has meant the development of ethics committees (Minogue, 1996). The modern committee is often a multidisciplinary group that includes physicians, nurses, social workers, philosophers, laypersons, lawyers, administrators, and religious leaders. In recent years health care providers have become increasingly sophisticated regarding ethical issues and processes through the means of readings, conferences, seminars, and so forth. In that ethical training is increasing in all health care programs, in the future more health care professionals will be prepared to participate in the IECs.

Often the philosophy of the committee will reflect the nature of the institution. For example, a Catholic hospital will generally reflect the tenants of that faith. The refinements in policies concerning brain death determinations, DNR orders, and patient rights have been a great strength of the ethics committees. Given our movement toward health care reform and the use of market forces to assist in cost containment, it is likely that new areas of policy will include issues involving care of the uninsured, care for the medically indigent, organ procurement, rights of the incompetent elderly patient, and problems of premature discharge. Although the development of ethics committees is a rather recent phenomena, it appears that they will continue to play an important role in American health care delivery.

CONCLUSION

The provision of health care is a shared practice, where the expert and the consumer both work to ensure that what is delivered is satisfactory to each. Although there is some room in particular cases for paternalism, the trend is toward placing the principle of patient autonomy over that of provider beneficence. As the expert, the practitioner knows what is needed in a pure medical sense, but does not know how the value preferences of the patient will affect what part of the care will be accepted. As a result of honoring patient autonomy in these situations, it is clear that the provider will find times when medical rationality will need to bend to the will of an authentic choice by the patient.

Because there is general agreement that the patient, through the exercise of personal autonomy, has the right to decide the nature of the care, it is vital that the practitioner ensures that the decision is based on appropriate information. Informed consent is required for all procedures that have the potential for harm. The physician must disclose pertinent details about the nature and purpose of the procedure, its risks and benefits, and any reasonable alternatives to the recommended treatment.

There have been several standards for this disclosure of information, but today most courts recognize the reasonable patient standard, which requires that the information be divulged in such a manner that a hypothetical reasonably prudent person, in similar circumstances, could understand and make decisions regarding the course of treatment. Because each individual has a unique set of values, it will take time to develop a more subjective standard than that of a reasonable person, to ensure understanding.

While there is general agreement that the autonomous adult has the right to decide these issues, there are times when the autonomy of the patient is limited by pain, trauma, age, and mental competency. A competency determination that assesses the patient's ability to appreciate the nature of the situation and the various options seems the best option, if we are to honor patient autonomy as it is focused not on community standard or diagnosis, but on the particular situation. In these assessments, we must first assume that the patient is competent until proven otherwise. As health care providers, we have a tendency to believe that patients are competent when they are agreeing with us, and incompetent when they refuse our counsel.

LEGAL CASE STUDY:*Cobb v. Grant*, 502 P. 2d 1 (Cal. 1972).

The patient was admitted to the hospital for the treatment of a duodenal ulcer. The surgeon went over the nature of the surgery but did not advise the patient regarding attendant risks. The patient signed the informed consent form, the surgery was performed, and the patient went home eight days later. Readmission of the patient to the hospital became necessary, due to internal bleeding caused by a severed artery in his spleen. Injuries to the spleen are not uncommon with this type of duodenal surgery and occur in about 5 percent of the cases. The problem created the need for a second surgery when the spleen was removed. The patient was later readmitted to the hospital after developing a gastric ulcer, which is another not uncommon risk inherent to the surgery performed. The patient was later readmitted again, when he began to bleed from premature absorption of a suture, which is also one of the attendant risks associated with this type of surgery.

At the trial, the **plaintiff** made allegations against the hospital and physician, charging both with malpractice and negligence. The malpractice claim was related to the way the surgery and later care were conducted, and the negligence to the lack of full disclosure. The court did not find sufficient justification against the surgeon, based on the theory of malpractice in the conduct of the surgery, but did so in the area of negligence, related to failure to adequately explain the collateral risks and hazards.

1. What was wrong with the informed consent obtained?
2. Did the disclosure satisfy the reasonable patient standard?
3. Define what is meant by a material risk.
4. Should a 5 percent incidence of occurrence be enough to trigger the requirement to tell the patient?

REVIEW EXERCISES

1. Decisions in regard to accepting or rejecting health care are often dependent, not on medical expertise, but on the value preferences of the patient. The following list of values may cause very different decisions in regard to health care. Rank (a–e) in the order of importance to you personally.
   a. "I want to live as long as possible."

    b. "I wouldn't want to live if I had to remain on a ventilator."

    c. "If I can't live an active life, I don't want to live at all."

    d. "I don't care what you do, or what condition I'm in, so long as I don't suffer from any pain."

    e. "I would rather die than live a life that doesn't allow me to be me."

    f. In regard to the case of the professional athlete found in the chapter, which of the above mentioned values best expresses her decision?

2. The following cases are examples of the struggle between patient autonomy and provider beneficence. State what you think should be done in each case.

    a. An 18-year-old woman of medium height and weight who is about ten pounds over her standard weight comes to your office. She has recently read that a new medication will assist her in weight control. After consulting the literature you note that the drug has the potential although remote side effect of primary pulmonary hypertension which is fatal in about 50 percent of the cases. You inform the patient of the problem; however, the woman wants to take the chance and demands the prescription.

    b. A study on Navajo culture indicates that there are problems associated with the legal requirements of the Patient Self-Determination Act. The problem lies in the fact that within the Navajo culture in times of illness there is a need to speak and think positively and avoid the negative. The requirements that health care providers discuss the presence of life-threatening conditions and seek to elicit answers regarding whether the patient would wish life-supporting technology go against the need for remaining positive in the face of illness. According to tradition, asking such questions could result in complications, perhaps even death. In that these questions are designed to promote patient autonomy and are legally required, what is the practitioner to do?

    c. You are a radiographer with a personal view favoring pro-life. You are doing an ultrasound examination on a pregnant patient to determine the week of gestation and gender of the fetus. She tells you that she is trying to determine the gender of the fetus so that she can legally request an abortion if the gender indicates female. Given your personal view, would you need to perform the test? What place does your professional autonomy play?

    d. A young man with AIDS died in a Midwest hospital in 1993. His physician had placed a DNR order on his chart. Prior to becoming incompetent, the patient had legally authorized a friend to make decisions for him if he was not in a position to make them himself. Twice during the last few weeks of the patient's life, the surrogate decision maker had requested that the DNR order be removed. The request to remove the DNR order was based on the history of the patient who had fought courageously against his disease and had on previous occasions of acute exacerbations, rallied, returning to an almost normal life. The DNR order remained in effect—no attempt at resuscitation was made.

3. What is the benefit to the patient of the legal requirement that we must first assume that the patient is competent until proven otherwise?

4. In the following three cases, indicate whether you think that it would be justified to overcome the autonomy of the patient under the principle of beneficence.

    a. In the intensive care unit, you are working on a patient in a very unstable state. The woman and her children (who were all killed), had been in an accident. It is clear that further emotional trauma would be disastrous to the patient and may cause her death. In a lucid moment, she looks at you and asks, "How are my children?" Is this an instance when therapeutic privilege seems reasonable? Whether you decide yes or no to the therapeutic privilege question, write a sentence that you think would be the most appropriate answer for the patient.

    b. You are working late and you enter the patient's room to find that she has climbed out on the window ledge. She appears to be crying and tells you to leave her alone.

    c. Your elderly patient hates to have the bed rails up and tells you to leave them down.

5. You have now made three decisions regarding whether you would use the principle of beneficence to overcome patient autonomy. Think about how you made these decisions and write two rules that you might adopt to assist in the decision. For an example you might adopt a rule such as: Only competent adults have autonomy.

6. In *Geddes v. Daughters of Charity* of St.Vincent DePaul Inc. (1965), an elderly woman was tricked into going to a mental institution by being told that she was entering a regular hospital. Once she discovered the nature of the institution, she requested that she be released. The physicians and nurses viewed her complaints as being customary and ignored her requests.
   a. What is the tort that is used in her claim known as?
   b. What type of criteria would have to have been in place to retain the woman against her will?
   c. This is clearly a legal problem, but in what ways did her providers fail in their ethical duty to this patient?

7. You are an RN who works with an excellent but busy surgeon who has problems relating to patients. In that you have excellent teaching and people skills, the surgeon asks that you go over the details of the impending surgery with the patients, provide the information required, and get the necessary written informed consent for the surgeon. Should you?

8. Quite often the ethics committee is responsible for drafting institutional policy. For your local area, collect all local institutional policies that relate to DNR orders. Working as a class, draft a consensus policy from those collected.

REFERENCES

Alpers, A., & Lo, B. (1995). When is CPR Futile? *JAMA, 273*, (2), 156–158.

American Thoracic Society. (1991). Withholding and withdrawing life sustaining therapy. *North American Review of Respiratory Disease, 144,* 728.

Anderson, G., & Anderson, V. (1987). *Health care ethics* (pp. 199–200). Rockville, MD: Aspen Publication.

Brody, H. (1992). *The healers power.* New Haven, CT: Yale University Press.

Cobb v. Grant, 502 P. 2d I (Cal. 1972).

Canterbury v. Spence, 464 F.2d 772–7 (D.C. Cir. 1972).

Code of Ethics. (1984). American Medical Association.

Code of Medical Ethics. (1992). *Current opinions.* American Medical Association. Chicago: Council of Ethical and Judicial Affairs.

Council on Ethical and Judicial Affairs. (1992). *Current opinions.* Chicago: American Medical Association.

Emanuel, E., & Emanuel, L. (1992). Four models of the physician-patient relationship. *Journal of the American Medical Association, 267* (16) 2221–2226.

Geddes v. Daughters of Charity of St. Vincent DePaul Inc, 348 F.2d 144 (5th Cir. 1965).

Gert, B., & Culver, C. (1979). The justification of paternalism. In W. Robinson & M. Pritchard (Eds.), *Medical responsibility.* Clifton, NJ: Humana Press.

Holy Bible. (1984). Authorized King James Version, Old and New Testament. Salt Lake City: The Church of Jesus Christ of Latter-Day Saints.

In re Estate of Brooks, 205 N.E.2d 435 (Ill. 1965).

Katz, J. (1982). Informed consent—a fairy tale? In T. Beauchamp & L. Walters (Eds.), *Contemporary issues in bioethics (pp. 191–197).* Belmont, CA: Wadsworth Press.

Keeton, W., Dobbs, D., Keeton, R., & Owen, D. (1984). *Prosser and Keeton on the law of torts* (5th ed.) (p. 175). St. Paul: West Publishing.

Lane v. Candura, 376 N.E.2d 1232 (Mass. App Ct. 1979).

Lorys, O. (1994). Enhancing patient's autonomy. *Dimensions of Critical Care Nursing, 13* (2).

Mill, J. S. (1976). In G. Himmelfarb (Ed.), *On liberty* (pp. 68–69). New York: Penguin Books.

Minneapolis Star Tribune. 26, May 1991, 18A.

Minogue, B. (1996). *Bioethics: A committee approach.* Boston, MA: Jones and Bartlet Publishers.

Natanson v. Kline, 350 P. 2d 1093 (Kan. 1960).

President's Commission for the Study of Ethical Problems in Medicine and Biomedical and Behavioral Research (1982). Washington, DC: U.S. Printing Office.

Prince v. Massachusetts, 321 U.S. 158 (1944).

Pozgar, G. (1993). *Legal aspects of health care administration.* Gaithersburg, MD: Aspen Publication.

Salgo v. Leland Stanford Jr. University Board of Trustees, 317 P. 2d 170 (1957).

Schloendorff v. The Society of New York Hospital, 211 N.Y. 125, 105 (1914).

Siegler, M. (1977). Critical illness: The limits of autonomy. *The Hastings Center Report,* (pp. 7, 12–15).

Southwick, A. (1978). *The law of hospital and health care administration.* Ann Arbor: Health Administration Press.

Stowers v. Wolodzko, 191 N.W. 2d 355 (Mich. 1971).

CHAPTER 5

Confidentiality and Veracity

Goal

The major instructional goal is to examine the problems associated with the ethical principles of confidentiality and veracity as they are applied in modern health care.

Objectives

At the conclusion of this chapter, the reader should understand and be able to:

1. Write a defense for the principle of confidentiality within health care from a utilitarian, duty-oriented, and virtue-ethics point of view.

2. Explain the rationale for the harm principle, as it relates to the *Tarasoff* case.

3. List the two basic ethical principles seemingly in conflict in the *Tarasoff* case.

4. Give five instances when the practitioner would have the legal requirement to report confidential matters that relate to health care.

5. Explain how vulnerability guides the decision-making process when confidentiality is overridden by the duty to warn.

6. List five groups who are not involved in direct patient care that have a legitimate interest in the medical record.

7. List six safeguards that should be considered in regard to allowing access to confidential patient information.

8. Explain why confidentiality is considered a principle with qualifications.

9. List the four classes of torts involving invasion of privacy.

10. Explain the error in the *DeMay v. Roberts* case.

11. Differentiate between privilege and qualified privilege, and give examples.

12. Explain how being newsworthy affects an individual's right to privacy.

13. Differentiate between libel and slander.

14. Write a defense for the principle of veracity using duty-oriented, consequence-oriented, and virtue-ethics reasoning.

15. Explain the ethical problem associated with the use of placebos in clinical practice. Cite the ethical principles that appear to be in conflict with placebo usage.

16. Using the Gert and Culver criteria justifying paternalism, identify those circumstances when lying to a patient may be justified.

17. List four exceptions to the need to prove harm in a defamation case.

18. Explain the two basic defense postures against a charge of defamation of character.

Key Terms

alleged

defamation

fraud

harm principle

institutional review board (IRB)

libel

placebo

plaintiff

primum non nocere

right to privacy

slander

third-party payers

ETHICAL BASIS FOR CONFIDENTIALITY

The patient has a right to every consideration of privacy concerning his own medical care program. Case discussion, consultation, examination, and treatment are confidential and should be conducted discreetly. Those not directly involved in his care must have the permission of the patient to be present. The patient has the right to expect that all communications and records pertaining to his care should be treated as confidential.

A Patient's Bill of Rights (1975)

Who could deny that privacy is a jewel? It has always been the mark of privilege, the distinguishing feature of a truly urbane culture. Out of the cave, the tribal teepee, the pueblo, the community fortress, man emerged to build himself a house of his own with a shelter in it for himself and his diversions. Every age has seen it so. The poor might have to huddle together in cities for need's sake, and the frontiersman cling to his neighbors for the sake of protection. But in each civilization, as it advanced, those who could afford it chose the luxury of a withdrawing-place.

Phyllis McGinley (1905–78), U.S. poet, author (1959)

Confidentiality is an expectation of the patient-provider relationship. The value of this principle can be arrived at and defended using any of the three systematic approaches to ethical decision making outlined in Chapter 2. Whether the reasoning is from a utilitarian, duty-oriented, or virtue-ethics standpoint, confidentiality seems to be a settled issue. It is, perhaps, the most ubiquitous admonition found in the codes of health care professional ethics.

From a utilitarian point of view, the long-term consequences of making public personal information gained as a result of the practitioner-patient relationship would be a chilling effect upon the truth-telling in that relationship. Because health care practice is normally conducted under a tacit agreement of confidentiality, practitioners who breach this trust are in violation of an agreed upon expectation. This expectation is especially critical in psychotherapy, where the patient is encouraged to take risks in personal disclosure. If the patient loses confidence in the process, and fails to discuss personal issues with the practitioner, the amount of care that could be provided is severely limited. Regardless of the health care setting, if the patients knew that their personal information was the daily fare of the cafeteria, along with the mashed potatoes, our ability to provide care would be severely curtailed by this breach of trust.

From a duty-oriented perspective, personal privacy is a basic right with its foundations firmly based not only in long-standing codes of professional practice, but also in common law. The unwarranted disclosure of a patient's private affairs, the unauthorized use of a person's photograph, or exploitation of a person's name have been considered traditionally as acts that might give rise to legal action on the grounds of invasion of an individual's right to privacy. The legal standard for judging a breach of confidence is clear: you may be found liable for any unauthorized breach of confidentiality that "offends the sensibilities of an ordinary person." The medical duty to protect the confidentiality of patients could be argued from our general rights as citizens to be free from invasion of privacy. The individual in our society has the autonomous right to control personal information, and to protect personal privacy. In some sense privacy can be viewed as a person's right, whereas confidentiality is the professional's duty.

From the vantage point of virtue ethics, the practice of patient confidentiality has been a mainstay of health care practice and forms one of the virtues that a patient expects of the "good practitioner." Regardless of specialty or practice, the envisioned good practitioner could not be thought to be cavalier in regard to protecting the patient's confidences. While it is obvious that confidential information must be shared among practitioners so that the best care be provided for the patient, or that the body of knowledge within health care be extended, it is equally obvious that this does not take the form of talks in elevators, cafeterias, or to friends at a party. Even Hippocrates, the father of medicine, understood the need for maintaining confidentiality and made it an important part of this oath of practice.

> What I may see or hear in the course of the treatment or even outside of the treatment in regard to the life of men, which on no account one must noise abroad. I will keep to myself holding such things shameful to be spoken about.

The real question then is not whether confidentiality is good regardless of what form of ethical reasoning you use, but whether it is a moral absolute, or rather one that should be overridden by other considerations. In the classic and precedent setting, 1976 California Supreme Court decided the *Tarasoff* case, which involved a young man by the name of Prosenjit Poddar. Prosenjit confided to his clinical psychologist that he intended to kill a young woman he readily identified as Tatiana. The psychologist, understanding that his patient presented a real danger to the young woman, decided that Prosenjit should be committed for seventy-two hours to allow further evaluation and notified security to assist in securing the patient's confinement.

The patient, however, convinced the security officers that he was rational, and was released following his promise to stay away from the young woman. The health care providers rescinded the orders to place Prosenjit in confinement for evaluation. No effort was made to warn either Tatiana or her family of the potential danger. Within weeks of this event, Prosenjit murdered the young woman.

The health care practitioners later defended their decisions to maintain patient confidentiality on the basis that they had a duty only to their patient and, in the absence of duty, they were not required to protect the life and safety of others. To whom did the caregivers owe duty—to the real patient or to the potential victim? They had chosen to serve the one and ignore the other. Arguments used in their defense were that effective treatment required the patient's full disclosure of his innermost thoughts and that without the promise of confidentiality, patients needing psychiatric treatment would fail to seek care.

The court, in its decision, recognized the difficulty that a practitioner may have in attempting to accurately forecast whether statements made by a patient would be carried out. It ruled, however, that the specialist would be held to the standard of reasonable practice and, where that standard indicated a foreseeable danger to another, a duty to warn was created. The protective privilege of confidentiality is limited when the health and safety of others is involved. The breaching of this obligation to maintain confidentiality is recognized and allowed by the current Principles of Medical Ethics of the American Medical Association (1992) which states that:

> A physician may not reveal the confidences entrusted to him in the course of medical attendance . . . , unless he is required to do so by law or unless it becomes necessary in order to protect the welfare of the individual or of the community.

The balance between protecting the confidentiality of the patients we serve and yet, safeguarding the community, has found its way into many specialties' codes of ethics. This balance can be seen in the guideline for confidentiality for the Colorado Society of Clinical Specialists in Psychiatric Nursing (1990).

Confidentiality Guidelines
1. Keep all client records secure.

2. Consider carefully the content to be entered into the record.

3. Release information only with written consent and full discussion of the information to be shared, except when release is required by law.

4. Use professional judgment deliberately regarding confidentiality when the client is a danger to self or others.

5. Use professional judgment deliberately when deciding how to maintain the confidentiality of a minor. The rights of the parent or guardian must also be considered.

6. Disguise clinical material when used professionally for teaching and writing.

THE HARM PRINCIPLE

In her book, *Secrets: On the Ethics of Concealment and Revelation,* Sissela Bok (1983) cites several instances when confidentiality is overridden by more compelling obligations. Many of these have found their way into legal statutes and practitioners are generally required to report cases involving child abuse, contagious diseases, sexually transmitted diseases, wounds caused by guns or knives, and other cases when identifiable third parties would be placed at risk by failure to disclose the information. Bok believes that the personal protective privilege of confidentiality is limited by the **harm principle.** This principle requires that health care providers refrain from acts or omissions that would foreseeably result in harm to others, especially in those cases when the individuals are particularly vulnerable to the risk.

An example of how harm principle is modified by vulnerability might be what is required in a case of a married man who tested HIV positive. In that the risk to the community at large is rather minimal, and the risks to the man in regard to discrimination, deprivation of rights, and occupational and social harm are great, the practitioner would have a legal and ethical obligation to be discrete in regard to confidentiality, and do little more than what was legally required in reporting the test results. In the case of the wife, however, who is far more vulnerable than the community at large, the practitioners must assure themselves that the situation is modified to lessen the woman's vulnerability or disclose the information themselves to the woman. It would seem then that the practitioner's observance of the principle of confidentiality must always be balanced by the need to protect others from foreseeable harm, especially if the other individual is particularly vulnerable to that harm.

MODERN MEDICINE AND CONFIDENTIALITY

In the early 1900s, maintaining confidentiality was a much easier task as 85 percent of the direct medical care services were delivered by physicians. Access to and the obligation to maintain confidentiality, in regard to medical records, was limited to the physician and a small direct staff. The records kept were maintained as paper charts, usually poorly indexed, and with little opportunity for access outside of the particular clinic or hospital. In some sense, patient confidentiality was easier to maintain, as systems were simpler. Today over 80 percent of the direct patient care is provided by allied health and nursing professionals. In hospitals today, approximately one-third of a patient's record is maintained by physicians with the rest being recorded by other members of the health care team.

The patient record is not only accessible to the attending physicians, but is readily available to a whole host of technical and administrative staff who generate and handle patient data. Following the complaint of one patient in regard to confidentiality, a survey revealed that at least seventy-five individuals had legitimate access to the patient's record by virtue of the fact that they were involved in providing either direct care or support services to the patient.

TABLE 5–1
Health records and legitimate access

Level One—Direct Patient Care	
Physicians	Institutional Services
Nurses	Therapists/Technologists
Level Two—Supportive Services	
Service Payers	Quality Care Reviews
Risk Management	
Level Three—Social Services	
Insurance	Research
Licensing	Education
Employment Decisions	Media
Civil/Criminal Judicial Review	Law Enforcement
Public Health Reporting	Rehabilitation

The complexities of modern medicine and health information systems make the fulfilling of patient confidentiality a major task. Table 5–1 provides some indication of the multitude of possible legitimate access to health care information.

The problem of access to patient information has been exacerbated by the growing use of computerized information systems. The enormous scale on which information can be stored and ease of access to this data has made distribution of information outside the arena of the patient and health care practitioner interface a daily routine as patient data is used for administration, payment, utilization review, teaching, and research. In addition to the health care providers, patient files may be available to insurance companies (because they pay the bills), public health agencies (to assist in monitoring and investigating disease outbreak patterns), employers (to assess job-related injuries), federal, state, and local government (to develop health care plans and to allocate resources), attorneys and law enforcement agencies (as evidence to settle civil and/or criminal matters), media (to report health hazards and to help report medical research development), and accreditation, licensing, and certification agencies (to assess compliance with various criteria and standards). Table 5–2 provides a listing of common legal reporting requirements found in most American jurisdictions (Pozgar, 1993).

The interests of these **third-party payers** with access to medical information may coincide with the patient's best interests, as confidentiality and privacy are not necessarily a high priority with groups such as governmental regulators, third-party payers, insurers, or utilization reviewers. Given the tasks they perform, they may favor safety, truth, and knowledge far more than they value the personal privacy of a single patient. This accumulation, analysis, and storage of rather unlimited quantities of medical information has overwhelmed the health information management professionals who are ethically entrusted with protecting patient privacy and confidentiality (Siegler, 1982). Siegler, who is director of the Center for Clinical Medical Ethics at the University of Chicago,

TABLE 5–2
Common legal reporting requirements

- Newborn Disease (e.g., diarrhea and staphylococcal infections)
- Child Abuse
- Elder Abuse
- Communicable Diseases
- Births and Deaths
- Suspicious Deaths
- Wounds made with Guns or Knives
- Criminal Acts (e.g., attempted suicide, assault, rape, drug use)

argues that, in hospital medicine, the existence of third-party interests and the development of team medicine have made confidentiality a "decrepit concept."

ETHICAL BASIS FOR THE PRINCIPLE OF VERACITY

There is no alleviation for the sufferings of mankind except veracity of thought and of action, and the resolute facing of the world as it is when the garment of make-believe by which pious hands have hidden its uglier features is stripped off.

Thomas Henry Huxley (1825–95)

While everyone may agree that honesty is the best policy, the principle of truth-telling as an absolute is often difficult to fulfill. What of the fragile patient when truth-telling would potentially cause mental or physical harm? Whereas we are bound to truth-telling, we are also bound to nonmaleficence. ***Primum non nocere,*** Latin for "first, do no harm," is the principle that seems to be most often in conflict with the absolute requirement for veracity. And yet, while there may be conflict, it is clear that the special relationship between the practitioner and the patient is such that the patient has a right to expect a higher level of truthfulness from us than others with whom they deal. When one buys a used car you may in fact hope the dealer tells you the truth. If asked a direct question in regard to a specific problem and the dealer lies, he is committing **fraud.** In most jurisdictions, however, if the direct question is not asked, it is not required for the dealer to volunteer the information. The practitioner, however, is bound within the limitations imposed by their role to disclose all relevant information.

Veracity binds both the patient and practitioner in an association of truth. The patient must tell the truth to the practitioner if rational care is to be provided. The practitioner must disclose factual information to the patient so that the patient can exercise personal autonomy.

Although it is conceivable that lying to the patient may become necessary to avoid some greater harm, it cannot be entered into lightly as it interferes directly with the patient's autonomy. Tolerance for lying damages health care delivery. Patients believe lies only because truthfulness is expected from health care providers. Once patients begin to look for deceit, an essential element of good health care delivery will be lost.

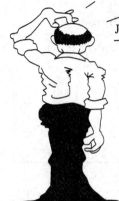

Justification Criteria for a Paternalistic Lie

- The lie benefits the person lied to; that is, the lie prevents more evil than it causes for that particular person.
- It must be possible to describe the greater good that occurs.
- The individual should want to be lied to if the evil avoided by the lie is greater than the evil caused by it, a person would be irrational not to want to be lied to.

FIGURE 5–1 Justification Criteria for a Paternalistic Lie

Even under the guise of benevolent deception, the idea of not telling the truth to patients is suspect. The excuse often put forward is that the patient is not strong enough to tolerate the truth, or more time is needed to prepare the patient for an unpleasant fact. Unfortunately, this lack of truth-telling is somewhat like skipping a pebble across a still pond. While the deceit may provide temporary comfort to the one individual, the ripples reach out and teach all others involved—for example, friends, family, housekeeping staff, and volunteers—that health care providers lie to their patients. When these individuals become ill themselves, they remember the previous deception and feel that they cannot depend upon the word of health care providers.

It would be a rare occasion that truly justified the lying to a patient. Figure 5–1 is taken from *The Justification of Paternalism* by Gert and Culver (1979), which provides criteria to determine whether a paternalistic lie is justified.

THE PLACEBO PROBLEM

One gray area involved in the principle of truth-telling is the use of substances known as **placebos.** Placebos are biologically inert substances without therapeutic value. Fundamental to their use is that the practitioner must engage in nondisclosure and deception in order for the practice to work. The defense of the practice is that the deception is solely for the benefit of the patient. This is a triumph of doing good (beneficence) over patient autonomy, which virtually forms the definition of paternalism. Whereas the use of placebos may form a necessary part of a research study, their use in clinical practice is suspect. Figure 5–2 suggests rules to be considered and questions asked prior to participating in placebo therapy (Desmarais, 1988).

Health care providers should be committed to the truth. When faced with situations in which lying seems a rational solution, other alternatives must be sought. The harm to patient autonomy and loss of practitioner credibility make lying to patients a practice that in almost all cases should be avoided.

- Placebos with active agents which may have harmful side effects are not acceptable.
- Placebos should not be given to patients without their consent.

- What is the condition being treated?
- What are the motives for the therapy?
- What is the placebo supposed to do?
- Are there alternatives that are less misleading?
- What is the patient-provider relationship?

FIGURE 5–2 Placebo Therapy Rules and Questions

DEFAMATION OF CHARACTER

In general, defamation takes two basic forms, **libel** and **slander.** Libel is false or malicious writing that is intended to defame or dishonor another, and is published so that someone other than the one defamed will observe it. Libel can also be presented in signs, photographs, cartoons, etc. Slander, on the other hand, is a false oral statement made in the presence of a third person, that injures the character or reputation of another. Defamatory statements communicated only to the injured party are not grounds for actions.

Normally, to be actionable, injury must result from the slander or libel. However, there are four classes of exceptions when the courts have held that no proof of actual harm is required to recover damages: (1) accusing someone of a crime, (2) accusing someone of having a loathsome disease, (3) calling a woman unchaste, and (4) using words that affect a person's professional reputation (Pozgar, 1993).

Truth and privilege are the two main defenses against the charge of defamation of character. When someone is charged with defamation after making statements that harmed someone's reputation, that person cannot be held for slander if it can be proven that the statements were true. The defense of privilege is also used in those cases when statements, which would ordinarily be considered defamatory, are made in circumstances under which the individual is charged with a higher duty. Examples of this might be the legal requirements to report certain health problems or when the state has provided immunity for those involved in peer review processes.

Absolute Privilege and Qualified Privilege

Information shared by patients with their physicians during treatment is private and is legally recognized as privileged communication. Besides physicians, some states have adopted privileged communication statutes for social workers and psychotherapists.

The law generally recognizes two forms of privilege, absolute privilege and qualified privilege, which permit the publication of privileged communication even if it is proven to be false statement and injurious to an individual's reputation. Examples of absolute privilege would include instances when the statements were made in legislative, judicial, or administrative proceedings (e.g., disclosure of medical records containing defamatory information to a court would therefore not be actionable). An illustrative case might be *Gilson v. Knickerbocker Hospital* (1952), when the hospital had in response to a lawful subpoena released records stating that the plaintiff had been under the influence of alcohol. The plaintiff sued the hospital for libel, claiming that the hospital had maliciously allowed the publication of false and defamatory material.

Qualified privilege is provided for communications made in good faith, with probable grounds for belief usually, by one who is acting in an official capacity. It is not tainted with malice, and regards a subject in which the speaker has an interest, or in respect to which he has a legal, moral, or social duty. The communication is made by the speaker to a person having a corresponding interest or duty. A request for information by a totally disinterested party would never create a situation of qualified privilege.

The courts have generally held that providers have a duty to not disclose information acquired during treatment, unless the information was necessary to protect the patient or another individual from serious harm. An example of a situation when the provider would find it necessary to break the patient's privacy might be in a case similar to the *Tarasoff v. Regents of the University* case. Because the young woman represented a vulnerable individual whose life was at risk, the courts held that the providers had a duty to breach the confidential patient-provider relationship. Confidentiality and patient privacy are qualified rights in that the state requires the reporting of wounds from knives and guns, child abuse situations, venereal diseases, and other contagious diseases. There is room for caution in the reporting of these instances, however, in that concern must be taken to report the information only to the appropriate social or health agency. The state protects these communications so long as the communication is in good faith, under the appropriate circumstances, and given only to the appropriate individuals. The courts have not allowed individuals to hide behind the shield of privilege to carry out personal vendettas based on some hatred, spite, or ill will.

LEGAL FOUNDATION OF PRIVACY

The right to be left alone, free from unwarranted publicity is considered an important freedom in American society, and has found its way into both state and federal statutes. The phrase **"right to privacy"** is a generic concept encompassing a variety of rights thought to be necessary for an ordered democracy. American law has sought to prevent governmental interference into intimate personal relationships, activities, and decision making. In 1965, the U.S. Supreme Court struck down a Connecticut ban on the sale of contraceptives in the landmark *Griswold v. Connecticut* case. Justice Douglas described a "zone of privacy" created by several constitutional guarantees, which forbade governmental intrusion into the homes and lives of citizens. This constitutional recognition of a right to privacy and self-determination formed the basis of the *Roe v. Wade* (1973) decision on abortion. The Supreme Court of the United States determined that a woman's right to make this personal choice rested first, on the avoidance of disclosing personal matters and second, on the need to provide for an arena where independent decision making could take place.

In general, we have the right to make fundamental choices involving ourselves, our families, and our relationships with others free from the scrutiny of others, so long as our assertion of these rights is consistent with law or public policy. We have the right to maintain our private life and to restrict the collection, processing, use, and dissemination of data about our personal attributes and activities. The law provides legal redress against those who would infringe upon our legitimate privacy from motives of malice, curiosity, or gain.

The standard to determine whether an invasion of privacy has taken place is that of a "person of ordinary sensibilities." If such a hypothetical individual would find that the appropriation or exploitation of one's personality, publicizing one's private affairs, or wrongful intrusion into one's private activities was unwarranted and brought about mental suffering, shame, or humiliation, then there would be grounds for action based on invasion of privacy.

INVASION OF PRIVACY CATEGORIES

Generally, tort actions involving invasion of privacy involve one or more of four classes. The first is misappropriation, which usually deals with the unpermitted use of an individual's name or likeness for another's benefit or advantage. In the *Clayman v. Bernstein* (1940) case, a physician who took pictures of the patient's disfigurement and planned to use them for instructional purposes was forbidden to use the pictures in this manner. The second class of tort action is intrusion, which usually involves the intrusion upon another's solitude or seclusion; for example, invasion of an individual's home, persistent unwanted telephone calls, or eavesdropping. Case examples of this class might be the allowance of unessential or lay personnel to be present during a surgical procedure or physical examination. Teaching hospitals should make it clear to the patients that students may be involved in these processes, and that their presence is an integral and necessary part of the educational experience. The third class is public disclosure of private facts. Publicity of an objectionable nature of private information may give rise to legal action even if the information is true. An illustrative case is that of *Hetter v. The Eighth Judicial Court* (1994), which involved a plastic surgeon photographing a before-and-after picture of a patient. The courts held that this public disclosure was objectionable to the patient and, although true, violated the patient's right to privacy. The fourth class of tort action is false light in the public eye. These cases usually involve the publication of information that leads to the public regarding the plaintiff falsely. An example of this might be the use of an unrelated picture of a surgical team in an article about Medicare fraud. The intent was to show a generic picture of physicians; however, the implication would place them in a false light.

COMMON ERRORS IN CLINICAL PRACTICE

Health care providers are often involved in areas of patients' lives that they would most like kept private, and at a time when they are most vulnerable. Consider the common practice of having patients disrobe during examinations and treatments. Problems arise when through a lack of sensitivity or in the pressure of the moment, the practitioner does not ensure that others are absent during the procedure. When an examination is being done and the radiographer comes in to take an X ray or housekeeping comes in to clean the sink, how do we ensure patient privacy? Without the expressed consent of the patient, unessential personnel not involved with the procedure are not allowed to be present. Anyone who has experienced the hospital environment, either as a patient or practitioner, has seen many instances when the patient's comfort zone of privacy has been invaded. Do we really believe that patients do not mind being paraded down halls with the backs of their gowns open, or moved through public areas on gurneys covered only by thin garments? It is possible that through these activities, so common in the hospital setting, and the thousands of other times in which we take shortcuts in transporting, examining, and treating patients, we have crossed the border into the realm where a "person of ordinary sensibilities" might be deeply offended. Unless the patient has given consent, most of these instances could possibly form the basis of a claim for invasion of privacy. An early example of this lack of thought and sensitivity is the case of *DeMay v. Roberts* (1881). In this case the physician was called to the home of a female patient in labor. The physician was accompanied by a nonphysician friend who remained in the delivery area and held the woman's hand providing her comfort during her labor. When the woman became aware that the individual was not a health care provider, she sued the physician for a breach of individual privacy. The court held that having a nonessential person present during the labor violated the woman's legal right to privacy at the time of her child's birth.

LEGAL PERSPECTIVE TO MEDICAL RECORD ACCESS

As a general rule, a patient's medical records are to remain confidential and only be disclosed upon obtaining patient consent. However, as previously identified, there are several instances when health care providers are required to breach patient privacy for the public good. This qualified privilege of disclosure provides a defense against a claim based on **defamation** of character or violation of an individual's right to privacy.

Many state statutes and a few federal regulations require the reporting of certain types of information from the medical record to appropriate agencies with or without the patient's authorization. The child abuse statutes in most states require that hospitals and practitioners report incidents of suspected abuse. If the reported child abuse is later found to be untrue, and so long as the statements are made without ill will or malice toward the individual, the practitioner is generally protected from liability for defamation of character, invasion of privacy, or other civil wrong. In fact, the failure to report a suspected case of child abuse could potentially make the physician and clinical unit liable for a malpractice action for negligence in failing to recognize the "battered child syndrome." An Illinois statute (1984) is illustrative:

> Any physician, hospital administrator and personnel engaged in examination, care and treatments of persons, ... having reasonable cause to believe a child known to them in their professional or official capacity may be an abused child or a neglected child shall immediately report or cause a report to be made .... The privileged quality of communication between any professional person required to report and his patient or client shall not apply to situations involving abused or neglected children and shall not constitute grounds for failure to report as required by this Act.

Some states maintain a registry of the names and addresses of all patients who obtain drugs that are subject to abuse. These reporting regulations have been upheld as a reasonable exercise of an individual state's broad police powers. In the absence of a legal regulation to provide patient information, a police agency has no authority to examine a medical record without the patient's authorization.

LEGITIMATE INTEREST

The medical record goes far beyond only medical information, and contains personal data of a financial and social nature. It is generally the property of the hospital or clinic, but the patient has a legal interest and right to the information. The record is generally considered confidential and access to it should be limited to the patient, authorized representatives of the patient, the attending physician, and hospital staff members who have a legitimate interest. The exact specification of who has a legitimate interest is a great concern to health care practitioners, but some general guidelines are accepted when there is need for patient care, professional education, administrative functions, auditing functions, research, public health reporting, and criminal law requirements.

In regard to patient care, any information may be shared among health care providers who are responsible for the patient within the treating facility. Modern medicine is a team practice, with adequate exchange of information necessary for patient care. The need for professional education usually permits for information in regard to in-house patients to be exchanged for these purposes. This generally includes medicine, nursing, allied health, psychology, social services, or any other professional group involved in the patient care. If the information is to be disseminated outside the treating facility (as in a patient case study), this may not be done without prior patient consent or unless it is in a form that precludes all possible patient identification.

Limited amounts of information as needed for the administrative functions of appointments, admissions, discharges, billing, compiling census data, etc. are necessarily shared among clerical and administrative staff. Duly appointed quality-of-care auditors, governmental third-party payers, and professional review organizations have a legitimate access to the patient record.

Data, in regard to the conduct of research, can generally be shared with the researchers involved, provided that the patient is not identified directly or indirectly in the process, or subsequently in any other report or presentation. Hospitals that permit their staff to engage in research generally have research committees set up to screen the protocols. These **institutional review boards (IRBs)** attempt to balance the potential risk to the patient against the potential benefits of the research. In the absence of more stringent standards, the research committees should require the following as minimum standards (Roach, Chernoff, & Esley, 1985):

1. The research results should be presented in such a fashion as to protect the anonymity of the patients.
2. Only those involved in the study will have access to the raw data.
3. Safeguards to protect the patient's privacy will be part of the research protocol.
4. The same level of obligation to maintain patient confidentiality in the practice of health care is expected in the conduct of medical research.

A Patient's Bill of Rights, provided by the American Hospital Association (1975), outlines the patients' right to inspect their own charts and to receive complete information concerning their treatment in the hospital. In some states, the rules governing access to the medical records of mental health patients differ from those of the general patient population. In the past, these patients were not given access to their records. This practice was based on the assumption that access would be injurious to their health. Recent court cases have tended toward the allowance of this patient group to have greater access to their records and, in some states, mental health patients have the same right to inspect their records as do other patient populations.

It is essential that hospitals establish effective procedures to protect the content of medical records, not only from a standpoint of patient confidentiality, but also from the possibility of intentional falsification or alteration of the record. Unfortunately, records have been doctored by both patients and practitioners, who wished to improve their chances in pending legal actions. With the advent of computerized records, the following steps should be taken to protect the security of patient medical records:

- Access codes for the various categories of personnel that differentiate between those who may only view the records, from those who may view, delete, enter, or modify the records.
- Automatic deletion of access code in cases of employee termination, suspension, or resignation.
- Internal measures to detect unauthorized tampering or entry into the system.
- Competent medical records or risk management personnel to review a record before it is examined by the patient or the patient's representative.
- No removal of a medical record from the hospital except pursuant to legal process or a defined hospital procedure such as allowing an accompanied patient to take personal records to another facility for testing.
- No private examination of the medical records by either the patient or the patient's authorized representative.

QUALIFIED PRIVACY FOR THE NEWSWORTHY

In that inquiring minds want to know, we have a double standard in regard to the privacy of newsworthy or public figures, as they do not have the same protection under the law as do ordinary citizens. When the national tabloids report intimate details of the lives of famous individuals that go well beyond what would offend the sensibility of an ordinary person, the individual would only have a claim if the assertion was untrue. This doctrine is stated in the California case of *Cohen v. Mark* (1950), which held that a "person by his accomplishments, fame or mode of life, or by adopting a profession or calling which gives the public a legitimate interest in his doings, affairs, or character, is said to become a public personage, and thereby relinquishes a part of his right to privacy." This loss of personal rights by the famous or notorious has led in a recent case, to where those having evidence pertaining to a murder were more interested in reporting this to the tabloids than police. Being newsworthy, unfortunately for the patient, forms a complete defense against an action based on invasion of privacy.

The issue then becomes what is newsworthy? If, for instance, a national figure were in the hospital and pictures were taken of his admissions and, perhaps his gurney ride into the surgery suite, it would be hard to bring an action based on an invasion of privacy. Clearly, the admission and surgery would be something that the citizens may have a legitimate interest in knowing. If, however, following the surgery you took a picture of the individual walking down the hall with their backsides exposed, it is likely that this would go beyond the nature of newsworthy and would provide for a possible action.

CONCLUSION

The principles of veracity and confidentiality are important to the practice of health care. Not only are these important ethical principles, failure to maintain appropriate practice standards have grave legal ramifications. In the United States, citizens have a remedy under law for invasion of personal privacy under the 1974 Privacy Act. In addition, the First, Third, Fourth, Fifth, Ninth, and Fourteenth Amendments to the Constitution provide some legal recourse. Because the Constitution does not specifically identify privacy as a personal right, the interpretations have varied over time.

In health care, the general patient population still places a great deal of faith in the truthfulness of practitioners and in our maintenance of the principle of confidentiality. These principles seem to serve two basic purposes. First, they acknowledge a respect for the individual's right to personal autonomy as guaranteed by our legal system and enshrined in our cultural values. Second, and perhaps more importantly to the health of the patient, our observance of these principles provides a bond between the practitioner and patient which allows for a full and honest disclosure of information. In those rare cases when disclosure is necessary to protect a community interest, confidentiality must be balanced by a duty to warn, especially with vulnerable third parties.

Although the establishment of hospital team medicine and bureaucratic interventions have eroded the principle of confidentiality, it is imperative that to the fullest possible extent, health care providers should take meticulous care to guarantee that patient medical and personal information be kept confidential. To the degree that health care providers must breach confidentiality to third parties, it would seem that the patient should be notified of the nature and ramifications of these disclosures. If patients understand what will happen to the information, they then would be in a better position to decide which of their personal matters they would choose to relate and which they would prefer to keep private.

Policies must be designed to balance the right to legitimate personal privacy, while not offsetting the institutional need to make necessary information quickly and easily available to those who have a legitimate claim to it. It would seem that, at a minimum, these privacy safeguards should (1) define circumstances under which medical information is disclosed to other parties; (2) provide procedures by which patients may gain access to their records; (3) allow access to records to others only on a "need to know" basis; (4) ensure anonymity in aggregating data for research or statistical purposes; (5) carefully balance society's long-term goals and the legitimate need of organizations to have access to medical records with the patient's short-term desire for and right to privacy; and (6) inform the patient of what is meant by confidentiality in the context of current practice.

These safeguards would be in the spirit of informed consent and patient autonomy, and would offer some protection against misuse and abuse of patient information. In addition, if patients have access to their records, they can ensure that the information contained therein is accurate, complete, and relevant to their care. Patient advocacy is a significant responsibility of health care practitioners. Practitioners must work toward the restoration of some semblance of institutional responsibility in the area of confidentiality if our patients are to continue to believe in the process.

Modern technology has vastly improved our access to information. Large amounts of data can be stored on small disks, whisked across cyberspace via the information superhighway. It is, as Charles Dickens suggested, "the best and worst of times." In 1993, computer disks containing information on 8,000 patients of a Florida AIDS clinic were stolen. The private medical records relating to a congressional candidate's suicide attempt were released to the media and made headline news (Frawley, 1994). Our health information system is becoming more computerized and centralized, thus making all health histories more accessible. The Joint Commission on Accreditation of Healthcare Organizations (JCAHO) requires that institutions have policies in place to safeguard the security of computer and paper-based records. We are in a time of great transition in regard to health care information. As we make our way through this period of rapid development of computerized data retrieval systems, health care will benefit from the process and become more vulnerable to exploitation.

Veracity and confidentiality are important legal and ethical elements in the provision of health care. The individual in our society has the autonomous right to control personal information, and to be free from libel and slander. It is clear that the observance of these principles frames the environment necessary to create an appropriate patient-provider trust relationship. If the patient felt that the provider could not be trusted to tell the truth or that information regarding the patient's body or condition was the subject of public conversation used to brighten the coffee break in the cafeteria, or was subject to release to publications, a great barrier between practitioner and patient would exist. This fear of disclosure has, in the past, led minors with sexually transmitted diseases to suffer without care rather than seek aid, knowing that the health care system required parental notification. With the advent of computer technology and sophisticated information systems, personal privacy is beset in all aspects of our lives. This is especially true with medical information systems where patient information can be brought up on a CRT screen in a variety of areas throughout the hospital, making this information available to all who have access. Health care providers must come to understand the profound legal and ethical implications involved in the principles of confidentiality and veracity.

LEGAL CASE STUDY 1: *Martin v. Baehler,* No. 91-C11-008, 1993 WL 258843 (Del Supr. Ct. May 20, 1993).

This action arises out of an **alleged** and unauthorized release of confidential information regarding the plaintiff Stephanie Dempsey Martin. The **plaintiff** alleges that on December 5, 1989, while a patient of Dr. Baehler, she was found to be with child. On December 19, 1989, Idella L. Fontana, an employee of Dr. Baehler contacted the plaintiff's grandmother, and without consent or justification informed the grandmother of the pregnancy. On the same day also without consent or justification the **defendant** Idella Fontana also informed the plaintiff's mother and stepfather.

1. In that the defendant told only family members of the plaintiff about the pregnancy and did not broadcast the information to the general public do you feel that there is sufficient cause of action for invasion of privacy?

2. Even if you decided that there was insufficient cause for an action based on invasion of privacy, could the action of telling the family be ethically justified?

3. In that the physician was not involved in the telling of the family, why was she listed as a plaintiff? What legal principle justifies her being listed?

LEGAL CASE STUDY 2: The Confidentiality of HIV-Related Information Act. (Ref. 35 P.S. § 7607(a) (1990).

The Pennsylvania legislature, in 1990, recognized the need to protect the confidentiality of those infected with HIV and diagnosed with AIDS. The legislature passed the Confidentiality of HIV-Related Information Act with the intent of promoting confidential testing so as to encourage those who need it the most to obtain testing and the appropriate counseling. The act specifically prohibited any "person or employee, or agent of such person, who obtains confidential HIV-related information in the course of providing any health or social service . . . . may not disclose or be compelled to disclose the information."

1. How would this law relate to the harm principle?

2. In your opinion would such a law promote or harm the public health?

3. Does such a law presume that allied health and nursing professionals cannot be trusted to act with ethical integrity?

REVIEW EXERCISES

1. Unauthorized vs. authorized disclosure: In this exercise state whether you think the disclosure of information was appropriate or inappropriate and defend your position.

    a. A young woman who states she has just been raped comes into the emergency room requesting a pelvic examination and a morning-after pill, but insists that the staff not call the police. The staff reports the incident.

    b. A young man brings his child into the emergency room for an arm injury. The family has brought the child in several times of late for similar injuries with the excuse that the child is somewhat clumsy and is having difficulty learning to ride her bike. The child shows no fear of the parent and upon questioning confirms the parent's version of the events. The staff reports the injury as a possible child abuse case.

    c. You are a nursing student on a pediatrics rotation within the hospital and you notice that the neighbor of your parents has been admitted to the surgery unit. During your lunch break you review her record before you drop in to see her.

    d. You are a technical nurse who has completed post-op care of a young woman who is a fellow church member who has just had an abortion. You are very concerned for the young woman and decide to confide this information to your minister.

    e. A young man who lives in the same housing complex as you, comes into the hospital's clinical laboratory for tests and is confirmed as being HIV positive. As the manager of that laboratory, you feel it a duty to tell the manager of the housing complex that, in fact, the person in Unit Five has an infectious disease.

    f. You are a respiratory therapist and the patient states that she would like to tell you something, but only if you would hold it in strictest confidence. She then relates to you that she is very depressed and is thinking about taking her own life once she is discharged from the hospital. You relate this information to the attending physician.

    g. You are a medical records technician and are in the department when two men come in and flash badges indicating that they are from the FBI and need to see the Hiram Jones record as a matter of national security. You cooperate and allow them access to the files.

    h. As a result of caring for a patient, the physician notes that a patient who works as a bus driver is at risk for having a heart attack and recommends that the driver cease driving, as he may be placing the children at risk. The driver asks that the physician not notify the school district as it would put the driver at risk of losing his job. The physician notifies the district.

    i. During the course of a patient evaluation you find that the family of the patient has incest problems. You recommend the notification of the police.

2. In the article "Giving the Patient His Medical Record," Shenkin and Warner (1973) propose the following:

> We propose that legislation be passed to require that complete and unexpurgated copy of all medical records both inpatient and outpatient, be issued routinely and automatically to patients as soon as the services provided are recorded. The legislation should also require that physician and hospital qualifications and charges be recorded. Hospital

records should be available regularly to patients on the ward, and copies sent to them upon termination of hospitalization.

   a. In this exercise, list four positive consequences that you think would come from such a law (e.g., better communication between health care providers and patients).

   b. List four potential negative consequences (e.g., increased litigation).

3. You are working with someone who you find reprehensible and suspect of stealing from the department's coffee fund. On your way out to the parking lot one day, you stop the person and express yourself in the strongest terms, you accuse him of theft, call him a bitter name, and remark about his ancestry. Have you committed an actionable defamation of character? If you had, of which form of defamation are you guilty? Have you committed a breach of health care ethics?

4. As the pharmacist of the local community pharmacy, you have been filling prescriptions for Mrs. Arthur for several years. She has an extensive medication profile which suggests that she has several chronic illnesses including a psychiatric disorder. In her dealings with you there has been nothing that indicated an inability to make competent decisions or to authorize appropriate treatment decisions. One day her husband, Bob, comes into the pharmacy and requests that you give him a copy of his wife's medication profile. He indicates that he wanted to be sure that his wife was receiving the correct medications and was being compliant in taking the drugs as prescribed. What shall you do?

5. You are a local primary care physician in a small community. The Conrads are an important family within the community and are your friends. Joe Conrad, the patriarch of the family, comes in for a routine examination and tests positive for gonorrhea. It is a form that is very susceptible to a common antibiotic, which is your planned treatment. Joe asks you as a friend, not to place this information on his medical record, or report the information to the public health department. What is the legal and ethical thing to do?

6. You really do not like a co-worker who is working on his licensure. You find out that during the last state examination he took, he failed to pass the test. You post his grades on the department bulletin board. Have you created the tort of defamation of character? What about invasion of privacy?

7. Using the Gert and Culver (1979) criteria for justification of paternalism, determine whether it would be ethical to lie to the patient in the following situations. Be prepared to defend your choices.

   a. Mrs. Jones is in the unit and waiting for laboratory tests. She is planning to go home over the weekend to spend time with her family and will return to the unit first thing Monday morning. You receive her tests in the early afternoon prior to her leaving, and it shows that she has metastatic cancer which has spread throughout her body. It is clear that this may be the last trip home for Mrs. Jones. When you enter her room she asks you whether the tests have come back.

   You tell her that her tests will probably come back after she leaves and for her to have a great weekend and you will see her Monday. Was your deception ethical?

   b. Mrs. Smith was in an accident in which she was terribly injured and her three children were killed. She is in the intensive care unit and her cardiovascular status is very unstable. It appears to you that any additional shock or stress could place her life in danger. While you are standing beside her, she becomes lucid, looks at you, and asks how her children are.

   You tell her that everything that can be done for the children is being done and that she needs to focus on herself getting well now. Was your reply ethical?

   c. The Sneads are a wonderful elderly couple who live together in the nursing home. While Mrs. Snead is out visiting friends in the unit, Mr. Snead has a heart attack. The code is called but the staff is unable to restore the pulse. The staff likes Mrs. Snead and decides not to tell her that her husband has died. When she comes in the staff continues the code. In that the room is dark and her eyesight poor, Mrs. Snead does not know that her husband is dead. The staff waits a few minutes and then tells her that he is beginning to fade. The staff also tells her that it was as if he had waited for her to say goodbye. With tears in her eyes, Mrs. Snead thanks the staff saying, "I am so glad he waited." Was the deception ethical?

REFERENCES

American Hospital Association. (1975). *A patient's bill of rights.*

American Medical Association. (1992). *1992 Code of medical ethics current opinions.* Chicago, IL: Council on Ethical and Judicial Affairs.

Bok, S. (1983). *Secrets: On the ethics of concealment and revelation.* New York: Vintage Books.

Clayman v. Bernstein, 38 Pa. D.C. 543 (1940).

Cohen v. Mark, 211 P.2d 320 (Cal. Dist. Ct. App. 1950).

Colorado Society of Clinical Specialists in Psychiatric Nursing. (1990). Ethical guidelines for confidentiality. *Journal of Psychosocial Nursing, 28* (3), 43–44.

De May v. Roberts, 46 Mich. 160, 9 N.W. 146 (1881).

Desmarais, M. (1988). The nurse's ethical guide to placebo giving. *California Nurse,*

Frawley, K. (1994). Confidentiality in the computer age. *RN,* 59–60.

Gilson v. Knickerbocker Hospital, 116 N.Y.S. 2d 745 (N.Y. App. Div. 1952).

Gert, B., & Culver, C. (1979). The justification of paternalism, 1–9. In W. Robinson & M. Pritchard (Eds.), *Medical responsibility.* Clifton, NJ: The Humana Press.

Griswold v. Connecticut, 381 U.S. 479 (1965).

Hetter v. Eighth Judical District, 874 P. 2d 762, 110 Nev. 513 (Nev. 1994).

Huxley, T. *Collected essays* Vol I. Westport, CT: Greenwood Publishing Group 1970.

Ill Ann Stat Ch. 232054 (Smith-Hurd Supp. 1983–1984).

Martin v. Baehler, No. 91C-11-008, 1993 WL 258843 (Del Supr. Ct. May 20, 1993).

McGinley, P. *Province of the heart.* N.Y.: Viking Press 1959.

Pozgar, G. (1993). *Legal aspects of health care administration.* Gaithersburg, MD: Aspen Publications.

Roach, W., Chernoff, S., & Esley, C. (1985). *Medical records and the law.* Rockville, MD: Aspen Publications.

Roe v. Wade. 410 U.S. 113 (1973).

Shenkin, B., & Warner, D. (1973). Giving the patient his medical record: A proposal to improve the system. *New England Journal of Medicine, 289*(13), 688–699.

Siegler, M. (1982). Confidentiality in medicine—A decrepit concept. *New England Journal of Medicine, 307,* 1518–1521.

Tarasoff v. Regents of the University of California, 551 P.2d 334 (Cal. 1976). (July, 1976).

---- CHAPTER 6 ----

Role Fidelity

Goal

The major instructional goal is to come to an understanding of the obligations imposed under the principle of role fidelity upon members of the health professions.

Objectives

At the conclusion of this chapter, the reader should understand and be able to:

1. List the rationale for a profession's creating a code of ethics.
2. Outline the ethical obligations we have toward impaired colleagues.
3. Outline the importance of the scope of practice as it relates to practitioner activities.
4. Outline the problems associated with joint venturing and kickbacks.
5. State an ethically based rationale for forbidding sexual relations between patients and health care providers.
6. Outline the professional's obligations that make whistle-blowing an appropriate albeit unpleasant aspect of practice.
7. Explain the nature of *qui tam* actions.

Key Terms

agency	**False Claims Act**	**joint venturing**
alleged	**fiduciary**	**respondiat superior**
caveat aeger	**fraud**	**scope of practice**
disparagement	**gatekeeping**	**self-referral**

PROFESSIONAL CODES OF ETHICS

In ethical terms, to be a professional is to be dedicated to a distinctive set of ideals and standards of conduct. It is to lead a certain kind of life defined by special virtues and norms of character. It is to enter into a subcommunity with a characteristic moral ethos and outlook.

Don Welch (1995)

A code of ethics is primarily a convention between professionals. According to this explanation, a profession is a group of persons who want to cooperate in serving the same ideal better than if they did not cooperate. A code protects members of a profession from certain consequences of competition. A code is a solution to a coordination problem.

Michael Davis (1993)

Historically the essential characteristics of the learned professions (education, clergy, law, health care) are self-regulation, a specialized body of knowledge, standards of education and practice, a **fiduciary** relationship with those served, and the provision of a particular service to society. Most often the professional groups operate under a legal practice act and develop a code of ethics to assist in self-regulation. Codes of ethics are common within the many specialties of the health professions. The language within these codes is usually vague as to levels of expected performance, and therefore the fair enforcement of the rules is difficult. In addition to set statements listing minimum criteria for ethical performance, codes usually include a section outlining the profession's mission and objectives. It is toward these ideals that the profession moves. Common problems associated with professional codes are:

- Vagueness as to duties and prohibitions
- Incompleteness as to duties
- Excessive concern with promotion and prestige of profession
- Vagueness in regard to self-regulation and peer enforcement
- Excessive concern with financial and business interests

Although most health education curricula have coursework that examines ethical and legal issues, the stress placed on these areas is generally less than the technical aspects of the field. Yet, when we enter practice, it is often the human elements contained within legal and ethical practice that are the most difficult to master. When we review the profession's code, we often fail to find a solution to the problem among the listed rules, and must turn to ethical theory and reason for answers. Professional codes are often as much concerned with professional etiquette as with matters of important ethical concern. This is not to say that the codes of our professions do not have a legitimate place. They have, as a purpose, the binding of a group of practitioners and the expressing of the aims and aspirations of that group. They speak to our better selves in the area of personal integrity, dedication, and principled behavior.

As a member of a health profession, you take upon yourself the obligation to be a peer to others on the health care team. Part of these obligations can be considered **gatekeeping** functions, whereby one looks out for the interests of the profession and of others in a similar practice. These obligations flow naturally as a result of our professional obligations and education, which lead to a strong sense of collegiality with others in our practice. This sense of collegiality and mutual support is found in the earliest of codes when new practitioners undertook obligations to their teachers and the professional guild. The following statement is found in the standard English translation of the Hippocratic Oath.

> *I swear by Apollo Physician and Asclepius and Hygieia and Panaceia and all the gods and goddesses, making them my witnesses, that I will fulfill according to my ability and judgment this oath and covenant: To hold him who has taught me this art as equal to my parents and to live my life in partnership with him, and if he is in need of money to give him a share of mine, and to regard his offspring as equal to my brothers in male lineage and to teach them this art—if they desire to learn it—without fee and covenant; to give a share of precepts and oral instruction to all the other learning to my sons and to the sons of him who has instructed me and to pupils who have signed the covenant and have taken an oath according to the medical law, but to no one else.*

Hippocratic Oath

The new practitioner, in taking the oath, bound himself to share knowledge only with those within the guild, and to treat other practitioners equal to members of one's own family. From these early practices have come a series of traditions within the professions, to avoid the **disparagement** of other practitioners, to share new therapies and technologies, to offer professional courtesy for services, and to look after the general welfare of the profession and those in practice. This chapter will focus on the special duties and roles that are attendant to being a member of a health specialty.

GATEKEEPING

Although some health care practitioners are independent entrepreneurs, the principle of **caveat aeger** (the patient beware) cannot be allowed to govern the interactions between clients and health care providers. A fiduciary relationship exists between the provider and the patient. This relationship of responsibility is based on the disparity of information and vulnerability on the part of the patient. It is the trust component of the therapeutic relationship that causes individuals to feel betrayed and outraged when abuses occur. To ensure that vulnerable patients are not exploited, society and the professions have adopted regulatory licensing mechanisms, legal remedies, and peer review systems.

Not only are we responsible for our individual actions in regard to the patient, but we are also charged with the duty to ensure that the rest of the team is practicing appropriate care. Many professional codes echo the statement found in the American Nurses Association's (ANA's) *Code for Nurses with Interpretive Statements* (1985) which states, the "nurse acts to safeguard the client and the public when health care and safety are affected by incompetent, unethical, or illegal practice by any person." This essentially means that a duty is imposed that requires the nurse to assume the role of patient advocate—to take action against anyone, any practice, or any system that is prejudicial to the patient's best interests. This statement may be easy to say but difficult to practice, and requires that health care providers be prepared to monitor their peers and to whistle-blow if needed to correct a state of injustice, neglect, or abuse.

TABLE 6–1
Justification of Whistle-Blowing

- The wrongdoing in question is grave and has created, or is likely to create, serious harm.
- The professional who is contemplating blowing the whistle has appropriate information and is competent to make a judgment about the wrongdoing.
- The professional has consulted others to confirm information and judgment.
- All other internal resources to resolve the problem have been exhausted.
- The whistle-blowing will most likely serve a useful purpose.
- The harm created by the whistle-blowing is less than the harm done by a continuation of the wrongdoing.

The only obligation which I have a right to assume is to do at any time what I think is right. It is truly enough said, that a corporation has no conscience; but a corporation of conscientious men is a corporation with a conscience.

Henry David Thoreau (1849)

For many, whistle-blowing is an issue that is somehow culturally wrapped in terms such as informer, squealer, rat, etc. The very thought of whistle-blowing among professionals seems contradictory to the normal standard of loyalty to colleagues and the institution, which are important aspects of professional practice. Obviously, if whistle-blowing were commonplace within an organization, it would create a climate hostile to mutual trust, interdependent practice, and ethical conduct, all of which are vital if we are to practice in health care teams. The correction of problems through whistle-blowing will often cost money, embarrass colleagues, or embarrass the institution in which one works. Individuals and institutions do not usually appreciate being embarrassed, and as a result, even if the reported problems are true instances of abuse, the whistle-blower may find that, as their reward, they are harassed, avoided, demoted, and even terminated. It is because of the seriousness of the effects of whistle-blowing on the practitioners, the institution, and the community of colleagues that whistle-blowing should be reserved only for serious issues. Table 6–1 offers guidance on when whistle-blowing is justified.

Regardless of the risk, the professional must also recognize that to not report serious misconduct is to become an accessory to the conduct. Whistle-blowing is an obligation of role duty that cannot be ignored. Peter Raven-Hansen (1980), an attorney, has outlined a series of defensive strategies for those who have come to the conclusion that whistle-blowing is necessary.

1. Write a clear, short summary of the problem, describe what it means and why action is necessary.

2. Avoid personalization, focus on the nature of the incident.

3. When possible, have your statements corroborated by other health care providers. Sticking to the facts of the incident should assist you in avoiding charges of slander and libel.

4. Make every effort to settle the matter internally. The media should be your last, rather than first, channel of communication.

5. Do not believe that you can remain anonymous. The nature of the incident and the details of the disclosure will more than likely reveal the source.

6. The nature of bureaucratic institutions creates barriers to change. Expect a slow process.

7. Expect retaliation. The whistle-blower must expect to be characterized as a snitch and disloyal troublemaker. You must either be prepared to live with these attitudes or be prepared to move on to another position.

In 1986 the Congress of the United States enacted the **False Claims Act.** This act strengthened the protection for those who reported fraud in federally funded programs and provided an incentive for whistle-blowing. Under the act an individual may sue in the name of the federal government and receive 15 to 30 percent of any triple damages and fines that are imposed. These suits are known by the Latin phrase *qui tam,* which means "Who as well as the King sues in the matter." In health care programs such as Medicare and Medicaid, which have massive federal funding, the potential for fraud is great.

Whistle-blowing is not a task to be entered into casually. Even under the best of circumstances, the individual must understand that, though necessary, the position of whistle-blower is high risk, often lonely, and rarely appreciated. As health care professionals committed to patient advocacy, we must at times assume these risks, but perhaps more importantly, we must consider how we can support others who take on this important aspect of role duty. One important aspect of this role is the predisposition to suspend judgment until enough facts are known. Not all whistle-blowers are correct in their allegations (Darr, 1991).

IMPAIRED COLLEAGUES

The provision of health care is stressful, and it is not surprising that certain providers have found themselves susceptible to alcohol and drugs. Caring for critically ill patients, being surrounded by their families, and practicing in an age of increased litigation and cost containment are sources of moral conflict and distress. The ANA has estimated that 6 to 8 percent of nurses use alcohol or other drugs to the extent sufficient to impair their professional performance (Hughes & Smith, 1994). The most commonly abused drug is alcohol. Signs of chemical dependency often include a decline in job performance, mental status changes, and a decline in professional image. Among the most common signs are:

1. Excessive use of sick time

2. Sloppy, illogical charting

3. Long breaks

4. Excessive use of mints; alcohol on breath

5. Lowered clinical performance, increased mistakes

6. Inappropriate emotional responses

7. Diminished alertness

Often the practitioners who are caught up in these destructive practices are bright, hard working, and hold responsible positions. Addicted individuals seem to have an infinite supply of rationalizations, prevarications, and subterfuges to show that the truth is untrue. What is to be done when you find that a colleague is impaired?

Guided by the principle of role fidelity and nonmaleficence, the question that must be faced is not whether the practitioner has a duty to intervene, but rather the manner of intervention. It is a lesser error to express a concern that later proves to be wrong than it is to do nothing in the face of a pattern of behaviors that suggest that a colleague has a difficulty. It is hard to imagine a more unpleasant task than confronting a colleague with regard to substance abuse. When possible, it is best that the individual be encouraged to seek effective help independently. When this is not possible, help still must be obtained to protect the patients and salvage the practitioner. Regardless of how the process goes, the basic elements are that the practitioner receives effective help, and that those with knowledge of the situation treat the impaired colleague humanely, as we would any patient who needed our assistance. It seems that these instances can be guided by the following two questions: Are the patients being protected from unnecessary harm? and Is the practitioner being treated with due process and the respect that is owed a colleague?

SEXUAL MISCONDUCT IN HEALTH CARE PRACTICE

Whatever houses I may visit, I will come for the benefit of the sick, remaining free from all intentional injustice, of all mischief and in particular of sexual relations with both female and male persons, be they free or slave.

Hippocratic Oath

It is generally held among health care providers, that sexual relations between practitioners and patients are unethical. The failure to handle the emotional content of the therapeutic relationship is universally condemned by the professions. Most studies regarding sexual contact with patients have involved the field of psychiatry. One major problem with sexual contact between practitioners and patients is that the relationship is never equal. The nature of the provider-patient relationship always places the practitioner in a position of advantage in the critical areas of knowledge, vulnerability, power, and status. Anyone who has worked in health care knows that the environment is at times emotionally confusing. The emotions of caring, admiration, trust, and affection are part of the relationship. These emotions can become quite intense when either party is experiencing pressures or traumatic events. It is not unusual for sexual attraction to be one emotion that comes to the surface.

Because of the inequality of position, sexual relations under these conditions cannot be considered, nor can they be understood as representing true consent on the part of the patient. Inasmuch as practitioners have an obligation to treat the needs of the patient first, their own personal gratification cannot become a consideration. The therapeutic relationship rests on the premise that the provider is dedicated to the patient's welfare and has no other conflicting motives or considerations. This belief by the patients is so strong that some will tolerate uncomfortable situations in the belief that the provider would not betray their trust (Rapp, 1987). Although some in the professions excuse the conduct, women who have experienced the practice view it as negative and destructive. Victims report feeling angry, abandoned, humiliated, and exploited (*Boston Globe,* 1990). Whether these events are due to a temporary failure to manage the therapeutic relationship or to crass exploitation of the professional situation, these relationships are neither ethically excusable nor condonable, and under certain situations are illegal.

The provider who begins to feel that a potential for misunderstanding is possible, or feels that there is a potential for mutual feelings of romantic interest, is best advised to end the professional relationship. In that the patient's feelings are formed during a time of illness, they often extend beyond the health care situation. For this reason, the termination of the care in and of itself does not provide an ethics-neutral basis for allowing such a relationship to blossom into sexual contact. In regard to the obvious question of how long is an acceptable period of interruption of association, the answer is whatever time it takes for the emotions derived from the therapeutic relationship to weaken to the point that the patient cannot be exploited or manipulated. This principle forms the basis for the ruling in the *Heineche v. Department of Commerce* (1991) case in which a male nurse's license was suspended for having sexual relations with a patient. The fact that he had resigned his position and was living with the woman was not sufficient to excuse his behavior.

SCOPE OF PRACTICE

All allied health and nursing personnel work within a **scope of practice.** Figure 6–1 lists the elements usually found in a scope of practice act. Practitioners who stray outside the bounds of legitimate practice not only call upon themselves censorship from their peers and colleagues but also may face loss of credentials and litigation. In this era of health care reform, when change is occurring at a dizzying rate, providers are being asked to assume additional duties. Prior to stepping beyond their traditional roles, providers would do well to review the appropriate state practice act to determine if the service being requested exceeds the boundaries of professional practice as defined by state statute (Abeln, 1994). The principle of role fidelity requires that we remain within our scope of practice. In most cases, the scope of practice is clearly defined, and one does not cross the line without willful intention. For example, the nurse or allied health professional who is performing physicals and pretending to be a physician has not made an honest error. One hallmark of a professional is to know the limits of one's own professional knowledge.

> - Scope of professional practice
> - Requirements and qualifications for licensure
> - Exemptions
> - Grounds for administrative action
> - Creation of an examination board and process
> - Penalties and sanctions for
>   unauthorized practice

FIGURE 6–1 Basic Elements of a Practice Act

The case of *Stahlin v. Hilton Hotel Corporation* (1973) is precisely the type of scope of practice error that is easy to fall into and difficult to defend. In this case a guest of the Hilton Hotel fell while dressing, striking his head against the wall. A call was placed to the hotel desk for help and Mrs. Anderson, the house physician's secretary, went to the room and identified herself as a nurse. She took the individual's vital signs and examined his head. When she noticed that he had medications for a heart condition, she advised him to stay in bed for twelve hours. The next day, the patient's condition worsened and he was transferred to the hospital where he was diagnosed as having a subdural hematoma. Surgery was immediately performed to relieve the condition, but the patient was left with residual brain damage. The patient sued the hotel for negligence, and the physician and the secretary for malpractice.

RESPONDIAT SUPERIOR

The doctrine of **respondiat superior** comes from an historical period in England when peasant farmers served on large estates. The farmers usually worked for room and board and received few if any wages. The wealth and power was concentrated in the hands of the masters of the estates. Much of the law of this period consisted of proclamations (writs) set down by the royal family. These writs usually were specific to a particular problem and might require that an individual provide compensation for intentionally injuring another.

The need for the doctrine of respondiat superior came about as a result of the disparity of power and wealth between landlords and peasants. A landholder could order the peasant farmers working on his estate to do injury to the estate of a neighboring landlord. Once the damage had been done, the neighboring landlord had little recourse as the individual who did the damage was poor and no monetary compensation could be gained.

The intent of the doctrine was to make the landlord liable for the acts of his servants. Respondiat superior literally means "let the master answer." The doctrine has evolved to include liability assessment against employers for negligent acts of employees, if the negligent conduct occurred within the course and scope of their employment duties. This vicarious liability is assessed when a master-servant relationship exists between the employer and employee and when the wrongful act occurs within the scope of the employee's employment. Liability is often assessed against a hospital or physician for the negligent conduct of allied health and nursing personnel based on the fact that the employer placed these individuals in a position that gave them the apparent authority to act on the employer's behalf.

Although respondiat superior allows for hospitals and physicians to be held liable for certain wrongful acts committed by allied health and nursing personnel, it in no way exempts these health care providers from responsibility for their individual acts. Health care is practiced at many levels, from routine tasks that can essentially be done by anyone with a small amount of training to advanced skills requiring years of education and intensive internships. Each level of practice is held to the standard of care for that specialty. Physicians, nurses, and allied health specialists are held to the level of practice that meets the prevailing standard for their individual specialties. For example, a pharmacist who assumes the care of a client has the duty to exercise in that care that degree of skill, care, and knowledge ordinarily possessed and exercised by other pharmacists.

Often in cases of negligence more than one person may be involved in causing a patient's total injury. Under a doctrine known as joint and several liability, several different parties can be held liable for contributing to the injury. In these cases the plaintiff may recover damages from one or all.

CONFLICTS OF INTEREST

Under no circumstances may physicians place their own financial interests above the welfare of their patients. The primary objective of the medical profession is to render service to humanity; reward or financial gain is a subordinate consideration. For a physician unnecessarily to hospitalize a patient, prescribe a drug, or conduct diagnostic tests for the physician's financial benefit would be unethical. If a conflict develops between the physician's financial interest and the physician's responsibilities to the patient, the conflict must be resolved to the patient's benefit.

Council on Ethical and Judicial Affairs (1992)

Recently in the literature the practice of **joint venturing** and **self-referral** practices have been questioned. Most of these criticisms have been directed at physicians who have joint ventured into health care services such as physical therapy, ambulatory surgical centers, and durable medical equipment companies. Surveys in regard to this practice have shown that with ownership, there is often increased utilization and self-referral (Scott & Ahern, 1992).

Nothing is inherently wrong with joint ventures and in many cases the patients are well served. It seems clear, however, that to self-refer to an establishment where you do not provide service but have an economic interest is at least suspect and perhaps unethical. Whereas self-referral is suspect, kickbacks are criminal acts punishable under federal and state laws (Pozgar, 1993). The Medicare Fraud and Abuse Anti-Kickback Law provides that whoever knowingly and willfully solicits or receives a bribe or rebate shall be guilty of a felony.

Although the spotlight has been pointed at joint venturing and kickbacks, we are all surrounded by the troubling small conflicts of interests that are more ubiquitous and more subtle. What of the pens, writing pads, free texts, medical equipment, and drug samples that at times seem a normal part of the delivery of health care? Does the fact that the gift is small make it more ethical to take?

The practitioner who changes the way of practice through any motive other than patient benefit, has embarked on a slippery slope of compromised ethics. As a health care provider, each practitioner will need to evaluate and prioritize to determine the point at which a service, a managed care incentive, or provided gift ceases to be merely good advertisement, good business, or continuing education and begins to be a favor offered to compromise the client-centered nature of our health care practice.

CONCLUSION

This has been a chapter involved with issues often thought of as "small ethics." There were no life and death consequences, and yet, in some ways it is the maintenance of appropriate professional behavior that creates the atmosphere of trust. It is from this wellspring of trust that we manage the "large ethics" issues of life and death. If our patients begin to doubt our ability to maintain their confidences, to fear that we will exploit them in their weaknesses, to believe that the advice they receive from us is based solely on economic incentives, then the practice of health care will have lost much of its status as a profession. The duties described in this chapter come to us as a function of role fidelity and are the price that one pays for being a professional health care provider. As practitioners of health professions, we have an obligation not only to our patients and communities, but also to our colleagues with whom we share practice.

LEGAL CASE STUDY 1: *Stewart v. Midiani*, 525 F. Supp. 843 (N.D. Ga. 1981).

This case, set before a Federal District Court of Georgia, illuminates some of the complex issues that surround the apportionment of liability in an action for respondiat superior. In the *Stewart v. Midiani* case, a wrongful death action was filed by the decedent's wife against the hospital and the emergency room attending physician. The wife claimed that a misdiagnosis and failure to order further tests on the part of the attending physician in the emergency room cost her her husband's life. Interestingly enough, the doctor was part of a group of doctors who independently contracted with the hospital to provide emergency room services.

The court wrestled with the distinction between an employee and an independent contractor. The court agreed as a general rule that when "the employer assumes the right to control the time, and manner, and method of executing the work, as distinguished from the right merely to require certain definite results in conformity to the contract" there is an employer-employee relationship for which the employer will be held liable. The court recognized that it could easily hold the hospital not liable because it did not control the manner in which the doctor diagnosed and treated the patients in the emergency room. The court used eight separate factors determinative of whether a person was an independent contractor or an employee; (1) the right of the employer to impose will upon the employed and direct the work step by step, (2) a contract for a service rather than for one entire task, (3) the employer's ability to control the employed's time, (4) the employer's right to inspect the employed's work, (5) whether the employed or the employer supplied the equipment, (6) who has the right to terminate the contract, (7) the nature and level of skill required by the employed to accomplish the work, and (8) the method of payment (hourly, monthly, or lump sum). The court concluded, based on these factors, that the hospital would not be liable, but the group of doctors could be held liable under the doctrine of respondiat superior. The court's analysis, however, did not end with that conclusion.

The court went a step further and held that a hospital could not escape liability by employing independent contractors. The court looked to the principle of **agency** law and reasoned that the normal, reasonable patient would probably seek medical help at a particular hospital based upon its reputation and based upon the assumption that the hospital would only provide competent medical personnel in its facility. The hospital could therefore be held liable for the acts or omissions of its independent contractors if it did not provide a disclaimer or notice to the general public of the employment status of the various professions who worked therein.

LEGAL CASE STUDY 2: Moving Beyond Simple Conflict of Interest (ref. *United States v. Greber,* 1985).

The *Greber* case involved an osteopathic physician, board certified in cardiology. The physician formed a company that provided diagnostic services such as holter monitoring. The diagnostic company would bill Medicare for the services provided and when payment was received forward a portion of the fee to the referring physicians. The rebate was described as an interpretation fee but was greater than that permitted by Medicare. In practice, the physicians receiving the rebates generally allowed the company to perform the interpretation.

In the Greber case the court ruled that the payments made to the physicians were made to induce referrals rather than to perform professional services; that even in those cases when some interpretation was done by the physicians, the sum provided was greater than the services provided; and that a secondary intent was to induce future referrals.

1. How do criminal and civil law differ?

2. In what way did this differ from simple joint venturing?

3. Do you feel that any of the physicians involved dishonored their fiduciary relationship with their patients? If so how?

REVIEW EXERCISES

1. Consider the following situations in light of the doctrine of respondiat superior.
    a. The physician allows her office assistant to give medications. While the physician is at lunch, a patient in the waiting room complains of a headache and asks if the assistant has any aspirin. The assistant looks in the desk, sees some aspirin samples given by a pharmaceutical representative during her last visit, and gives them to the patient. The patient suffers a severe reaction to the nonaspirin ingredients in the drug.
    b. Following surgery the patient complains of abdominal distress. An X ray taken shows that surgical clamps have been left in the abdomen. Using the doctrine of res ipsa loquitur (the thing speaks for itself) you could conclude that negligence occurred. If the negligent act was on the part of the surgical nurse, could you use the doctrine of respondiat superior to hold the surgeon and hospital liable as well?
    c. The medical assistant who works in the office of Dr. Jones is allowed to dispense medications to the doctor's patients. While the assistant is at church one of the parishioners tells her that she is having headaches and asks her advice. The medical assistant tells her friend that Dr. Jones generally has his patients take two aspirin. The friend takes this advice but due to a preexisting ulcer begins to vomit blood and is taken to the hospital. Is Dr. Jones liable for the advice given by his medical assistant?

2. Use this decision-making format for the following case.
    Steps to Problem Solving
    a. Problem sensing—gather information, review facts
    b. Formulate the problem
    c. List all solutions of initial credibility
    d. Evaluate each solution in terms of its consequences for individuals involved
    e. Evaluate solutions in terms of upholding or sacrificing the basic principles of health care
    f. Select the solution with best consequences and least sacrifice of basic principles
    g. Prepare a defense for the choice
    Take each step as a separate exercise and work through the problem.

    You and Joe have been friends since you met while in school. Following graduation you both took positions within a local clinical department. Lately Joe has been going through a difficult and emotional divorce. At work he has begun to act erratic, often talking a mile a minute and at other times being very quiet. You wonder whether he has begun to abuse drugs.

    One day Joe confirms your fears when he tells you that he is needing to take pills to go to sleep and that he takes others in the day to stay awake. He asks you as his friend to not tell anyone and tells you that he will get a handle on his problem once the divorce is final.

    The next morning during report Joe appears to fall asleep. After report your supervisor who knows that you and Joe are friends comes to you and asks, "What is the matter with Joe?"

    You respond, "......."

3. In the mid 1970s, a nursing educator in Idaho had contact, through a student, with a female client who had chronic myelogenous leukemia. This form of leukemia can often be managed for years with little or no chemotherapy. The woman had done well for about twelve years and ascribed her good condition to health foods and a strict nutritional regime. However, her

condition had turned worse several weeks before and her physician had advised her that she needed chemotherapy if she were to have any chance at survival. The physician had also advised her of the potential side effects of the therapy including hair loss, nausea, fever, and immune system suppression.

The woman consented to the therapy and signed the appropriate forms, but later began to have second thoughts. The nursing educator and student had given the patient one dose of the therapy when the woman began to cry and to express her reservations about the therapy. She questioned the nurse about alternative treatments to the use of chemotherapy. The patient related that she had accepted the therapy because her son had advised her that this was the best treatment. She related that she had not asked about alternate forms of treatment as the physician had indicated that the chemotherapy was the only treatment indicated. The nurse did not discuss the patient's concerns with the physician, and later that evening talked to the patient about alternative therapies. In the discussion, rather nontraditional and controversial therapies were covered including reflexology and the use of laetrile. During the talk the nurse made it very clear that the treatments under discussion were not sanctioned by the medical community.

The patient's feelings toward alternative therapies were strengthened by the evening's conversation; however, she continued with chemotherapy. The treatments, however, did not bring remission to her crisis and she died two weeks later. Upon hearing about the conversation between the off duty nurse educator and his patient, the physician brought charges against the nurse for unprofessional conduct and interfering with the patient-physician relationship (*In re Tuma*, 1977).

a. What if anything did the nurse do wrong?
b. Had she moved beyond her scope of practice?
c. Could the nurse's conduct be justified under the patient advocate portion of her role?
d. If you were a member of the state board for nursing and had to decide the issue of unprofessional conduct and interference with the patient-physician relationship, would you sanction the nurse?

REFERENCES

Abeln, S. (1994). Stepping beyond traditional roles. *Rehabilitation Management, vol. 5* pp. 44–50.

ANA code for nurses with interpretative statements. (1985). *American Nurses Association.* (1990, June 18). *Boston Globe,* Health Science Section.

Council on Ethical and Judicial Affairs. (1992). Opinions on practice matters, 8.03. *American Medical Association.*

Darr, K. (1991). *Ethics in health services management.* Baltimore: Health Professions Press.

Davis, M. (1993). Thinking like an engineer: The place of a code of ethics in professional practice. *Philosophy and Public Affairs, 20*(2), pp. 150–167.

Heineche v. Department of Commerce, 810 P.2d 459 (Utah, Ct. App. 1991).

Hughes, T., & Smith, L. (1994). Is your colleague chemically dependent? *American Journal of Nursing.*

Pozgar, G. (1993). *Legal aspects of health care administration.* Gaithersburg, MD.: Aspen Publication.

Rapp, M. S. (1987). Sexual misconduct. *Journal of the Canadian Medical Association, 137,* pp. 193–194.

Raven-Hansen, P. (1980). Dos and don'ts for whistle-blowers. *Technology Review, 82,* p. 34.

Scott, E., & Ahern, M. (1992). Effects of joint venturing on health care costs. *Nursing Economics, 10* (2).

Stahlin v. Hilton Corporation, 484 F.2d 580 (7th Cir. 1973).

Stewart v. Midiani, 525 F. Supp. 843 (N.D.Ga. 1981).

Thoreau, H. D. (1970). On the duty of civil disobedience. In R. Bavrizio, E. Karas, & R. Menmum (Eds.), *The Rhetoric of Dissent.* New York: Holt, Rinehart and Winston, Inc. (Original work published 1849).

Tuma v. Board of Nursing, 593 P.2d 711 (Idaho 1979).

United States v. Greber, 760 F. 2d 711 (Idaho 1979).

Welch, D. (1995). Just an ordinary day at the office. *Professional Ethics, 2* (3), p. 3.

———————— C H A P T E R 7 ————————

AIDS and Health Care Practice

Goal

The major instructional goal is to gain an understanding of the nature of the AIDS epidemic and to examine selected ethical and legal problems associated with this crisis.

Objectives

At the conclusion of this chapter, the reader should understand and be able to:

1. Discuss the nature of the disease process and how it is acquired.

2. List the major infection control methods that have been used to bring the epidemic under control.

3. Explain how standard precautions have reduced the risk of infection for health care providers and what place the precautions play in affirming a duty to treat.

4. List the high risk behaviors associated with the spread of this disease.

5. List the reasons why confidentiality is perhaps more important for this patient group than for others we treat.

6. Write a rationale for the duty to treat this patient group.

7. List the conditions under which the moral duty to treat would cease to be a duty and become only a moral option. How would this relate to a virus such as the Eboli?

8. Write a series of guidelines that would provide the patient protection from AIDS-infected health care providers.

9. Provide a rationale for both a policy to tell and a policy to not tell the non-physician health care providers the HIV status of their patients.

10. Explain the nature and function of the "reasonable person."

11. List three measures that a unit could take to reduce the claim of discrimination brought by an HIV-infected health care provider.

12. Differentiate between the risk standard used in the *Bradley* and *Precourt* cases.

13. Write a pro or con rationale as to whether you feel that HIV-infected providers should be allowed to continue to practice. Use the *Behringer, Bradley,* and *Almaraz* cases in your decision.

Key Terms

acquired immunode-
ficiency syndrome
(AIDS)

"emergency
exception"

high risk behaviors

human immunodefi-
ciency virus (HIV)

materiality test

moral duty

moral option

prima facie case

randomized clinical
trials

safe sex

standard precautions

THE NATURE OF THE DISEASE

Both the Moral Majority, who are recycling medieval language to explain AIDS, and those ultra-leftists who attribute AIDS to some sort of conspiracy, have a clearly political analysis of the epidemic. But even if one attributes its cause to a microorganism rather than the wrath of God, or the workings of the CIA, it is clear that the way in which AIDS has been perceived, conceptualized, imagined, researched and financed makes this the most political of diseases.

Dennis Altman, author, activist (1986)

It's the virus Stupid!

Dr. David Ho, Aaron Diamond AIDS Research Center

In the early 1980s health care institutions within the United States began to report patients with overwhelming and unusual opportunistic infections. These patients began to present an identifiable syndrome characterized by general swelling of lymph nodes, substantial weight loss of 10 percent or more of body weight, profound malaise, night sweats, prolonged low grade fever intractable to aspirin or similar products, persistent skin irritations on various parts of the body, persistent diarrhea, and thrush mouth.

One striking element of these cases was that the patients were mostly young white men living in urban centers. These young men were being diagnosed with conditions thought to be rare and normally seen only in severely debilitated individuals or in textbooks. Relatively rare entities such as candidiasis of the esophagus, extra pulmonary cryptococcosis, Kaposi's sarcoma affecting a patient less than 60 years of age, progressive multifocal leukoencephalopathy, and pneumocystitis carinii became

TABLE 7–1
AIDS Cases by Exposure Category

	Subtotals
Men who have sex with men	259,672
Injecting drug use	128,696
Men who have sex with men and inject drugs	33,195
Hemophilia/coagulation disorder	4,107
Heterosexual cases	40,037
Receipt of blood, components, tissue	7,433
Children—Exposure Category	
Infected mother	6,256
Hemophilia/coagulation disorder	227
Receipt of blood, components, tissue	366

indicator diseases for what later became known as **acquired immunodeficiency syndrome** or **AIDS.** The **human immunodeficiency virus (HIV)** that causes AIDS is transmitted through sexual contact and exposure to infected blood or blood components and perinatally from mothers to infants. Although the HIV has been isolated from blood, vaginal secretions, semen, breast milk, saliva, tears, and cerebrospinal fluid, epidemiological evidence has implicated only blood, semen, vaginal secretions, and possibly breast milk in transmission. Table 7-1 lists the AIDS cases by exposure category (Center for Disease Control (CDC), 1995).

With the recognition of the syndrome came the hunt for the cause, and for a short time there were several competing theories. For some members of society, AIDS was seen as a righteous judgment from God upon those who committed the sins of drug abuse and homosexuality. As increased numbers of women, infants, children, and hemophiliacs became ill with the syndrome, this view of the disease lost credibility. For a time, the attention was focused on Gaetan Dugas, a flight attendant for Air Canada, with numerous romantic liaisons across the nation. Mr. Dugas became known as Patient Zero. It is now known that Mr. Dugas was only the best known of the early cases, and not the first. His identification did not provide information as to the cause of the disease although it helped explain how it spread so rapidly among the gay male population. Because many of the early patients used drugs and stimulants such as amil nitrate poppers, it was thought that perhaps these were cofactors involved in lowering the resistance of the body to the virus. The cofactor theory holds that a combination of factors such as lifestyle and diet causes a decrease in the immune system. Perhaps the theory that seems most in keeping with the American society and its love of a good conspiracy was the view that the virus was a result of biological or chemical warfare research gone awry. Depending on the political bent of the advocates of these theories, the virus either escaped or was released as a plot against gays or African-Americans.

The theory that seems to have the most acceptance is that AIDS began as a mutant virus, which was picked up from a species of African monkeys and transferred to humans by way of bites. It was then transmitted among the African populations via direct mucous-to-mucous contact, through semen, and perhaps during blood exchange. From Africa the disease spread to Haiti, and was later carried to the United States probably by homosexual males. The heterosexual population became infected as blood supplies became contaminated and as a result of intravenous drug use and the sharing of contaminated needles. Female sexual partners of those infected through contaminated blood or needles contracted the disease through semen and spread the disease to other partners and perinatally to their infants. Currently 6 percent of the reported cases are linked to heterosexual contact and 19 percent to intravenous drug use. Up to one million Americans are HIV infected, and AIDS has become the leading cause of death in those 25 to 44 years of age. As many as 40,000 to 80,000 new cases of HIV infection occur each year, even in the face of a clear understanding of how this disease is transmitted (Stryker et al., 1995).

Several high profile cases were important in providing a human dimension to the disease for most Americans. Ryan White, an Indiana teenager and hemophiliac who contracted the disease from contaminated blood products; Kimberly Bergalis, the Florida teen who was thought to have contracted the disease from her dentist; and Rock Hudson, the actor and friend of then President and Mrs. Reagan all reinforced the notion that AIDS was not confined to a specific portion of our population and that the disease deserved concerted national attention. This humanization of the epidemic did much to bring the disease into focus as a public health issue.

INFECTION CONTROL METHODS

Figure 7-1 lists the six elements known as the chain of infection. If any element is missing, the infection will not spread. As with other epidemics, those working for national infection control for AIDS have sought to control the disease by breaking the chain of events causing the spread of the infection. This work usually is done at three basic levels: by decreasing the susceptibility of the host, by eliminating the source of the organisms, and by interrupting the mode of transmission. Although positive reports have come from researchers seeking a vaccine for the HIV, no widely available vaccine exists and most researchers believe that it will be years before a safe and effective vaccine is developed for general use (Fox, 1996). The major efforts toward eliminating the source of the infection have been through an active educational program, legal notification requirements, and special techniques in providing barriers at the point of direct and indirect contact.

Between 26 May and 30 June 1988 the U.S. Department of Health and Human Services distributed over 107 million copies of the brochure "Understanding AIDS." With this mailing the government attempted to contact virtually every home and residential box office in regard to this public health problem. The efforts directed toward breaking the chain of infection through special techniques to reduce its spread in the general public have taken many forms. These range from the rather controversial methods such as clean needle exchange programs for intravenous drug users and provision of free condoms to high school students, to those less controversial such as screening prospective blood donors for high risk behaviors, increased testing of blood supplies, and the promotion of **"safe sex"** or abstinence in high risk situations. Some

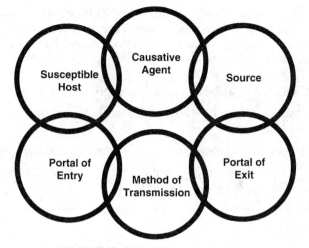

FIGURE 7–1 Chain of Infection

High Risk Behaviors

- Sharing drug needles and syringes
- Anal sex, with or without a condom
- Vaginal or oral sex with someone who injects drugs or engages in anal sex
- Sex with someone you do not know well (a pickup or prostitute) or with someone you know has several sex partners
- Unprotected sex (without a condom) with an infected person

Safe Behaviors

- Not having sex
- Sex with one mutually faithful, uninfected partner
- Not abusing drugs

FIGURE 7–2 High Risk and Safe Behaviors

studies in regard to the use of condoms for safe sex have indicated that perhaps the safety is more illusionary than real. In married couples in which one partner was HIV infected and condoms were used, 10 percent of the healthy became infected within two years (Mishell, 1989). The Health and Human Services brochure listing of both safe and **high risk behaviors** is found in Figure 7-2.

In their writings, Milliken and Greenblatt (1988) suggested several specific criteria for an ethical social policy toward control of this epidemic. It was felt that only the adoption of such criteria would ensure the acceptance by the citizenry, which is a basic requisite for successful policy.

1. Methods selected must be efficacious and appropriate to the stated goals.

2. The goals selected must be ethical, and equal consideration of interest must be central to processes.

3. Implementation of the policy must avoid discrimination and be justly administered.

4. Harm to society or its subgroups that may result from the proposed policies must be identified and clearly understood.

5. The balance between harms and benefits must weigh heavily toward benefit.

OCCUPATIONAL RISK

In 1985 the Center for Disease Control (CDC) developed infection control guidelines called "universal precautions" in response to HIV and the AIDS epidemic. These precautions were designed to prevent the spread of bloodborne pathogens such as HIV and hepatitis B. These recommendations have recently been updated by the CDC into a new set of **standard precautions** published in 1996 (see Figure 7–3) (Acello, 1996). In that medical history and examination cannot reliably identify all patients infected with HIV or other bloodborne pathogens such as hepatitis B, standard precautions are recommended for all patients. This is especially critical for such practitioners as nurses, respiratory care specialists, and clinical laboratory technicians as their work brings them into medical situations where contact with blood is common and the infection status of the patient is unknown (National Safety Council, 1993).

In that great numbers of health care workers did not contract the disease in the early 1980s, it has become evident that the transmission modes for HIV are rather specific. Current practice calls not only for standard precautions but also employee training and postexposure evaluations. The virus is a rather fragile entity and involves little risk for practitioners who follow standard processes and who are otherwise not engaged in high risk behaviors (Henderson, 1988).

An exception to HIV infection being related to high risk behaviors is the hemophiliac patient. These patients acquired the disease in great numbers as a result of initial poor quality testing of needed medications used with their condition. Many of these individuals contracted the disease early in the epidemic. The 1987 *McKee v. Miles Laboratory Inc.* case is instructive in regard to how the courts viewed the matter. The patient, a hemophiliac, had contracted the disease as a result of contaminated blood products supplied by the defendants. The court explained that in 1983 when the patient contracted the disease, the medical community had still not come to a consensus on whether AIDS could be transmitted by blood or that HIV was the AIDS-causing virus. Hence the supplier was not guilty of violating a standard of care because there was not a standard that required testing or treatment of contaminated blood. Currently, in suits based on the receipt of contaminated blood products, the

STANDARD PRECAUTIONS FOR INFECTION CONTROL

Wash Hands (Plain soap)
Wash after touching blood, body fluids, secretions, excretions, and contaminated items. Wash immediately after gloves are removed and between patient contacts. Avoid transfer of microorganisms to other patients or environments.

Wear Gloves
Wear when touching blood, body fluids, secretions, excretions, and contaminated items. Put on clean gloves just before touching mucous membranes and nonintact skin. Change gloves between tasks and procedures on the same patient after contact with material that may contain high concentrations of microorganisms. Remove gloves promptly after use, before touching noncontaminated items and environmental surfaces, and before going to another patient, and wash hands immediately to avoid transfer of microorganisms to other patients or environments.

Wear Mask and Eye Protection or Face Shield
Protect mucous membranes of the eyes, nose, and mouth during procedures and patient-care activities that are likely to generate splashes or sprays of blood, body fluids, secretions, or excretions.

Wear Gown
Protect skin and prevent soiling of clothing during procedures that are likely to generate splashes or sprays of blood, body fluids, secretions, or excretions. Remove a soiled gown as promptly as possible and wash hands to avoid transfer of microorganisms to other patients or environments.

Patient-Care Equipment
Handle used patient-care equipment soiled with blood, body fluids, secretions, or excretions in a manner that prevents skin and mucous membrane exposures, contamination of clothing, and transfer of microorganisms to other patients and environments. Ensure that reusable equipment is not used for the care of another patient until it has been appropriately cleaned and reprocessed and single use items are properly discarded.

Environmental Control
Follow hospital procedures for routine care, cleaning, and disinfection of environmental surfaces, beds, bed-rails, bedside equipment, and other frequently touched surfaces.

Linen
Handle, transport, and process used linen soiled with blood, body fluids, secretions, or excretions in a manner that prevents exposure and contamination of clothing, and avoids transfer of microorganisms to other patients and environments.

Occupational Health and Bloodborne Pathogens
Prevent injuries when using needles, scalpels, and other sharp instruments or devices; when handling sharp instruments after procedures; when cleaning used instruments; and when disposing of used needles.

Never recap used needles using both hands or any other technique that involves directing the point of a needle toward any part of the body; rather, use either a one-handed "scoop" technique or a mechanical device designed for holding the needle sheath.

Do not remove used needles from disposable syringes by hand, and do not bend, break, or otherwise manipulate used needles by hand. Place used disposable syringes and needles, scalpels, blades, and other sharp items in puncture-resistant sharps containers located as close as practical to the area in which the items were used, and place reusable syringes and needles in a puncture-resistant container for transport to the reprocessing area.

Use resuscitation devices as an alternative to mouth-to-mouth resuscitation.

Patient Placement
Use a private room for a patient who contaminates the environment or who does not (or cannot be expected to) assist in maintaining appropriate hygiene or environmental control. Consult Infection Control if a private room is not available.

FIGURE 7–3 Standard Precautions (Courtesy of BREVIS Corporation, Salt Lake City, UT)

119

TABLE 7–2
CDC Data as of December 1995 listing reported
AIDS cases among health care providers

Profession	AIDS Cases
Nurses	1,358
Health Aides	1,101
Technicians	941
Physicians	703
Paramedics	116
Therapists	119
Dentists and Hygienists	171
Surgeons	47
Misc. Health Workers	1,680
Total	6,436

injured party must show that a standard of care existed, that the plaintiff's actions fell below the standard, and that this was the actual and proximate cause of the injury (Pozgar, 1993). In recent studies, Lackritz et al. (1995) estimated that the current risk of transmission of the human immunodeficiency virus by screened blood in the United States is 1 case per 450,000 to 660,000. Of the twelve million donations collected by the Red Cross blood centers each year, an estimated eighteen to twenty-seven infectious donations are potentially available for transfusion.

Table 7–2 gives a listing of all health care workers with documented and possible occupationally acquired AIDS-HIV infection, by occupation, reported through December 1995 in the United States (CDC, 1995). It is difficult to determine the occupational risk for health care providers. Obviously much depends on the nature of the duties. While the office worker is assuming virtually no risk, those involved in invasive procedures, emergency care, and childbirth are another matter. It is estimated that surgeons cut a glove during one in four procedures, and cut their own skin in one in forty.

Of the million cases of HIV infections in the United States, by the end of the first decade only the five involved with the Florida dentist are believed to have been infected by health care providers. These five Florida cases, however, and the media coverage, created an overwhelming public concern with regard to infected health care providers. A poll by Gallup showed a majority of the lay public (87 percent) desired mandatory testing and disclosure of HIV status by health care providers. A bill that would impose a ten-year prison sentence upon HIV-infected health care providers who continued to practice without informing their patients passed overwhelmingly in the Senate, but fortunately failed to become law (Seidl, 1994). Yet, at the present time, no documented case of a physician- or surgeon-transmitted infection exists. Retrospective studies completed by the CDC in 1993 reported that HIV tests and follow-up studies on 19,036 patients treated by fifty-seven infected health care providers showed no confirmed instances of seroconversion as a result of the health care contacts, (Deville, 1994). The CDC using statistical estimation techniques predicted that a patient undergoing a serious invasive procedure by an HIV-infected practitioner had between a 1:40,000 to 1:400,000 chance of contracting the virus. If standard precautions are used, the risk becomes essentially nonexistent. C. H. Fox (1991), a Harvard researcher, stated that the patient is in far more danger of being hit by a careless motorist or by lightning on the way to the clinic than of contracting HIV after arriving.

Apparently in the first decade of the epidemic, less than 100 care providers contracted the disease from patients (Grady, 1991). Of these, most were infected through deep needle sticks or were caused by blood splashes into the eyes, mouth, or nose. This is a relatively small number and shows that neither the patients nor the health care providers are at much risk, with the health care workers assuming the greater portion.

ETHICAL AND LEGAL ISSUES AND THE AIDS EPIDEMIC

AIDS is a devastating epidemic with the potential for killing all who become infected. Although the risk of acquiring a hepatitis B infection is far more likely, the deadly consequences of getting AIDS have made this disease a major ethical issue. In recent years the population group affected by the disease has extended into all groups so that it is best not described by high risk groups but rather by high risk behaviors. The economic implications of AIDS are staggering. When considering personal medical costs, direct costs of research, and indirect costs such as education, screening, and potential productivity losses, you are looking at a disease with a yearly price tag of over $66 billion. The economic implication of these numbers is overwhelming when you consider the already overburdened health care system. Added to these tangible costs are another set of factors that defy fiscal analysis—the loss of hopes, dreams, and future potential of its victims. What is the cost of these losses, when young people are handicapped during the time of their lives when they are at the peak of their productive work and childbearing years? One real problem with solving the AIDS dilemma is that many Americans appear to be experiencing a great deal of both fear and denial concerning their own risk of acquiring AIDS, and have rationalized the continuation of lifestyles that place them at risk (Spronson, McCartney, & Yesalis 1990). Perhaps an equally serious case of denial can be seen in the report by the *American Journal of Nursing,* which stated that 93 percent of the nurses surveyed indicated that they would wear protective gloves while performing a venipuncture on an HIV-infected patient; however, only 59 percent indicated that they would take the same precautions on a patient if the HIV status was unknown (Seidl, 1994).

The problems associated with this disease are many and cut to the very heart of what it means to be a health care practitioner. The fact that AIDS has no known cure or preventive vaccine makes it a disease that has caused the rethinking of basic fundamental issues. Do health care practitioners have a duty to treat? In a health care system already overburdened with the costs of health care, how much care should be allocated to a group of patients with a terminal disease? How much access to expensive technologies should terminal patients have? What is an acceptable risk for health care professionals? Should the patient be warned if the health care practitioner is HIV positive? Should the practitioner be warned if the patient is HIV positive? Should infected practitioners be allowed to continue practice? What is the meaning of confidentiality when it comes to AIDS and who should be told?

Duty to Treat

How much risk is an acceptable risk for health care practitioners? Although much of the public press has been directed toward patients who have been infected with the HIV virus by health care practitioners, the truth is that it is far more likely that the practitioner will be infected by the patient than vice versa (Lo, B. & Steinbrook, R. 1992). A 1987 study showed that 1,875 adults with AIDS were also employed in a health care setting. In comparison, almost seven million persons, representing about 5.6 percent of the population of the U.S. labor force were employed in the health services. Of the health care providers reporting infection, 95 percent of these have been reported to exhibit high risk behaviors; for the remaining 5 percent the means of HIV acquisition was undetermined. Health care workers were significantly more likely than other workers to have an undetermined risk of acquiring AIDS (5 percent versus 3 percent, respectively). Health care workers who have contracted the disease have included direct patient care groups such as physicians, dentists, nurses, nursing assistants, clinical laboratory technicians and therapists, but also groups such as housekeeping and maintenance which usually do not have direct patient contact.

Under common law, physicians and other health care providers have been free to accept or reject patients as they see fit under the general principle that the provider is under no obligation to act affirmatively to prevent injury to another except for special circumstances. The nature of the special circumstances is usually the establishment of the patient-provider relationship. Assuming no relationship, there is no legal obligation. At the scene of an accident, the health care provider has no greater legal duty to provide emergency care than does the layperson, although there is obviously a greater **moral duty.** If the health care provider does stop and begin to assist, then he would incur the legal duty to continue until either he was relieved by a response team, his own safety became in danger, or he was ordered from the scene by the police. Regardless, once you begin to render assistance, you have a duty to leave the victim in a state no worse than you found him, otherwise you will be held liable. In these circumstances, you are provided limited protection under the Good Samaritan statutes. To err on the side of caution, it is usually wise to carry malpractice insurance that covers you even when you are away from your usual place of practice (Owens, 1993). Conversely, the patient who has been admitted to your unit has accepted your offer for care and cannot legally be refused treatment.

The general principle of common law that allows the individual health care provider to not enter into a patient-provider relationship outside of the clinical setting was extended to include hospitals, and limited the duty owed to potential patients. AIDS is an expensive disease, and costs rise exponentially as these patients approach death. As a result, many long-term care facilities are reluctant to admit patients with AIDS and current legislation does not mandate admission (Huber, 1993). The exception to this principle is the **"emergency exception."** A seriously ill or injured patient who reports to the emergency room under most circumstances cannot be refused care. The basis for this exception is found in statutes such as the Hill-Burton Act of 1944, which tied available hospital construction and modernization funds to the provision of a reasonable volume of services to those who could not pay. The Consolidated Omnibus Budget Reconciliation Act (COBRA) of 1985 established an emergency room obligation for all hospitals who participated in

TABLE 7–3
Professional Duties in an Epidemic

- To provide service consistent with skills.
- To obtain skills if needed by the patient population as consistent with scope of practice.
- To provide accurate and up-to-date information.
- To promote the patient's best interests regardless of personal feelings toward the patient or the disease entity.

Medicare. Under COBRA, the hospital would be required to assess the patient in regard to the nature of the emergency. If an emergency condition did in fact exist, the hospital would be obligated to treat the patient until the condition stabilized. To maintain tax-exempt status the Internal Revenue Service requires hospitals to provide a level of gratis care. AIDS patients may benefit from the requirements for emergency care as many of its associated conditions, when in an acute phase, classify as medical emergencies. The Rehabilitation Act of 1973 and the Americans with Disabilities Act of 1990 also provide powerful legal barriers against a hospital refusing to treat patients with AIDS (Jarvis et al., 1991).

Once a patient is admitted to the unit, the potential risk posed to health care practitioners seems to be minimal. The use of universal precautions on all patients should provide an effective barrier and reduce the risk to a negligible level. It would seem then, that the small risk to the practitioner would not provide a suitable ethical rationale to refuse to treat patients with known HIV infections. In practice it is probably not the known HIV-infected patient that is most likely to spread the disease to health care workers. Table 7-3 lists recommended guidelines for practice in an epidemic provided by the Health and Public Policy Committee of the American College of Physicians and the Infectious Disease Society of America (1986). The bases of these guidelines are found in many of the health providers' codes of ethics; for example, the nursing code for the care of victims of communicable disease calls for the "provision of services with respect for human dignity and the uniqueness of the client unrestricted by considerations of social or economical status, personal attributes, or the nature of the health problem."

The nurse or allied health practitioner then has a duty to provide care commensurate with the defined scope of practice. Should the practitioner feel unsure with regard to universal precautions, there is an implied duty to obtain the needed skills and keep updated on all available information. Ignorance in this case might provide a short-term rationale for refusing to treat a patient with AIDS, but once trained in universal precautions, this would no longer provide a legitimate excuse. Western culture and health care practice provide historical precedence for the obligation to treat persons regardless of their social status, political affiliation, or whether they be enemy or friend. The Good Samaritan ethic endorsed by our culture also provides strong ethical precedence for coming to the aid of those in danger or in need of help. This ethic of assistance does not, however, require that the rescuer take unacceptable risks in the process. For example, the nonswimmer is not expected to jump into the pool to save a drowning victim, for clearly this would not be in the interest of the victim or the potential rescuer.

What then does our culture require of us in regard to AIDS patients? Although we are not required to risk our lives in futile and perhaps dangerous gestures, under most situations that is not what we face with this patient group. Although the potential for contracting AIDS within the workplace is a significant concern, it has occurred on an exceedingly infrequent basis. In general, this concern would not represent an acceptable rationale for refusing to treat but would instead create an obligation on the part of all health care workers to take appropriate protective actions.

The ANA Committee on Ethics (1985) offers some useful guidelines with regard to decision making and whether the practitioner has a moral duty to treat or whether the decision is left as a **moral option.** The four fundamental criteria are:

1. The patient is at significant risk of harm, loss, or damage if the practitioner does not assist.
2. The practitioner's intervention or care is directly relevant to preventing harm.
3. The practitioner's care will probably prevent harm, loss, or damage to the patient.
4. The benefit the patient will gain outweighs any harm the practitioner might incur and does not present more than a minimal risk to the health care provider.

If the practitioner can answer yes to all four criteria it would seem that a moral duty to treat would exist under the principle of beneficence. If the circumstances placed the practitioner in such a position that all criteria could not be answered with yes, then the decision to treat would become a moral option rather than a duty. An example of this might be an answer of no for the crucial fourth criteria, in a case when the practitioner finds a patient bleeding from the mouth and in respiratory failure requiring CPR. Assuming that no masks or airways were in place, the decision to perform mouth-to-mouth resuscitation would not be mandated by duty.

Most health provider codes of ethics give a clear directive in regard to the treatment of patients despite their disease status. These moral directives were often ignored and certain health care providers refused to treat HIV-infected patients. To overcome this reluctance to treat this patient group, the government moved those persons infected with AIDS under the federal legislation barring discriminatory practices.

This patient group is now afforded protection of Section 504 of the Rehabilitation Act of 1973 and the Americans with Disabilities Act of 1990. HIV serostatus and AIDS are now considered handicapping conditions covered under federal legislation prohibiting discriminatory practices. The failure to treat is no longer only a moral issue but also has potential legal consequences (Kolasa, 1993). The range of concerns that can be accommodated under these acts can be seen in the *Doe v. Centinela Hospital* (1988) case in which an asymptomatic, HIV-infected patient was refused admission to a hospital's federally funded residential drug and alcohol program. The individual was refused for fear of contagion and the hospital claimed that, because the patient was asymptomatic at the time, he was not handicapped by the disease. In its decision the court recognized that HIV-infected individuals are handicapped not only by their disease but also because others perceive them as being impaired.

Another interesting case in regard to protection afforded under the Rehabilitation Act of 1973 and the Americans with Disabilities Act of 1990 is that of *Bradley v. University of Texas M. D. Anderson Cancer Center* (1993). In this case a surgical technician revealed to a local paper that he was HIV positive. The hospital responded to the information by reassigning him to the purchasing department as a procurement assistant. Mr. Bradley sued the hospital and two supervisors claiming that the reassignment violated the Rehabilitation Act, the Americans with Disabilities Act, and his First Amendment rights to free speech.

To establish a **prima facie case** of discrimination, and according to the Rehabilitation Act, Mr. Bradley had to prove the following: First, that he was handicapped for the purposes of the statute. Second, that he was "otherwise qualified" to be a surgical technician. Third, that his reassignment had been based solely on his handicap. It was clear from previous cases that AIDS is a handicapping condition, so the court could narrow the issue to examine whether he was "otherwise qualified" to be a surgical technician. An important aspect of the definition of "otherwise qualified" is that individuals can perform the essential functions of their role without posing undue threat to the health and safety of others. To assist them in their decision the court relied on the findings in the *School Board of Nassau County v. Arline* (1987) case. In Arline, a noninfectious school teacher with tuberculosis alleged that the school board had fired her in violation of the Rehabilitation Act. In regard to employing a person with a contagious disease, the inquiry must include the medically relevant facts regarding the nature of the risk, the severity of the risk, and the probability of transmission. In the case of the school teacher, the teacher was noncontagious, which negated any probability of transmission.

In the *Bradley* case, however, although the court acknowledged that the risk was minimal, it was not so small as to nullify the catastrophic consequences of an accident. The disputed issue became the probability of transmission. The nature of the tasks which involved sharp instruments and open body cavities led the court to conclude that the plaintiff's HIV infection made him not "otherwise qualified" to perform the duties of a surgical technician.

Mr. Bradley continued to argue that even if he could not be assigned as a surgical technician, at least he should have been assigned to duties that included direct patient contact. The court responded that once the decision had been made that a reasonable accommodation within the surgical suite could not be made, the employer was not bound to assign him to any particular position, although they could not deny him alternative employment on the basis of the existing hospital policy.

The federal court granted summary judgment in favor of the hospital and the supervisors. Mr. Bradley appealed the decision but the appeals court affirmed the lower court opinion. One powerful message that comes from this case is that careful documentation of the process is critical to show that the hospital's actions were considered, reasoned, and based on sound medical evidence and legitimate patient concerns.

CONFIDENTIALITY IN AN AGE OF AIDS

What I may see or hear in the course of the treatment or even outside of the treatment in regard to the life of men, which on no account one must spread abroad, I will keep to myself holding such things shameful to be noised about.

Hippocratic Oath

Confidentiality seems based on at least three foundations: (1) the duty-oriented acceptance of a personal right of self-determination that requires the control over privacy and personal information; (2) the utilitarian view that if confidentiality were commonly breached, patients would be deterred in seeking medical assistance for problems with sensitive or personal aspects; and (3) the long held virtue-oriented belief among health care providers that a special relationship exists between practitioner and client that calls for the tacit agreement of confidentiality and mutual trust.

It would seem that the first two foundations have a special importance when considering the AIDS epidemic. The nature of the illness and the recognition of its association with high risk populations such as homosexuals, drug users, and prostitutes creates an enhanced danger of harm should private information be revealed beyond appropriate circles of care. Discrimination in housing, insurance, employment, or even physical harm are very real consequences due to breaches of this patient group's confidentiality. Although rarely talked about in the press and in the national call for the screening of health care workers for AIDS, these same potential outcomes to a breach in confidentiality in regard to a health care provider's HIV status must be equally considered. Given the potential for personal harm, it is not hard to see that the belief of confidentiality is important if this patient group is to be forthcoming in providing health care providers with the necessary information needed to contain the epidemic and provide adequate care. Because AIDS is universally fatal, protection of the uninfected must take precedence over other concerns, and those vulnerable must be warned. Unlike other infectious diseases, AIDS is also associated with a form of dementia where the infected individual may feel vindictive and intentionally try to transmit the virus.

When considering AIDS cases, the principle of confidentiality must be balanced between our obligations to provide appropriate disease control within the community and to protect vulnerable populations. Should a health care worker in the emergency department and an EMT be notified that a patient who came into their care and whose bleeding they controlled was later confirmed to be HIV positive? In that all practitioners at this level should practice standard precautions for all patients, and if practiced these precautions reduce the vulnerability to a negligible risk, at first glance, the answer would seem to be no. If the risk was minimal, and the practitioners were not vulnerable, confidentiality should not be broken. As autonomous moral agents who have accepted the role of health care provider, the practitioners have a duty to protect themselves in these cases, and if protected would not be a particularly vulnerable population. Yet on second consideration, anyone who has practiced in these situations knows that it is often less controlled than one might wish. The EMT reaching into the car to remove the bleeding patient often tears the gloves that are to provide the barrier; the emergency room worker is subject to needle or sharp sticks and barrier loss. Although the postevent findings that a patient was HIV positive may not be of use in preventing the health care provider from contracting the disease, it may provide needed information regarding treatment and may possibly save the family or other contacts of the health care provider from the infection. It is for these reasons that special categories of health care workers who are subject to direct body fluid contact have a right to know about the HIV status of their patients.

Currently AIDS is a reportable disease in every state of the union. Physicians and hospitals must report every case to the public authorities including the names. Cases reported are also reported to the Centers for Disease Control with the names encoded by a system known as Soundex. All CDC records fall within the protection of the Federal Privacy Act of 1974, but under statute permission, are available to other federal agencies (Pozgar, 1993).

Recent surveys among practitioners show a general belief that those who are directly working with AIDS patients should be informed of their diagnosis. This information is not so much to allow them to minimize personal risk as universal precautions are expected for all patients. The need to know has more to do with the professional tasks at hand as it is difficult to provide adequate care without an accurate diagnosis. It is hard to imagine that physicians would feel comfortable treating patients for whom others have decided that they should not be given the correct diagnosis. The level of professionalism of allied health practitioners and nurses would seem to make it reasonable that indeed they also need to know the diagnosis of the patients they treat. HIV-positive status and the diagnosis of AIDS should be treated like any other disease; it should be part of the medical record. If this were to become the policy of hospitals and clinics, it then becomes far more important that the charts be stored in a safe place so that patient confidentiality can be assured.

THE INFECTED HEALTH CARE PROVIDER

There are legitimate reasons for mandatory testing for everyone. Early diagnosis would perhaps allow for early counseling and assist in curbing the spread of the infection. Early treatment is thought to slow the progress from the HIV antibody to full blown AIDS. Early use of drugs such as AZT is thought to delay the onset of dementia and retard the resistance to AZT. And finally, having a mandatory system of testing would provide the types of statistics that would allow agencies to better follow the spread of the disease and allow for more reasoned allocations of resources (Seidl, 1994). Public health research has shown that a majority of physicians (57 percent) and nurses (63 percent) support mandatory testing (Fox, 1991).

Yet a real concern exists in regard to the cost:benefit ratio of mandatory testing. The cost of these programs would not only be the cost of the individual tests but also the cost of enforcement of rules, and the pretest and posttest counseling. Activities would also include increased levels of segregation, education, and prevention efforts. One example of broad based screening that may prove illustrative is the experience of the testing of 159,000 marriage license applicants in Illinois. Of these 23 were found to be HIV positive, and the program had an estimated cost of $5.6 million, which translates into $243,000 per positive test (Field, 1990). One need ask if this money could not have been better spent in education, treatment, or research. The CDC does not advocate mandatory testing—the Center estimates that the chance for transmission of the HIV virus by an infected surgeon to a patient is about 1:41,600 to 1:416,000 surgical procedures. This places the risk much lower than that of driving cars, smoking cigarettes, or even from dying from the anesthesia used for the surgery (Daniels, 1992).

The courts have been rather unclear in the area of mandatory testing of select populations. In the *Local 1812 American Federation of Government Employees v. U.S. Department of State* (1987) case, the employees argued that the requirement for tests infringed upon their constitutional rights to privacy. The court ruled that the testing did not abridge constitutional rights, and that the department had a practical need to know the HIV status of its diplomats and thus avoid complications that might occur if an individual became ill in a foreign land. In *Glover v. Eastern Nebraska Community Office of Retardation* (1989), a group of employees challenged the mandatory requirement for HIV testing. The court held that the risk to patients or providers in this situation was negligible and therefore did not warrant the intrusive process of mandatory testing. The premise for the decision was based on the Fourth Amendment which protects persons from unreasonable search.

The *Behringer v. Medical Center at Princeton, New Jersey* (1991) case dealt with the practice restrictions placed on an HIV-infected surgeon. The hospital upon finding out that the staff member was infected allowed the physician to continue practice but limited his performance to procedures that posed no risk for HIV transmission. They also required that the physician obtain a written informed consent from the patients. This decision to inform the patients of the provider's condition was justified on the basis of patient autonomy and the duty of beneficence and nonmaleficence.

The ethical requirement of informed consent is well established under the principle of patient autonomy. The legal precedents include the watershed case of *Cantebury v. Spence* (1972) which provides for a **materiality test** to make the determination. Physicians are required to provide to the patient information with regard to any material risk or hazard inherent to the procedure or therapy. Material in this sense is any risk that a hypothetical, reasonable person in the patient's condition ought to know in deciding whether to submit to the treatment. This hypothetical person is not to be confused with the average individual. This is a being who overcomes the natural tendency to prefer personal interests over others, who is able to give an impartial judgment as to the likely harm to be done. This is a being who is prudent, careful, and always up to standard (Keeton et al., 1984).

Under the principle of the reasonable person, the physician is not required to inform a patient of all potential risks but only those that a reasonable person would find material. The reasonable person standard serves both the patients and providers, as it provides some objectivity to the process, protects the patient's right to know, and frees the providers from an unrealistic burden of disclosure. Courts in several cases have held that a low risk could be used to determine whether a particular piece of information was material. One court held that a 1:100,000 chance that a patient would lose sensation to the face following a tooth extraction was of such a remote possibility that it was immaterial and did not need disclosure.

We at the moment are in the hands of two sets of extremes—libertarians who desire no restrictions to practice, and communitarians who call for mandatory testing and prison sentences for those who fail to disclose. In his research, Gostin (1989) proposed some middle ground that seems to protect the legitimate interests of patients and providers alike.

- Health care providers should report their HIV status to their personal physician and their employer. In both cases, the information would be held in strict confidence.

- HIV-infected providers should be carefully monitored in the performance of their functions. This monitoring would include the state of their disease, and their compliance with rigorous infection control procedures.

- HIV-infected providers should refrain from performing seriously invasive procedures.

- Health care facilities should develop policies and resources for retraining, support, counseling, and compensation.

Yet, in recent cases such as the Maryland case of *Faya v. Almaraz* (1993), the test of materiality was challenged. Dr. Almaraz was diagnosed as being HIV infected in 1986 and decided to not inform his patients. Dr. Almaraz performed a partial mastectomy and axillary dissection on Sonja Faya in surgeries that took place in 1988 and 1989. Both surgeries were successful, and in 1990 Dr. Almaraz informed all of his patients that he was leaving practice to pursue research. Following his death on 16 November 1990 a newspaper attributed his death to complications associated with AIDS. Ms. Faya learned of his death on 6 December 1990 and immediately underwent testing for the virus. The results of the enzyme-linked immunosorbent assay (ELISA) tests were returned negative on 10 December 1990.

In her suit, Ms. Faya claimed that Dr. Almaraz had failed to provide an adequate informed consent because he failed to provide information regarding his HIV status. Her other claims included intentional infliction of emotional distress, fraud, negligent misrepresentation, breach of contract, battery, and breach of fiduciary duty. Ms. Faya argued that she was injured because she was exposed to the virus unjustifiably, that she would suffer for years to come in regard to potential seroconversion, and that his conduct exposed her to the expense and pain of future testing. However, because there had never been a reported case of transmission of the HIV virus by a surgeon to a patient, and given that such a transmission was unlikely if barrier precautions were used, the Baltimore trial judge dismissed the case.

Ms. Faya appealed the case to the Maryland Court of Appeals. The court addressed two central issues in its decision. First, whether HIV-infected surgeons have a duty to inform their patients of their status, and second, whether a patient can recover damages for the fear induced by a failure to disclose one's AIDS status.

To decide these issues, the court outlined the legal standards for a claim of negligence. In deciding the issue of a duty to inform, the judge relied upon a case involving sexually transmitted diseases. The case held that because the transmission of the disease was foreseeable, the sexual partner had a duty to warn of its potential transmission. The court also relied on a 1992 document of the American Medical Association's Council on Ethical and Judicial Affairs, which recommended that HIV-infected surgeons inform their patients of their status or refrain from performing invasive procedures. The AMA has since changed the wording of its recommendation to lessen the directionality of the statement.

The important aspect of the decision, however, was the movement away from the material risk basis for the judgment. Although the court agreed that the risk was minimal, the fact that transmission would eventually result in the death of the patient, moved the judge to rule that the severity of the situation places the physician under a duty to disclose. This was a substantial departure from previous cases such as *Precourt v. Frederick* (1985), when the court held that even the risk of a severe injury may be found to be immaterial if the probability was so low as to make it negligible. The court in the *Faya* case, however, did limit the potential injury to the four days during which the patient became aware of the physician's HIV status and received the negative test results. This narrowing the window of vulnerability came as a result of the fact that a negative test would usually indicate with a 95 percent certainty that there would be no future seroconversion.

The appeals court reversed the trial judge's dismissal of charges and held that the woman's fear was not unreasonable and might constitute a compensable injury. He ruled that a jury should be allowed to evaluate whether Dr. Almaraz's actions were appropriate, and whether the actions constituted a breach of his duty to provide informed consent. In that Dr. Almaraz treated over 1,800 patients while he was in practice at Johns Hopkins, this creates the potential for a great number of litigations. It will be cases such as this that will drive the hospitals away from liberal allowances in regard to HIV-infected practitioners.

The decision on how infected practitioners are to be treated in these cases for the most part seems to have been left up to the individual states so long as their guidelines are at least equal to those promulgated by the CDC (Kuntz, 1992). At this time, of those states that have complied with the call for guidelines, most have not required mandatory testing for health care workers nor have they required that practitioners limit their practice. The decision to not require mandatory testing seems to have been made on the basis of high cost and low effectiveness.

Although mandatory testing of all health care workers would seem like a good solution, it is ineffective as there can be a six-month lag between infection and the development of antibodies that can be found on the test. This lag time may provide a false sense of security for the patient. In that it can take up to six months to detect the virus, for employees with annual screening, the virus could go undetected for up to eighteen months. Mandatory testing seems to offer more of an illusion of security than real substance. These tests also provide a certain level of false positives, which have the potential of destroying a practitioner's career. Most health care providers feel that rigorously enforced infection control methods would be more useful in protecting patients and providers than mandatory testing.

Rather than require immediate cessation of practice or the limits of practice to noninvasive techniques, the CDC has recommended expert review panels be set up to decide on a case-by-case basis whether seropositive health care workers should continue to perform invasive procedures (*McKee,* 1987). The practitioner is required to notify the health department of the positive HIV status which is then charged with setting up an individual review of cases and a monitoring process. The review process would call for counseling of the infected practitioner and would rate the danger to the patient. If it was decided that the infected practitioner posed a threat to the patients, he would be advised to notify all affiliated institutions of his status. In that a certain amount of these patients have a period of dementia as part of their disease process, strict practice limitations or close monitoring seem appropriate. There are indications that the Florida dentist that infected Bergalis and others may have done so on purpose, perhaps as a result of paranoia brought on by his disease.

EXPERIMENTAL TREATMENT

In the early 1960s, Americans were both horrified and mesmerized in regard to the "thalidomide babies" (Munson, 1979). These infants, often born with severe deformities were the result of pregnant women taking a tranquilizer widely used in Europe which could be purchased there without a prescription. In that this drug had not been approved for use in the United States, most often the American babies born with the thalidomide effects were from women traveling in Europe who had purchased the drug overseas. Partially in response to this tragedy, the Food and Drug Act adopted the Kefauver Amendments which required that investigational and new drugs (INDs) obtain premarket approval. This was to assure the public that drugs would not reach the market without well-controlled studies proving that they were efficacious and safe.

Although criticized by physicians, patients, and drug companies for slowing the process of pharmaceuticals reaching the market, the Food and Drug Administration guidelines maintained these standards throughout the 1960s and 1970s. Although there was a great deal of individual discomfort and frustration with the slowness of these processes, the public in general felt that they were well served and protected.

These standards came under severe criticism in the 1980s as two rather divergent forces found common cause in speeding up the processes and began to advocate for loosening restrictions. In the Reagan era, the Council on Competitiveness (1982), which was designed to make recommendations necessary to create a freer and more responsive business climate, advocated for "accelerated approval" for INDs needed to treat life-threatening conditions or for those when no alternate therapy existed. This loosening of the rules would allow for drugs to reach the market still in the development stage, with some of the studies to be completed postmarketing. The second voice for change came from AIDS activists such as the AIDS Coalition to Unleash Power (ACT UP) (1989) who advocated for initiatives to find new drugs as well as the right of patients to have free access to new experimental therapies.

On the surface, the idea of making experimental drugs available to dying patients seems cold but rational, especially if they are part of the premarket studies. It seems a marriage made in heaven; the HIV-infected patients get experimental and perhaps useful drugs, and the pharmaceutical companies get volunteers for their studies.

Yet, there could be no legal obligation to provide these drugs, as the law holds physicians to the standard of customary care. Customary care by definition is that which one could expect from a competent and reasonable physician. In that the drugs in question are unproved, potentially dangerous, and experimental, they could hardly be included under the umbrella of customary care.

A secondary concern in the approach of providing experimental drugs to this group of patients is that of free choice. How free is the individual in selecting to be part of the clinical study, when the choice is being coerced by the lack of options? The option of a sure death as compared with a small hope is perhaps no option at all. In some way it is similar to the burn patient who pleads to be left alone or allowed to die in the emergency room. How much of this choice is self-determination and how much is being coerced by pain?

Finally, there is a serious scientific problem associated with the use of HIV-infected patients in the clinical studies. According to published reports and television documentaries, this group of patients is desperately seeking remedies from whatever source. Lack of compliance with clinical research protocols has always been a minor problem in research, but what is to be done in a situation when patients are so desperate that they will lie, cheat, or essentially do anything to gain access to what may be their only hope to personal survival? How would one do a serious study in a community that is self-medicating with whatever drugs can be found on any market? **Randomized clinical trials** depend upon therapeutic control of the experimental clinical groups. In uncontrolled circumstances when unauthorized drugs are being taken by the group assigned either the IND or the placebo, the possibility of nonscientific and erroneous conclusions is magnified.

In the *United States v. Rutherford* (1979) ruling concerning laetrile, the U.S. Supreme Court ruled that the Food and Drug Administration had the legal duty to protect the terminally ill from unsafe and unproved drugs. Fatally ill patients do not have a legal right on the basis of their illness to receive experimental and potentially unsafe drugs. Although the FDA processes need to be streamlined, safeguards must be maintained. What is not clear is where the compromise is to be cut, so as to accommodate the free market and AIDS activists and still protect the public. What is clear is that this is a decision when social prudence is perhaps the best policy.

CONCLUSION

Acquired immunodeficiency syndrome (AIDS) continues to grow as a worldwide epidemic. The disease virtually unknown prior to 1981 is now present in almost all countries and has today infected over 4.5 million individuals. About 18 million adults and 1.5 million children have been infected with HIV. The disease which at one time was centered within certain high risk groups has now spread into all segments of the population. In 1993, AIDS was the fourth leading cause of death among women aged 25 to 44. AIDS is increasing among women faster than it is among men. Heterosexual contact is the most rapidly increasing transmission category for women. Data from 1993 indicate that 7,000 infants were born to HIV-infected mothers. If one used an estimated perinatal transmission rate of 15 to 30%, then 1,000 to 2,000 infants were perinatally infected (CDC, 1995b).

The use of high risk groups is no longer the best way to identify those at risk for the disease but rather risk should be measured by the practice of certain high risk behaviors. Due to the frightening consequences of the disease and its relative newness, the public has reacted negatively toward those infected. Victims of the disease have been stigmatized and exposed to humiliation and loss of work, insurance, and housing. The issue of confidentiality and an attempt to provide a level of privacy beyond that which is provided for other diseases often create problems for the patient and the health care provider. This is the only condition that creates any question as to whether the nonphysician health care providers should be told the diagnosis of the patients they care for when on duty.

Ethical issues involved with this disease include confidentiality, the duty to treat infected individuals, the need for universal screening, the duty of infected health care providers to warn patients, and the need for equitable distribution of medical care and research dollars. It is clear that the resources that will need to be brought forward to care for these patients threaten to overwhelm an already burdened health care delivery system. Along with the ethical issues involved with the care of AIDS patients, the legal system has been particularly intrusive, and AIDS has generated more litigation than any other disease in the history of the American legal system (Gostin, 1991).

The current information with regard to HIV infections is both encouraging and discouraging. It is discouraging to note that a number of cultural and attitudinal barriers prevent the full implementation of an HIV risk reduction educational program and as many as 40,000 new infections occur each year. Yet the number of new HIV infections among the San Francisco gay population was estimated to be 1,000, down from the 6,000 to 8,000 infections reported in 1982 to 1983. While one may argue that 1,000 is too high given our current knowledge of how the disease is transmitted, it also shows that significant changes in behavior can occur and demonstrates the impact of behavioral interventions in reducing the risk of infection (Stryker et al., 1995). During 1994 health departments reported 80,691 cases of AIDS to the CDC. This report confirms a decline in AIDS cases reported when compared with 1993 data; however, the 1994 data unfortunately confirmed the continuation of the trend of increased cases among women and children (CDC, 1995a).

Allied health and nursing personnel are in the forefront for risk of exposure. The courts have recognized that those exposed due to negligence of their employers should be compensated; however, courts have drawn a firm distinction between AIDS phobia and true exposures. This can be seen in the *Stepp v. Review Board* case when a laboratory technician was discharged for refusing to process blood from HIV-infected patients even though the laboratory followed CDC guidelines. The technician stated that she feared contamination and that the disease was a plague sent from God. The court held that the technician had been discharged for just cause and was rightly denied unemployment compensation.

On the encouraging side, recent changes in therapeutic regimes offer some hope for those infected. People with HIV are living longer, healthier lives thanks to a new combination of drugs, including the new protease inhibitors. Dr. Peter Pilot, director of the United Nations Project on AIDS, has said that new research suggests that

AIDS is not "an inevitably fatal, incurable disease any more. We have not got a cure yet, but the new combinations of anti-retroviral drugs are holding out new hope" (SoRelle, 1996).

AIDS in a very real sense is just another infectious disease. Yet, it appears a disease with a difference, a disease that has made us reexamine who we are as practitioners. Even as we struggle to find a cure to the disease, as a society we also struggle with the ethical, legal, and health care issues associated with the condition. How we finally address and resolve these problems will either speak well or ill of the ethical and legal foundations of the American health care system. Because of the scope of the problems associated with this epidemic, our actions in response to it will leave either a proud or shameful heritage for future health care providers.

LEGAL CASE STUDY: *Estate of William Behringer v. Medical Center at Princeton, 592 A.2d 1251 (N.J. Super. Ct. Law Div. 1991).*

This case involves an otolaryngologist and plastic surgeon who was diagnosed as suffering from AIDS while an inpatient at the hospital where he practiced. Within hours of his discharge, he began to receive calls from members of the staff at the hospital wishing him well and expressing their concern for his condition. Other calls were received from friends in the community. Within several weeks of his discharge, his surgical privileges at the medical center were suspended.

The plaintiff brought suit against the hospital and named employees alleging breach of duty to maintain confidentiality of diagnosis and test results and violation of the New Jersey law against discrimination through the hospital's imposition of rules restricting his practice. The court held that:

- Failure of the hospital and laboratory director to take reasonable steps to maintain confidentiality was a breach of duty.

- The relationship between the hospital and physician was such that the suspension of surgical privileges was sufficient to bring the case within the scope of the New Jersey law against discrimination.

- The hospital acted properly in initially suspending the surgeon's privileges and thereafter imposing requirements of informed consent.

- In the context of informed consent, risk of surgical accident, and implications thereof, the fact that a surgeon was infected would be a legitimate concern to a surgical patient, warranting a disclosure of the risk.

This case is interesting in that it raises not only the issue of informed consent with an HIV-infected health care practitioner, but also the requirements needed to protect the confidentiality of the practitioner while he is a patient. Although the hospital had policies stating that charts were limited to those persons having patient care responsibility, in practical terms the charts were available to any doctor, nurse, or other hospital personnel. Ensuring confidentiality in these cases requires more than simply instructing employees that medical records are confidential.

The standard followed by the court in measuring the conduct of the hospital was:

> The dissemination of a patient's records and information is limited to qualified personnel involved in the diagnosis and treatment of the person who is the subject of the record. Disclosure is limited to only personnel directly involved in the diagnosis and treatment of the person.

The standard used to determine whether the hospital was correct in requiring that the surgeon disclose his health status was:

> Medical information or a risk of a medical procedure is material when a reasonable patient would be likely to attach significance to it in deciding whether or not to submit to treatment.

It has been calculated that the risk of contracting HIV in a single surgical operation on an HIV-infected patient is in the range of 1:130,000 to 1:400,000. It is impossible to accurately calculate the risk of HIV transmission from an infected surgeon to a patient, although it is thought to be infinitesimal.

1. Do you think that an infected health care practitioner should be required to inform the patient given the low risk?

2. Create a policy that would have protected this health care provider from the loss of confidentiality that he suffered as a patient. Do you think that a higher standard of confidentiality is due health care workers?

3. How does the advent of computerized records affect the access and confidentiality issue described in this case study?

REVIEW EXERCISES

1. In the following scenarios determine the correct provider response. Justify your answer.
   a. If the nurse attending the patient was herself immune suppressed, would this be enough to move the duty to treat an HIV-infected patient to the moral option of treating or not treating?
   b. You are a respiratory therapist and have been assigned to a floor unit. You find that your department head has decided to reuse patient suction traps on the basis of saving money. This is breach of universal precautions. What should your response be?
   c. As an EMT you punctured your gloves while removing an auto wreck victim from her car. In this case would you have a legitimate right to know her HIV status?
   d. You are a physical therapist and have been seeing Mr. Jones for months as a result of a referral from Dr. Smith. Over this time period your relationship has grown until the patient has a better relationship with you than with his physician. One day he tells you that he is HIV positive and asks that you not tell Dr. Smith. What is your obligation to the patient? What is your obligation to Dr. Smith?
   e. You are a dental hygienist and have found out that you are pregnant. Is this rationale for refusing to treat HIV-infected patients?
   f. In that Dr. Acer has caused alarm among dental patients, your clinic has decided to advertise in the local paper that all your staff is "HIV free." Is this ethical?
2. Recently in order to improve the immune system of an AIDS patient, cells from a primate were implanted into the patient to stimulate the human's immune system. Some scientists were critical of the process stating that it opened the possibility for the transmission of certain virus types that were not normally pathogenic to humans to the patient and then into the human population. Assuming that the criticism was true and that there was a risk, even if minimal, was the practice ethical?

3. In Israel the migrants from Ethiopia have recently protested the government policy of not accepting their blood donations. The policy is based on the fact that this particular population has a high incidence of HIV infection.

    The migrants see this as stigmatizing to their community which includes both infected and noninfected individuals. This appears to be a conflict between the right to give a gift and the right of the individual who receives the blood to know that the gift of blood is pure.

    State your opinion in regard to the argument. Is there a compromise position that would be satisfactory to both groups?

4. In one case a nurse sued the physician with whom she was working claiming that his failure to inform her of the positive HIV status of a patient on which they performed an invasive procedure was negligent and caused emotional trauma. The nurse had performed the procedure without protective gloves, and with a cut on her hand. The court dismissed the petition. It is clear that the nurse was in the wrong for not using universal precautions. Do you think that the physician had a legal or moral obligation (or both) to warn her of the risk?

5. Evaluate the following statements. Determine which are legal. State reasons, why or why not.
    a. Refuse treatment to an AIDS patient on the basis of the disease.
    b. Require all practitioners in your department to take mandatory AIDS tests.
    c. Refuse to take an AIDS test.
    d. Report that a patient has AIDS to outside authorities.
    e. Sue an HIV-infected physician for not informing you that he has tested positive for the virus.

6. New York State has perhaps had the greatest experience with AIDS-infected practitioners. The following is a 1991 New York State recommendation in regard to HIV-infected professionals. In light of the cases such as *Bradley* and *Almaraz,* do you think that the 1991 policy would still provide enough legal protection for the hospitals?

    HIV-infected professionals should continue all professional practice for which they are qualified, with rigorous adherence to universal precautions and scientifically accepted infection control practices. Decisions about work responsibilities of HIV-infected individuals with evidence of functional impairment or lack of infection control competence should continue to be made on a case-by-case basis involving the worker's personal physician.

REFERENCES

Acello, B. (1996). *Infection control update.* Albany, N.Y. Delmar Publishers.

AIDS Coalition to Unleash Power (ACT UP). (1989, June 4–9). A national AIDS treatment research agenda. Issued by ACT UP and distributed at the Fifth International Conference on AIDS. Montreal, Canada.

Altman, D. (1986). *AIDS in the mind of America.* Des Plaines, Ill: Anchor Books.

American Nurses' Association: *Code for nurses with interpretative statements.* (1985). American Nurses Association. Kansas City, MO.

Estate of *Behringer v. Medical Center at Princeton,* 592 A.2d 1251 (N.J. Super. Ct. Law Div. 1991).

Bradley v. University of Texas M.D. Anderson Cancer Center, 3 F. 3d 922 (5th Cir. 1993).

Canterbury v. Spence, 464 F.2d 772, (D.C. Circ. 1972).

Center for Disease Control (CDC). (1995a). Update: Acquired immunodeficiency syndrome—United States, 1994. *JAMA, 273* (9).

CDC. (1995b). Update: AIDS among women—United States, 1994. *JAMA, 273* (10).

CDC. (1995c). *HIV/AIDS surveillance report.* Division of HIV/AIDS Prevention, National Center for HIV/Aids Prevention STD, & TB Prevention Atlanta, Ga.

Council on Competitiveness Fact Sheet: Improving the nation's drug approval process. (1982). *Milbank Quarterly, 68* (Suppl. 1), 111–142.

Daniels, N. (1992). HIV-infected health care professionals: Public threat or public sacrifice. *Milbank Quarterly, 7* (1), p. 17.

DeVille, K. A. (1994, Summer). Nothing to fear but fear itself: HIV-infected physicians and the laws of informed consent. *Journal of Law, Medicine and Ethics, 22* (2), pp. 163–175.

Doe v. Centinela Hospital, No. CV87-2514, 1988 WL 8177b (C.D. Cal. June 30, 1988).

Faya v. Almarez, 620 A. 2d 327 (Md. 1993).

Field, M. (1990). Testing for AIDS: Uses and abuses. *American Journal of Law and Medicine, 16,* pp. 34–106.

Fox, C. H. (1991). AIDS transmission: Hazardous health care? *Harvard Health Letter, 17,* pp. 4–6.

Fox, M. (1996, September 10). Vaccine for HIV works on monkeys. *Washington Times.*

Glenn, P., Spronson, L., McCartney, M., & Yesalis, C. (1990). Attitudes toward AIDS among a low risk group of women. *JOGNN Clinical Studies, 20* (5), pp. 398–405.

Glover v. Eastern Nebraska Community Office of Retardation, 867 F. 2d 461 (8th Cir. 1989).

Gostin, L. (1989). HIV-infected physicians and the practice of seriously invasive procedures. *Hastings Center Report, 19.*

Gostin, L. (1991). The HIV-infected health care professional: Public policy discrimination and patient safety. *Archives of Internal Medicine, 151,* pp. 663–665.

Grady, D. (1991). Infected healers. *American Health* vol. 10 Issue 3, pp. 30–33.

Health and Human Services. Understanding AIDS. *HHS Publication* (CDC), HHS-88-8404. Horty, J. (1994). The legal view. *OR Manager, 10* (2), pp. 18–19.

Health and Public Policy Committee, American College of Physicians, and the Infectious Disease Society of America. (1986). Position paper on acquired immunodeficiency syndrome. *Annals of Internal Medicine, 104,* pp. 575–581.

Henderson, D. (1988). HIV infection: Risks to health care workers and infection control. *Nursing Clinics of North America, 23* (4), pp. 767–775.

Huber, J. (1993). Death and AIDS: A review of the medico-legal literature. *Death Studies, 17* (3), pp. 225–232.

Jarvis, R., Closen, M., Hermann, D., & Leonard, A. (1991). *AIDS Law* (p. 154). St. Paul, MN: West Publishing Company.

Keeton, P. et al. (1984). *Prosser and Keeton on the law of torts* (5th ed.). (p. 175). St. Paul, MN: West Publishing Company.

Kolasa, E. (1993). HIV vs. a nurse's right to work. *RN,* vol 56 (1) pp. 63–66.

Kuntz, L. A. (1992). CDC shifts control. *RT Image, 6* (29).

Lackritz, E. et al. (1995). Estimated risk of transmission of the human immunodeficiency virus by screened blood in the United States. *The New England Journal of Medicine, 333* (26), pp. 1721–1725.

Lo, B., & Steinbrook, R. (1992). Health care workers infected with the human immunodeficiency virus. *Journal of the American Medical Association, 267* (8), pp. 1100–1105.

Local 1812, American Federation of Government Employees v. U.S. Department of State. (1987). 662 F. Supp. 5 (D.C. Cir. 1987).

McKee v. Miles Laboratory Inc. (1987). 675 F. Supp. 1060 (E.D. Ky. 1987).

Milliken, N., & Greenblatt, R. (1988). *Ethical issues of the AIDS epidemic.* Rockville, MD: Aspen Publication.

Mishell, D. R. (1989). Contraception. *The New England Journal of Medicine, 320,* pp. 777–787.

Morbity & Mortality Weekly Report (1992). Reported cases of HIV infection and AIDS in the United States, 1990. *MMWR, 41* (15).

Munson, R. (1979). *Intervention and reflection* (pp. 50–51). Belmont, CA: Wadsworth Publishing Company.

National Safety Council. (1993). *Bloodborne pathogens.* Boston, MA: Jones and Bartlett Publishers.

Owens, B. (1993). Suits happen. *Emergency Medical Services, 22* (8), pp. 51–75.

Pozgar, G. (1993). *Legal aspects of health care administration* (pp. 180–184). Rockville, MD: Aspen Publication.

Precourt v. Frederick. (1985). 481 N.E. 2d 1144 (Mass).

School Board of Nassau County v. Arline, 480 U.S. 273 (1987).

Seidl, A. (1994). HIV testing: Patients' rights versus nurses' rights. *Nursing Issues of the Nineties and Beyond* (pp. 139–157). New York: Springer Publishing.

SoRelle, R. (1996, September 9). Triple play on HIV. *Houston Chronicle.*

Stepp v. Review Board of the Indiana Employment Security Division, 521 N.E. 2d, 350 (Ind. Ct. App. 1988).

Stryker, J. et al. (1995). Prevention of HIV infection. *JAMA, 273* (14).

United States v. Rutherford, 442 U.S. 544. (1979).

—————— C H A P T E R   8 ——————

Abortion

Goal

The general goal of this chapter is to outline the nature of the conflict between the pro-life (antiabortion) position and the pro-choice (not necessarily proaboration, but against legislation outlawing abortion) position and to update the current legal position of abortion in the United States.

Objectives

At the end of this chapter, the reader should understand and be able to:

1. Outline the distinction between "human" and "person" and the dispute regarding personhood criteria.
2. List the basic facts of fetal development.
3. Outline the sanctity of life argument.
4. List the elements of the doctrine of double effect.
5. Explain the pro-choice position from a life plan point of view.
6. Explain the pro-choice position from an environmental perspective.
7. Explain the reasoning of the Supreme Court regarding the 1973 *Roe v. Wade* case.
8. Explain the effects of the Hyde Amendment.
9. Explain how the *Roe v. Wade* case created a negative right to an abortion.
10. Explain both the pro-choice and pro-life positions.
11. Outline the current status of abortion in the United States today.
12. Explain the place of professional autonomy in the issue of abortion.

Key Terms

abortifacient	**abortionist**	**embryo**
abortion	**doctrine of double effect**	**fetus**

negative right	pro–life	therapeutic abortion
person	quickening	viability
potential life	RU 486	zygote
pro-choice	sufficing solution	

THE ABORTION ISSUE

The emphasis must be not on the right to abortion but on the right to privacy and reproductive control.

> Ruth Bader Ginsberg, U.S. educator, Supreme Court justice.

The greatest destroyer of peace is abortion because if a mother can kill her own child, what is left for me to kill you and you to kill me? There is nothing between.

> Mother Teresa, Albanian-born Roman Catholic nun, Nobel Peace Prize lecture, 1979

If men were equally at risk from this condition—if they knew that their bellies might swell as if they were suffering from end-stage cirrhosis, that they would have to go nearly a year without a stiff drink, a cigarette, or even an aspirin, that they would be subject to fainting spells and unable to fight their way onto commuter trains—then I am sure that pregnancy would be classified as a sexually transmitted disease and abortions would be no more controversial than emergency appendectomies.

> Barbara Ehrenreich , U.S. author, columnist.

As we approach the year 2000, the issue of abortion seems as current as this morning's newspaper, yet it has been under consideration at least for the full extent of Western civilization. In 335 B.C., no less a light than Aristotle himself promoted **abortion** as a form of birth control for parents with too many children. In *Politics* he wrote *". . . neglect of an effective birth control policy is a never failing source of poverty which in turn is the parent of revolution and crime."* Through the ages, societies either banned or promoted abortion depending upon size of the population and their social needs. The Greeks (and later the Romans) would encourage large families in order to supply recruits for their armies. The father of medicine, Hippocrates (429 B.C.) in his oath of practice bound his followers to avoid the process stating, *"Similarly I will not give a pessary to a woman to cause abortion."*

In the 1800s, the practice of abortion as a means of birth control came under severe pressure from the Roman Catholic Church and changing public opinion which led to strict antiabortion laws. In the United States, from the Victorian era until the middle of this century, the overwhelming position of state statutes was that all but **therapeutic abortions** were forbidden. An example of this cultural attitude toward abortion can be seen in the 1872 Comstock Law which made it a criminal offense to import, mail, or transport in interstate commerce "any article of medicine for the prevention of conception or for causing abortion" (Faux, 1988). Under common law, however, abortion was generally not considered an indictable offense before the time of **quickening.**

The arguments used to justify the criminal statutes of the nineteenth and twentieth centuries revolved around three issues. First, to discourage illicit sexual behavior; second, to restrain a woman from exposure to a potentially harmful medical procedure; and third, to protect prenatal life. In the watershed 1973 case of *Roe v. Wade,* the first two of these justifications had not been put forward, nor had they been considered seriously by any court or commentary. In its decision the court focused on the third issue.

ROE V. WADE

Until 1973, except in cases when the mother's life was in danger, abortion was a statutory crime in every state of the nation. The Supreme Court, relying on the constitutional right of privacy emanating from the word *liberty* in the due process clause of the Fourteenth Amendment, legalized a woman's right to have an abortion. This right, however, was not considered to be unrestricted, and the court recognized the state's legitimate interest in protecting health, the standards of medical practice, and prenatal life. The court's decision balanced the interests of the woman and the state, allowing the woman greater freedom of action in the beginning of the pregnancy and the state a greater right to regulate the process as the fetus developed. In the decision, the court divided pregnancy into three trimesters of twelve weeks each. In the first trimester, the state has little right to regulate the process, and the decision is that of the woman and her physician. During the second trimester, the state's interest increases, at least in the area of protecting the health of the woman (only those regulations directed toward this concern will be upheld as legitimate). This is somewhat problematic to those who feel that human life begins with quickening, as this usually occurs within the second trimester. One argument placed before the court against abortion was that fetuses, especially after quickening, are persons and deserve the protection under the Fourteenth Amendment. However, the court ruled that historically the term **person** was used only postnatally. The third trimester, which begins at twenty-five weeks' gestation, is when the court allowed the state to shift its interest to the protection of the fetus. The fetus has reached a point of potential **viability** outside the womb and the dominant interest of the state after twenty-eight weeks becomes the protection of this potential life. The court held that once viable, the fetus cannot be aborted except in those cases when the procedure is essential for the protection of the woman's life.

THE LEGAL STRUGGLE FOLLOWING ROE V. WADE

With this decision, the court set off a firestorm of public debate as citizens and state legislators attempted to gain an understanding of the dimensions of the ruling and either resist or embrace its potential outcomes. One important case which made clear the primacy of the woman's rights in the first trimester was the 1976 *Danforth v. Planned Parenthood of Central Missouri* case. In this case the Supreme Court examined a statutory provision which required a woman to receive her husband's, or if a minor her parent's or guardian's, permission prior to having an abortion. The court held that these requirements were unconstitutional given that they imposed restrictions within the first trimester, a time when the decision was left in the hands of the woman and her physician. In regard to the issue of minors, the court held that, like adults, minors had a constitutional right to privacy, although the scope of that protection might differ.

The *Roe v. Wade* decision, which provided women with a right to have an abortion, is essentially a **negative right** in that it provides liberty only from interference. This liberty is somewhat like having an equal right with all others, to determine what shall or shall not be done to or with one's body. The right to noninterference does not in itself create the reciprocal obligations for others to provide the means for an abortion. This has been an important battleground between **pro-life** and **pro-choice** advocates. In 1976 Congress enacted the Hyde Amendment which restricted the availability of Medicare funding for abortions. Under challenge, the Hyde Amendment was modified to allow funding for abortions in those cases when the mother's life was threatened by carrying the fetus full term, or in cases of incest or rape when the incidents had been reported to appropriate governmental agencies.

The Supreme Court reviewed the Hyde Amendment in *Harris v. McRae*(1980). There the court upheld in a six to three ruling the constitutionality of the amendment, reasoning that federal law did not mandate that states which participate in the Medicaid program provide funding for medically unnecessary abortions. The constitutional right of privacy, with its attendant right to abortion, did not, in the court's opinion, create an entitlement to governmental funding to take advantage of all aspects of the liberty granted. The court argued that the funding restriction was rationally related to the state's interest in protecting **potential life**and ensured the health of the mother. In that the state provided funding to those women who wished to have their children, and restricted funding to those who wished to have an abortion, the federal government was acting appropriately by making childbirth a more attractive alternative. Following the decision, abortions paid for by Medicaid funds fell from 295,000 in 1977 to only 2,100 in 1978 (Pozgar, 1993).

Pro-life forces took encouragement from the Hyde Amendment. They continued to mobilize campaigns to defeat politicians who supported legalized abortion. Critics of the amendment objected that while abortion was still legal, it had become the privilege of the rich. They asked what a "right" to an abortion meant, if you are too poor to afford the necessary services. When you ask this question you are making an appeal to consideration under the principle of justice. Accordingly, they felt that it was the responsibility of a just society to ensure the value of an individual's rights by guaranteeing access to necessary resources. The reality of the question was reinforced by the tragic death in McAllen, Texas, of Rosaura Jiminez, 27, a mother of a 5-year-old child. Unable to access Medicaid for an abortion, she died in pain at the hands of a local **abortionist**. Jiminez was the first recorded death by illegal abortion, following the passage of the Hyde Amendment.

In 1981 the Supreme Court again gave further direction as to the dimension of the liberty granted in *Roe v. Wade* in *H.L. v. Matheson* (1981). In the *Matheson* case, the Supreme Court upheld a Utah statute that required, under threat of fine or imprisonment, that the physician at least make a good faith effort to contact the parents of a minor prior to performing a requested abortion. The reasoning of the court was that the statute was designed to protect minors by encouraging parental involvement in decisions that had potentially permanent emotional and traumatic consequences. The court explained that the state has significant interest with regard to minors. Although the physician attempted to notify the parents, the statute did not give the parents a right to override the minor's decision in the matter. The Supreme Court again provided similar reasoning in the *Hodgson v. Minnesota* (1990) case when it sustained the state's right to require a pregnant minor to inform both her parents prior to having an abortion. Decisions such as the 1989 *Webster v. Reproductive Health Services* case, wherein the court held that a state could ban public employees and public health facilities from performing or assisting in performing nontherapeutic abortions, gave an indication that the Supreme Court was shifting toward a more conservative stance in regard to the abortion issue. This provided the pro-life advocates with hope that the Supreme Court would, in the future, further erode the 1973 *Roe v. Wade* decision.

The Bush administration on 29 January 1988 barred most family planning clinics that received federal funding from providing abortion assistance or counseling. This decision was reinforced by the U.S. Supreme Court in *Rust v. Sullivan* (1991), when it ruled that Congress did not violate the Constitution when it barred employees of family planning clinics that received federal funding from providing information with regard to the option of abortion. This gag order became a major ethical concern within the health care community as it interposed the government between the patient and the provider. The community began to question what effect this artificial barrier had on the principle of informed consent, and patient-provider autonomy. In response to the criticism of the policy, Congress passed a bill allowing abortion to be discussed as an option; however, this was vetoed by President Bush. One of the first actions of the Clinton presidency was to sign executive orders that partially overturned the gag rule; lifted the ban on the use of fetal tissue in federally funded research; and ordered a review of the prohibition on the French **abortifacient RU 486.** The Clinton administration lifted the barrier to foreign aid for family planning centers that offered abortion counseling; and ended the ban against overseas U.S. military hospitals performing abortions if they were paid for by private funds. In 1992, a panel of the U.S. Circuit Court of Appeals for the District of Columbia rejected the gag rule regulation issued by the Bush administration. The appeals court panel held that the administration had acted improperly and had issued the regulation without allowing for the traditional period of public comment (Pozgar, 1993).

The abortion issue still continues to be hotly contested, and it is likely to become even more explosive as positions are stated and restated, and patience and tolerance for the views of others wane. Civil disobedience, harassment, and vandalism are increasingly prevalent across the nation as more traditional methods of changing laws and minds have been exhausted. The confrontation between the groups reached a new level when Michael Griffin, a member of Rescue America, killed Dr. David Gunn outside an abortion clinic in Pensacola, Florida. The reaction across the nation was swift and polemic with pro-choice forces likening the pro-life activists to terrorists, while a minority of the pro-life proponents rejoiced in the murder. When questioned with regard to the tragedy, the national director of Rescue America stated that he considered the physician's death unfortunate, but that "we will not be outraged over the one death and not the other 4000 precious human beings being killed today by abortion . . ." (*Time*, 1993).

Currently the main framework of *Roe v. Wade* is still in place and is the law of the land, in spite of the fears of those who thought that judges appointed by Reagan and Bush would attempt to reopen the case and rethink the issue. We are in the midst of a struggle of titanic proportions with neither side being able to gain a clear victory. Rules that are promulgated by one group when it gains political power are often overturned when the political tide turns.

The recent level of violence with the death of physicians, attendants, and bystanders is an escalation that speaks poorly for all involved. It is a hollow moral victory when pro-life advocates proclaim that fewer physicians are willing to perform abortions when the basis for their decision may be fear of physical harm for themselves and their families. Conversely, there is little high ground when, on the basis of privacy, human life is trivialized by those who decide upon an abortion because they do not like the gender of the fetus. It must seem clear that after over two decades of political and legal struggle, the matter of abortion is one that cannot be decided by legal fiat or shifting political fortunes. We must in the end reason together if we are to bind our wounds. If either side is to truly "win," it should be by the force of their moral argument, not because they were able to coerce public opinion on a given day.

THE PROCESS

Currently the two common methods of abortion are uterine or vacuum aspiration, and dilatation and curettage. In the first, the cervix is widened by instruments, a tube is inserted, and the contents suctioned out. Dilatation and curettage is much the same; however, the contents are not suctioned but rather the fetal materials are scraped from the uterus with the use of surgical instruments. In late abortions, which are less common, the abortion is brought about by the instillation of saline solution which induces a miscarriage. Although rarely used, a cesarean section is also sometimes used to abort the fetus.

THE ADVOCATES

The opposing positions in the abortion controversy have taken the titles of pro-choice and pro-life. The pro-choice advocates believe that the decision to have an abortion is a personal choice protected by the constitutional guarantees of liberty and current law. Perhaps the bumper sticker that best fits their position is "If you don't like abortion! Don't have one." On the other hand, pro-life advocates are those that believe that the fetus is a human and abortion is tantamount to murder and regardless of *Roe v. Wade,* must be stopped. Perhaps the bumper sticker that best states their position is "It's a child not a choice."

It is important to examine the bumper sticker war between the two groups, because over time each has refined its position into absolutist, simplistic slogans, which do not allow for compromise or rational discussion. It is much like the old prayer, "Lord protect me from the man who has the truth." Each group seems only to state and restate its position with every indication that they are more interested in conversion than communication or the coming to a **sufficing solution.** If we examined both group's basic positions, we can come to understand their difficulties in finding areas for compromise.

- If we accept that the fetus is a child, then what are we to do? We know that children have special rights, not only as human beings, but as innocents. These rights create correlative obligations for all of us to protect them beyond the expectations of the normal protection that we would extend to other adults. Imagine that a 3-year-old child was playing in the street and we noticed that a bus was coming. If we rushed into the street, even at some risk to ourselves, and brought the child to safety, we would be considered heroes. If this is true, and if a fetus is an innocent child, then why is it so extraordinary that men and women are willing to lay in front of abortion clinics and block the way? In this light, perhaps it is not only not extraordinary but heroic. At least, I am sure that is how a pro-life advocate would view it.

- Conversely, what if we accept that a fetus is not a child, but a rather remarkable piece of tissue? Tissue, remarkable or not, is not generally something to which we assign rights, which then create correlative obligations. In this light, how can we criticize a woman for making a personal decision to do or not do whatever she decides is best for her with regard to this remarkable piece of tissue? When we consider the rights of others with regard to that piece of tissue, and compare them with the rights of the woman, there appears to be no contest. It would seem that the woman with her right to privacy and self-determination as an autonomous adult, is the only one who should be making the decision. If this is your view of the fetus, then it is extraordinary for people to block her way. At least, I am sure that is how a pro-choice advocate would view it.

SANCTITY OF LIFE ARGUMENT

At its most basic level, the argument for a sanctity of life position would be that the fetus is alive, and sacred, and therefore killing it is wrong. We do not proscribe all killing, as plants and vegetables are also alive, and yet there is very little hue and cry over their deaths and subsequent use for our tables. The argument's focus then, turns not on the issue of life itself, but rather on human life. Human life is thought to be sacred or at least inviolable on the basis of divine mandate, unalienable natural or human rights, or common collective decision. It seems a strange question, but it must be raised—What do we mean when we say "human"? Some argue that having a genetic code of a human being is what is essential. Others argue against this position, stating that the genetic code is not sufficient to establish humanity (acorns have the genetic code of the oak tree, yet we do not confuse the two). This dispute raises the question—Does the potential for becoming a human give an entity the same rights as a human being? Even if we accept that the fetus is a human, we often distinguish the rights of humans based on their age. A 12-year-old does not have a right to

TABLE 8–1
Stages of Human Embryo Development

- Conception—The penetration of the egg by the sperm is usually followed 22 hours later by syngamy, the alignment of maternal and paternal chromosomes to form a new genotype.
- Implantation Complete—In about 14 days the zygote settles into the uterine walls and enters a stage when it is described as an embryo.
- Fetus—At about 8 weeks the first neural cells start differentiating. The entity is known as a fetus; it will continue with this description until birth.
- Distinct Human Form—This occurs at about weeks 12 to 16. The fetus in this period responds to stimulation and may feel pain.
- Quickening—Occurs at about weeks 17 to 20.
- Viability—With modern technology viability is reached by weeks 22 to 24.
- Birth—Normally occurs at 9 months.

drive, although she certainly has the potential to do so. We do not generally provide for our children the rights and privileges that we allow the president of the United States, even though we teach them that they can potentially grow up to attain that position.

There are other problems with the genetic code argument. Down syndrome babies do not have the same genetic structure as other human beings; in fact, it is the cause of their condition. Does this mean that they do not have a right to life? The pro-life advocate would respond that a human genetic code is a sufficient but not a necessary condition of beings with a right to life. Thus, other entities may also have a right to life, but one with a human genetic code, in all its varieties, definitely has such a right. The question is whether the right to life is such a right and if so, when does it come into existence? Does the right to life come into existence with conception, with the establishment of measurable brain waves, at quickening, at viability, or upon entrance to the outside world? Table 8–1 lists the important stages in human embryo development. Some have decided that the defining moment is conception, the union of the sperm and egg. At that point the **zygote** has a full genetic code that will determine the gender, hair color, skin color, and a variety of other attributes. At about two or three weeks' gestation, the zygote settles into the uterine wall and enters the stage where it is described as an **embryo.** Yet, pro-choice advocates will point out that the embryo at this point is very dissimilar to what we consider human, having what appears to be a tail and gills. Pro-life advocates would quickly argue that it is a morally dangerous position taken when we base moral judgment upon appearance.

At about eight weeks' gestation, we call the entity a **fetus,** a term that will extend until birth. By the second trimester, the fetus will normally have begun to move and the mother will be able to sense the movement at a point that is known as quickening. It was once believed that the fetus gained a soul at the point of quickening, but given that the event does not correspond to any major medical changes, most have disregarded the moment of being able to sense the motion of the fetus as important

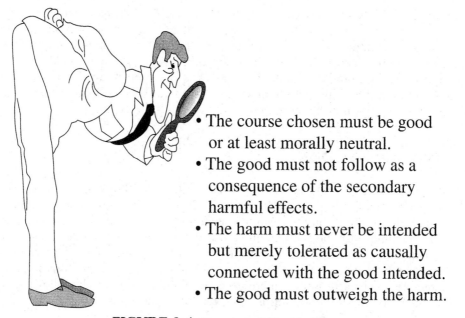

- The course chosen must be good or at least morally neutral.
- The good must not follow as a consequence of the secondary harmful effects.
- The harm must never be intended but merely tolerated as causally connected with the good intended.
- The good must outweigh the harm.

FIGURE 8–1 Doctrine of Double Effect

to the abortion issue. By the fifth month, neurologically the fetus can feel pain, and therefore at least enters into a status that we afford all creatures that feel pain. In the sixth month, the fetus enters a period of potential viability, when it could possibly survive apart from the mother. Neurologically the fetus also develops minimal consciousness during this last trimester. Birth generally occurs after nine months, but the infant at this point is still completely dependent on the mother, or at least some mother. Pro-life theorists argue that there is very little difference between the fetus prior to birth and the infant at the moment of birth. It is left to the pro-choice advocates to develop an argument that would explain how the newborn has a right to life that somehow was not present in a fetus five minutes prior to birth.

Even sanctity of life positions generally allow for a few exceptions. Self-defense is a widely accepted exception to the "thou shalt not kill" proscription. Generally it is held that if someone is trying to kill you, and the only way in which you can save yourself is by killing the other person first, that action of defense is justifiable. Some have used the self-defense argument as a reason to allow abortions in cases when the mother's life is endangered by the pregnancy. Others refute this by pointing out that self-defense is only permissible when the attacker is intending to kill you. If you were being attacked by a hungry man-eating lion, it would not be permissible to throw others in its path so as to satiate its hunger and escape being eaten.

The problem with the moral assessment of such actions arises from what we may call the "multiple character" of actions. To assess the correct moral action in cases with multiple consequences, the **doctrine of double effect** was developed. The doctrine, espoused by St. Thomas Aquinas, asks us to distinguish the intended effect of our actions from unintended effects. Figure 8-1 lists the determining criteria in deciding upon the morality of an action that has attendant negative consequences. This doctrine has been used to justify the death of fetuses under certain circumstances that threaten the death of the mother. Note that it would be impermissible, according to the doctrine, to perform an abortion to save a mother from death if the procedure involved the direct killing of the fetus. The doctrine would only provide justification in those cases when the death of the fetus resulted indirectly from the procedure and was not the intended result.

HUMAN OR PERSON?

Some would argue that the issue is not whether the fetus is human, but whether the fetus is a person. The Supreme Court ruled in *Roe v. Wade* that the liberties guaranteed to persons under the Fourteenth Amendment, dealt only with postnatal entities. Although one can be declared human on the basis of genetic code, a person is a member of the moral community on the basis of possessing certain characteristics recognized by that community as affording moral status. Several philosophers have created lists of characteristics that are necessary for personhood. The following is a listing of traits worth considering as being central to personhood:

1. Consciousness of objects and events
2. Ability to feel pain
3. Reasoning
4. Self-motivated activity
5. Capacity to communicate
6. Concept of the self.
7. Viability

With certain reservations, it appears that the list does indeed capture most people's understanding of personhood. For instance, it must be understood that criteria such as consciousness must deal exclusively with entities that are permanently unconscious. It is obviously not justifiable to kill a sleeping person. When one examines the criteria in regard to the fetus, it appears that they are not persons. Yet, what about the newborn infant? Newborns cannot really communicate and it is questionable whether they have a sense of self. So, if these are necessary conditions of personhood, then even infanticide may be permissible. Some philosophers, reasoning in regard to defective newborns, have justified infanticide based on the lack of essential personhood criteria (Warren, 1984). The major thrust of personhood reasoning in health care has been in deciding whether to withdraw life-sustaining technology. We will examine the personhood question in chapter nine; which is on these decisions. For this chapter, however, it is important to note that the fetus does not do well vis-á-vis traits defining personhood.

The viability question is important to the abortion debate, because many argue that the fetus gains standing when it can function independently from its mother. It can be seen from *Roe v. Wade* that the Supreme Court shifted the protection of the law from the mother to the fetus in the third trimester, a time when the fetus attains the potential for viability. One problem with using viability as a criteria is that it is technology dependent. Can one fetus become a person in the United States on the basis of advanced medical technology, yet another remain a nonperson for several more weeks in a developing nation? This may not be as problematic as it first appears, in that the status of personhood is a matter of cultural decision and not a natural property that one can discern like sodium in salt. In some places in the world, where infant mortality is high, the decision of personhood is often postponed for up to three years, after which the baby is given a name. Such a practice makes sense, given the emotional trauma that is caused by the loss of a child who is considered a person.

THE ARGUMENT REGARDING THE LIBERTY OF WOMEN

In the middle-class United States, a veneer of "alternative lifestyles" disguises the reality that, here as everywhere, women's apparent "choices" whether or not to have children are still dependent on the far from neutral will of male legislators, jurists, a male medical and pharmaceutical profession, well-financed lobbies, including the prelates of the Catholic Church, and the political reality that women do not as yet have self-determination over our bodies and still live mostly in ignorance of our authentic physicality, our possible choices, our eroticism itself.

Adrienne Rich, author (1929)

As described in this quote, much of the rhetoric of the pro-choice movement has been concerned with the issue of a woman's right to self-determination. For many women, it is unthinkable to imagine a woman not having the decision of whether to continue a pregnancy. They argue that if a woman is to be free, she must have control over her own reproduction. If a woman is to compete in the marketplace with men, then she cannot have an unwanted pregnancy interrupt her career. They argue that to regard a woman's career—or more importantly her life plan—as having so little importance that it must be set aside by the contingency of unwanted pregnancy is to regard women as less important than men. These women desire control over their life plan in the way a men have control. This is what has led many women to say, that if men could become pregnant, then there would be no controversy regarding a right to abortion.

If men could get pregnant, abortion would be a sacrament.

Florynce Kennedy, author (1973)

At this point, pro-life advocates usually argue that women can "just say no," that if the life plan is so important then the woman can refrain from sex or use any number of contraceptive systems that make pregnancy unlikely. In most instances, pregnancy is not the result of lack of available contraceptives, or lack of information as to how babies are created. They argue that adoption is an alternative to abortion and brings the obligation down to nine months, much of which does not really interfere with a person's life plan. As can be seen in the following quote, some pro-choice advocates will respond that even this is too much to ask.

Frankly, I adore your catchy slogan, "Adoption, not Abortion," although no one has been able to figure out, even with expert counseling, how to use adoption as a method of birth control, or at what time of the month it is most effective.

Barbara Ehrenreich, author (1991)

Quite often at this point the argument between the advocates shifts to include the issues concerning modern attitudes toward sex, which pro-life proponents see as being the root problem of the abortion issue. It is interesting to imagine the *Roe v. Wade* case in the context of America in 1935. In that context, would we see 1,500,000 fetuses aborted each year? Would there even be a debate? Would we see late trimester arguments for abortion? Notice that we are now in another area of intense and personal disagreement. What we find at this level of argument are differing ideas concerning sexuality and individual responsibility, ideas that ultimately come down to one's religious or most deeply held moral beliefs.

THE ENVIRONMENTAL PERSPECTIVE

Abortion throughout history has often been accepted or rejected based on considerations of societal needs. Early Greek and Roman societies encouraged large families to maintain the strengths of their armies. Even modern western nations such as France and Russia have attempted to curb abortions for societal ends often with mixed results.

In China today, the government restricts families in most instances to one child. Severe social sanctions are imposed upon couples who attempt to avoid this dictum, and abortion is considered patriotic. The Chinese government in this instance is attempting to control the nation's population growth so as to allow for a continued improvement of the quality of life for all citizens. Although the Chinese restrictions on individual reproduction are a severe example, many individuals throughout the world believe that an environmental perspective requires that we maintain and perhaps even encourage the use of abortion as a tool to control world population. One cannot derive a right to an abortion directly from the need to curb population growth—contraception seems better for a number of reasons—but an aggressive attitude toward family planning fits well with an attitude of respect for nature.

CONCLUSION

This chapter provides little information with regard to the health provider's role in abortions. The reason is that the abortion issue is not essentially a health issue but rather a social issue that takes place in the health care arena. Abortion in most instances when it is performed is legal. The American Medical Association in its Code of Medical Ethics, Current Opinions document (1992), 2.01 states:

> The Principles of Medical Ethics of the AMA do not prohibit a physician from performing an abortion in accordance with good medical practice and under circumstances that do not violate the law.

One's attitudes toward abortion are often intense, close, and personal. As a matter of professional autonomy, it would seem that health care providers with deeply held beliefs regarding this matter would not be required to participate in the process. However, this may require that the providers ascertain the philosophical views of the institutions where they desire employment prior to accepting the duty. It makes little sense to look at only the salary and fringe benefits of a hospital and then find yourself working at an institution where the daily practice of abortion creates for you severe moral distress.

Health care providers, regardless of their personal feelings toward abortion, cannot ignore the social realities of the time, such as the liberation of women and the problems of teenage mothers. There is little indication that the abortion controversy will end anytime soon. As a matter of role duty, we must come to understand that people of intellect and honor have come to very different decisions regarding the issue. As health care providers, we do not have the luxury of treating patients with whom we have formed a patient-provider relationship with anything but the highest level of professional concern, regardless how we may feel about their decisions in regard to this issue.

LEGAL CASE STUDY: *Roe v. Wade.* (1973). Landmark Supreme Court Case on Abortion

In this case a pregnant single woman brought a class action suit against Wade, the district attorney of Dallas County. Roe challenged the constitutionality of the Texas laws that made having or performing an abortion a criminal act except when medical advice determined that the mother's life was in danger. In an appeal to the Supreme Court of the United States, the justices ruled in a seven to two decision in favor of Roe. Justice Blackmun delivered the majority opinion. Regarding the question as to when life began, Justice Blackmun sidestepped the issue with the following:

> We need not resolve the difficult question of when life begins. When those trained in the respective disciplines of medicine, philosophy, and theology are unable to arrive at any consensus, the judiciary, at this point in the development of man's knowledge is not in the position to speculate as to the answer.

In regard to the status of the fetus as a person, the court wrote:

> The constitution does not define person in so many words. Section I of the Fourteenth Amendment contains three references to person . . . . . . in nearly all these instances, but in all these instances the use of the word is such that it can only have application postnatally. None indicates, with any assurance, that it has any possible prenatal application.

The court concluded that the right to personal privacy included the abortion decision, but that this is not an unqualified right and must be balanced against important state interests. The court created a sliding scale throughout the pregnancy that allowed the woman the predominate role in decision making during the first trimester and increased the state's interests as the pregnancy advanced.

First Trimester: The decision is a matter between the woman and her physician. The state may make regulations requiring that the procedure be performed by a licensed physician.

Second Trimester: During the fourth to sixth month the state, in promoting its interest in the health of the mother, if it chooses, may regulate the abortion procedures.

Third Trimester: During the final trimester the interest of the state increases in regard to the product of the conception, to a point which overrides the woman's right to privacy. Thus the state, if it chooses, may regulate and even prohibit abortion except when it is deemed medically necessary for the preservation of the life or health of the mother.

REVIEW EXERCISES

1. On 28 March 1992 the *Wall Street Journal* reported that the New Jersey Supreme Court had tossed out the appeal of a man seeking to stop his girlfriend from having an abortion. Much has been written about a woman's right to her body, but relatively little in regard to the father's rights. What legal case parallels this decision? If the man agreed to raise the child, would you think that he should be able to deny his girlfriend the right to have an abortion?

2. Review the personhood criteria and state when and if a fetus could become a person, based on each of the criteria.

3. Do health care providers have a duty to participate in abortions even if they find them morally repugnant? Defend your answer with either a legal or moral justification.

4. Rule utilitarianism regards rights as the product of human decision, merely good rules that yield the greatest happiness for the greatest number. Consider the abortion question in the perspective of rule utilitarianism and state which of the positions, pro-life or pro-choice, has the most utility.

5. Some state statutes require a waiting period and personal counseling prior to having an abortion. During this period the woman is required to view pictures of a fetus at the same stage as her fetus. Is this a good law? We generally do not require a surgical patient to view surgeries prior to entering the hospital. Justify your answer.

6. State your view in regard to abortions and justify it both legally and ethically. Did the Supreme Court use correct reasoning when it attached abortion to privacy? Defend your answer.

7. It is clear that the basic positions at the extremes within the pro-life and pro-choice camps are irreconcilable. Make a list of positions that you think might form the basis of a reasonable compromise between the two groups, which you think that a majority of Americans might support. (e.g., No abortions in the last trimester except in the case of danger to the woman's life).

8. Some state statutes require a good faith effort to notify parents if their unmarried minor child has requested an abortion. Generally these do not allow the parents to override the minor's decision, but let us suppose that it did. Imagine an addendum to the law that required the parents to accept the responsibility of raising the child if they overrode the minor's decision. Would this be a good law?

9. State whether you believe *Roe v. Wade* creates an obligation not only for society (as a just society) to not interfere with a woman's right to an abortion, but also to provide resources for poor women to implement this right if they so choose.

10. State which of the arguments presented in the chapter either for or against a right to an abortion is most persuasive for you personally.

11. It appears that an abortion pill will soon become available and thus the need for abortion clinics will lessen if not cease. Do you feel that this more private form of abortion will effect the abortion debate in the United States?

12. In that we have legally defined death in terms of brain function (brain death), without which one need no longer continue to work toward the preservation of life, would it be reasonable to define legally protected life in terms of measurable brain waves in the fetus?

13. Reflect on the legal and ethical implications of the following modest proposal. Prepare a list of the pros and cons for each side of the issue.

Abortion clinics are essentially businesses. If they could harvest and sell the fetal organs, they could lower costs and perhaps gain a competitive advantage. This might even allow them to offer their services at a lower price which might make it more available to poor women.

REFERENCES

American Medical Association (1992). *Code of Medical Ethics & Current Opinions.* Chicago: American Medical Association.

Danforth v. Planned Parenthood of Central Missouri, 428 U.S. 52 (1976).

Ehrenreich, B. (1989, 1991). The worst years of our lives, my reply to George (addressing George Bush).

Faux, M. (1988). *Roe v. Wade.* New York: New American Library.

Ginsberg, R. (1974). As quoted in Ms. New York: Ms Magazine, April 1974.

Harris v. McRae, 448 U.S. 297 (1980).

H.L. v. Matheson, 450 U.S. 398 (1981).

Hodgson v. Minnesota, 497 U.S. 417 (1990).

Kennedy, F.R. (1973). The verbal karate of Florynce R. Kennedy, Esq. *Ms Magazine.*

Pozgar, G. (1993). *Legal aspects of health care administration,* Gaithersburg, Maryland: Aspen Publication.

Rich, A. (1978, June 2). Motherhood: The contemporary emergency and the quantum leap (read at Future of Mothering Conference). *On lies, secrets, and silence,* 1980. Columbus, OH.

Roe v. Wade, 410 U.S. 113 (1973).

Rust v. Sullivan, 111 S. Ct. 175 (1991).

Time Magazine. (1993, March 2). One doctor down, how many more?

Tooley, M. (1984). A defense of abortion and infanticide. In J. Feinberg (Ed.), *The problem of abortion.* Belmont, CA: Wadsworth Books.

Warren, M.A. (1984). On the moral and legal status of abortion. In J. Feinberg (Ed.), *The problem of abortion.* Belmont, CA: Wadsworth Books.

Webster v. Reproductive Health Services, 492 U.S. 490 (1989).

CHAPTER 9

Decisions at the End of Life

Goal

At the end of this unit the reader will understand the various legal and ethical arguments used and the types of patients involved in the issues of withdrawing and withholding life support.

Objectives

At the conclusion of this chapter, the reader should understand and be able to:

1. Differentiate between "life" as defined in a biological and biographical sense.
2. State the necessity created by modern technology for redefining death beyond that of a loss of cardiac and pulmonary function.
3. Define the concept and criteria of brain death.
4. Outline the rationale for the proposal to redefine death with a neocortical definition.
5. Define persistent vegetative state and state the characteristics of the syndrome.
6. Differentiate between the best interest and substituted judgment standards as they relate to proxy decisions.
7. Define the difference between ordinary and extraordinary care.
8. Outline the problems associated with the standard differentiations given for ordinary and extraordinary care.
9. Differentiate between the various lines of reasoning and arguments needed to decide the following types of cases in regard to withdrawing or withholding care.
    a. Persistent vegetative state cases
    b. Profoundly retarded patient cases

    c. Baby Doe cases

    d. Informed non-consent cases

10. Outline the arguments for personhood criteria and state how it could be used in withdrawing treatment determinations.

11. Define what is meant by the clear and convincing evidence standard.

12. Explain the difference between the two major types of advanced directives, that of living wills and durable power of attorney.

13. Differentiate between active and passive euthanasia.

Key Terms

active euthanasia

advanced directive

assisted suicide

best interest standard

biographical life

biological life

brain death

clear and convincing
  evidence standard

cognitive sapient state

do-not-resuscitate
  (DNR) orders

durable power of
  attorney

euthanasia

living will

medicide

mercy killing

neocortical death

ordinary and
  extraordinary care

parens patria

passive euthanasia

Patient Self-
  Determination
  Act of 1990
  (PSDA)

persistent vegetative
  state (PVS)

personhood

quality of life

right-to-die
  movement

slippery slope
  argument

substituted judgment
  standard

wedge argument

REDEFINING THE CONCEPT OF DEATH

A physician can sometimes parry the scythe of death, but has no power over the sand in the hourglass.

                Hester Piozzi (1741–1821), English writer.

We have to ask ourselves whether medicine is to remain a humanitarian and respected profession or a new but depersonalized science in the service of prolonging life rather than diminishing human suffering.

           Elisabeth Kübler-Ross, Swiss-born U.S. psychiatrist.

Few legal or ethical problems within the arena of health care cause the same degree of moral anguish as that of withholding or withdrawing life support. There is usually a high level of consensus for those cases found at the extremes; for example, the well baby and the baby born without a brain. It is when you move toward a center point between these two case types that the issues become unclear and the level of consensus fades. The ability of modern technology to provide the means for life extension, but not for the restoration of a life free of pain and misery often makes the extended life seem more like an additional injury than a benefit. What is the duty of a patient advocate when the individual cannot be restored to some level of an awareness of his environment?

Health care providers assume a duty to respect life and preserve it when possible. Often in cases involving life support, the desire to preserve life comes into direct conflict with the duty to alleviate pain and suffering. Our most basic codes of health care ethics bind us to take upon ourselves the duty to adopt practices that benefit the patients and protect them from hurt or wrong. Yet modern health care providers must struggle for answers to the following questions.

- What is to be done when the care offered appears to have no value to the patient?

- What is to be done when not only does what we offer appear to have limited value, but is also in conflict with the desires of the patient with regard to an acceptable quality of life?

- What is to be done when the patient or the family desires from the health care providers treatments that are deemed to be futile?

In the face of modern technology, we must come to an agreement with regard to what is meant by the term "life." The term often means two very different things. Our language divides the world into two separate categories of living things—the generic category of living things that includes bugs, bushes, deer, and humans, and nonliving things that includes air, water, minerals, etc. When we ask the question "Is there life on other planets?" we are thinking of life in a basic biological sense. **Biological life** is not uniquely human.

In the second category we use the term "life" to differentiate human life from that which we share with bushes and other animals. We call this category **biographical life.** This is life that is captured in weddings, events, relationships, etc. The once popular television program *This Is Your Life,* used the term in this sense. It is our life events, our relationships, dreams, and expectations, that truly separate us from other life forms and make us uniquely human.

When we speak of the sanctity of life, there are some who speak to a reverence for all life forms. For most people, however, the concept is narrowed to a reverence for biographical human life. Yet this ambiguity of what we mean by the term "life," for which we have reverence, leads us into one of the truly troubling aspects of health care. Anyone involved in the practice of critical care can readily bring to mind patients who, due to injury, arrive in the ICU in a coma and are placed on life support systems. If the brain damage is extensive and the care is of high quality, some of these patients can survive in a **persistent vegetative state (PVS)** for months or even years. With current technology, often we can sustain life in a biological sense, but cannot restore the individual to an awareness of self or others. In many cases, an individual may survive for years without gaining consciousness.

What is the value of such a life? It is clear that the preservation of biological life at any cost leads to immense personal and social tragedies which consume individuals, human energies, and scarce resources. Yet, what is the ethical thing to do when all individual personality has irretrievably fled and all we can sustain is biological life?

Brain Death

Classically, the definition of death has been based on loss of cardiac and pulmonary function. Without a functioning heart or respiratory system, the body dies. With modern technology, even in cases of severe brain trauma, we can often with respiratory and cardiac support keep the remainder of the body's cells alive for days and months with no brain activity being present. Although these cases do not match the classic criteria for death, they are irretrievable. Technological advances have driven us from the classic definitions of death and a majority of jurisdictions within our nation have accepted the concept of **brain death.** Figure 9–1 lists the criteria for brain death given by the Ad Hoc Committee of the Harvard Medical School to Examine the Definition of Death (1981). The modern rules applied in these cases are derived from the Uniform Determination of Death Act (UDDA) (1981).

> An individual is dead when either (1) irreversible cessation of circulation and pulmonary function, or (2) irreversible cessation of all functions of the entire brain, including the brain stem occurs. These determinations must be made in accordance with acceptable medical standards.

Brain death cases are problematic to families as the use of technology provides the appearances of life. The patient appears to have natural warmth and color, the EKG may be in sinus rhythm, and the chest rises and falls with each cycle of the ventilator. Providers must counsel the family that these do not represent the true condition of the patient. It is during these periods of "cerebral silence" that providers often broach the question of organ donation, because the technology is merely maintaining the life of other organ systems within the body.

During these counseling sessions, a natural shift occurs from the provider's focus on the patient on the ventilator to a focus on the family. Nothing further can be done for the patient on the ventilator as they are in all reality deceased; however, it is critical that the family be supported in this time of personal loss. In reality, the family becomes the real patient. Great care and sensitivity must be taken as equipment is removed. Often the devices are turned down slowly so that cardiac failure takes place to simulate death. The removal of the equipment, however, is not an act of allowing to die, as in fact a corpse (as defined by brain death) cannot be thought to die. Practitioners may, out of respect to the families, or out of fear of legal issues, delay the removal of life-sustaining equipment but once brain death determination has been made, one is morally free to treat the remains as one treats other objects.

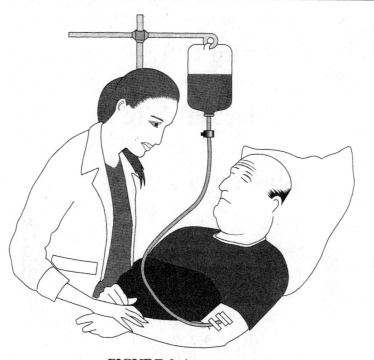

FIGURE 9–1 Brain Death Criteria
- Unreceptivity and unresponsiveness
- No movements or breathing
- No reflexes
- Flat EEG of confirmatory value

PERSISTENT VEGETATIVE STATE

If existence is determined by being capable of thought, patients in a persistent vegetative state (PVS) create a different set of ethical problems because they are not brain dead as defined by the loss of "whole-brain" function but, yet, they are incapable of thought. In brain death the body ceases to function once ventilatory support is discontinued. Often with PVS the patient will continue to breathe even with the loss of ventilatory support.

Patients in PVS have no recognizable cognitive function. The condition is characterized by a permanent eyes-open state of unconsciousness. Unlike the comatose patient, the PVS patient is awake but unaware. The eyes are often vacant and often the patient assumes a severely contracted body position. Clinically, PVS suggests the irreversible loss of all neocortical function. Many of these patients present with brain stem functions and the ability to breathe on their own; however, they do not meet the criteria of brain death because they have elicitable reflexes, spontaneous respirations, and reactions to external stimuli.

It is from this group that the occasional "miracle" occurs and the patient, after an extended period, awakens. One recent case is that of Gary Dockery, a Chattanooga,

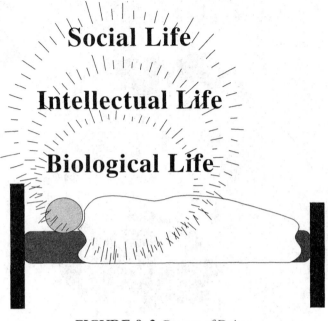

FIGURE 9–2 Process of Dying

Tennessee, policeman injured in the line of duty in 1988. Following his injury Dockery spent most of his time in a nursing home unable to communicate with anyone. Eight years later in February 1996 Mr. Dockery suddenly began to speak and proceeded to talk for eighteen hours, recalling friends and incidents in his past (Brodeur, 1996). Unfortunately these occurrences provide more of an illusion of hope than substance, as recovery from a persistent vegetative state is rather remote. Using the guidelines of waiting three months in cases of PVS following cardiac arrest, six months for patients below the age of 40 with head injury, and twelve months for patients below the age of 25 with head injuries, the chance of any sort of recovery is less than 1 in 1,000.

Due to the remoteness of recovery, some theorists have attempted to redefine death so that it includes some of the PVS patients or at least those whose lives are limited to biological life only. Under this criteria many patients in a persistent vegetative state who have the potential for years of vegetative life would be judged dead. However, real problems are involved in this thinking as some patients have come back from a PVS. Another serious problem is that PVS patients can often remain in that state for years, and to declare them dead would require a form of active euthanasia on the part of the health care provider to assist in the dying process.

One formulation of death is that provided by Thomas Furlow (1974) who explains death, not as an event, but rather as a process of withdrawal. According to his formulation, dying can be likened to three concentric circles as shown in Figure 9–2. The outermost ring comprises one's interpersonal relationships and is called the social life.

Being outermost, this is the most vulnerable of the aspects of our being and usually is the first to die. The individual then withdraws to the middle circle which represents human intellectual life, that part of ourselves that separates us from the rest of the biological world. Consciousness and interaction, deriving from the highest level of the brain or the cerebrum, characterize this level. Once dying has claimed this region, biographical death has occurred and only the innermost ring is left. This ring represents biological life and is largely controlled by the brain stem. This form of life is not uniquely human, because it shares common features with nonhuman life forms. Loss of function in this region constitutes biological death. Some authorities have argued that the time is near when medicine will need to revise the definition of death beyond the brain dead criteria to include **neocortical death** (Arras & Steinbock, 1995). A person would be considered dead by this criteria if only the higher brain centers, and not the entire brain, had irreversibly lost function. This still does not answer the next obvious question, what is to be done with a patient declared dead who continues to breathe?

FORGOING LIFE-SUSTAINING TREATMENT

One of the crucial initial court cases looking at the issue of withdrawing life support began in April 1975 when a 21-year-old woman, while with friends, ingested an undetermined amount of alcohol and tranquilizers. She arrived at hospital in a coma having suffered two periods of apnea (not breathing) lasting for at least fifteen minutes.

The patient remained in this state for a period of seven months being sustained by a ventilator and feeding tubes. After this time, the physicians in the case indicated to her parents and family that she had entered a chronic, persistent vegetative state and that it was their opinion that she would die if ventilatory support was removed. The parents were convinced that there was no hope she would ever regain consciousness. After hearing this grim prognosis, her father sought permission from the courts to disconnect the ventilator that was keeping her alive in the intensive care unit (*In re Quinlan*, 1976). It was her parents' view that this was in keeping with God's will and that they felt that their daughter would not have wanted to continue living this way. In its opinion the court advocated consultation with the hospital ethics committee in making the decision. This was one of the first legal enunciations for an ethics committee role in these matters and served as a stimulus for institutional ethics committees development across the country (Darr, 1991).

The case became a national issue and Karen Ann Quinlan became a name recognized throughout the nation. This brought an increased awareness of the need to create a process where extraordinary care could be withdrawn. On appeal, the New Jersey Supreme Court overturned the lower court decision and appointed Karen's father, Joseph, as her guardian with express authority to end all extraordinary medical procedures. The court ruled that when an individual has no chance of recovering to a **cognitive sapient state,** the state's interest in the protection of life was weakened and that the individual's right to privacy may call for discontinuance of burdensome life support as determined by a guardian. Unfortunately, Karen's nurses were not sympathetic to the concept of removing life support and, understanding that the court might grant discontinuance of the ventilators, began a weaning process from the device so that when removed she continued to breathe. Karen continued in a persistent vegetative state for an additional decade. In June 1985 she contracted acute pneumonia and died. Antibiotics that might have been used to continue her existence were not used.

When her ventilator was discontinued, the question was not asked whether all her life support systems could be disconnected. Karen Ann continued to live, sustained by feeding tubes and intravenous fluids. Had these been removed with her ventilator, she would have starved to death and of course died ten years earlier. The case of Karen Ann brings up many ethical problems not only in regard to removal of ventilators from patients with no chance of recovering but also what constitutes **ordinary and extraordinary care.**

Early discussions regarding the differentiation between ordinary and extraordinary care generally consisted of making lists with items such as oxygen, antibiotics, and intravenous fluids being considered ordinary, and ventilators, extracorporeal oxygenators, and dialysis devices being categorized as extraordinary. This view has two basic problems in that it does not take into consideration technological advancement or patient reference. It is clear that when a technology such as dialysis is new, often there is a shortage and the treatments are considered extraordinary. As technology advances and becomes more readily available, the extraordinary treatment then becomes ordinary.

The second issue is patient reference, for example, what might be extraordinary for a centenarian might be ordinary for a person 21 years old. A good example of lack of patient reference was the nasogastric feeding and intravenous fluids given to Karen Ann Quinlan. Under normal conditions, these are considered ordinary. In Karen's case, however, their continuance forced her to continue a life without personal value for another decade following the removal of the ventilator. In light of the fact that they offered no reasonable hope of benefit, perhaps these ordinary devices constituted extraordinary care.

One might argue that leaving someone in a state of unawareness for years ought to be done on the basis of the potential good that is derived. Even lives without personal value may at times have value beyond the individual. These cases surely offer universal opportunities to learn and practice the virtue of compassion. In the case of Karen Ann Quinlan, the health care profession and the society as a whole gained needed insights as a result of her case. The question that must be asked is whether our gain is a reasonable exchange for the suffering her family endured during the last decade of her life.

Figure 9–3 gives a formulation provided by Father Gerald Kelly, S. J. (1957) for ordinary and extraordinary care that allows for consideration of costs, pain, inconvenience, and potential benefit. Under this definition, the problems of technological change and patient reference are satisfied. Any form of care can be extraordinary if it offers no hope of benefit. Under this definition, intravenous fluids and nasogastric feedings would qualify for extraordinary care in patients with PVS as they offer no potential benefit. With this line of reasoning the focus is placed on the usefulness and burdensomeness of care, rather than on any characteristic of the treatment itself. Other scholars would argue that food and water are not, in a real sense, medical care at all, but rather "the sort of care that

> **Ordinary means** are all medications, treatments, and operations that offer a reasonable hope of benefit and that can be obtained without excessive expense, pain, or other inconvenience.
>
> **Extraordinary means** are all medications, treatments, and operations that cannot be obtained or used without excessive expense, pain, or other inconvenience or that if used, would not offer a reasonable hope of benefit.

FIGURE 9–3 Ordinary versus Extraordinary Means

all human beings owe each other" as a function of our common humanity (Meilaender, 1984). The removal of food and water seems more causally related to the death of the patient, than just standing aside and allowing the patient to die.

The Karen Ann Quinlan case brings to light the problem of what is to be done when the individual is no longer in a position to provide any direction as to personal care. In these cases, often the physician, hospital, or a family member may seek resolution of the problem from the courts prior to implementing a decision. Under the doctrine of **parens patria,** the state accepts these cases on the basis of a legitimate duty abiding in the principles of beneficence and nonmaleficence. This duty requires the protection of citizens under legal disability from harms they cannot themselves avoid. Within these patient groups, are two basic situations, one in which someone has been competent and then has lost the ability to make competent decisions, such as Karen Ann, and another when the individual was never in a position of competency. To decide these matters, the courts have adopted two proxy decision-making standards, that of **best interest** and **substituted judgment.**

For patients such as Karen Ann Quinlan, who were at one point competent, the courts have used the substituted judgment standard. These patients prior to their accidents or illness are autonomous adults with ideas, experiences, and relationships which give an indication as to what an authentic decision would be in the matter. Using the substituted judgment standard, an individual is selected who is required to act in proxy for the patient and to make the decision as the currently incompetent patient would have made if the patient had been competent. In the case of Karen Ann, her father could draw upon the experiences of her previous life to determine her wants in this particular case. If patients, while competent have clearly expressed their will through conversations or advanced directives as to their disposition in these cases, the substituted proxy judgment seems a rational approach.

Two groups, however, cannot benefit from the substituted judgment process—the patients who were competent and become incompetent without expressing themselves regarding such a tragic eventuality, and those patients who are mentally retarded and never meet the criteria for competency. What standard best serves these patients?

In cases when an authentic choice cannot be made due to a lack of information or lack of opportunity to make a choice, the best interest standard is used. This process takes into account such tangible factors as harms and benefits, physical and fiscal risks. In health care the courts might rely on such truisms as "Health is better than illness," and "Life is preferable to death." In cases when children have been denied life-preserving care by their parents, the state has often overturned the parental decisions based on the best interest standard. The courts base these decisions upon the principles of beneficence and nonmaleficence rather than patient autonomy.

An important case example of this process involves Joseph Saikewicz (*Superintendent of Belchertown State School v. Saikewicz,* 1977). Mr. Saikewicz, 67 years old, was profoundly retarded with the intellectual capacity of a 3-year-old and had lived his entire life in a mental institution. In 1976 he was diagnosed as having a terminal form of leukemia. Even with aggressive chemotherapy his chances for a remission would be only 30 percent, and the remission would only extend his life for a short period of perhaps another year. Without the chemotherapy he was expected to live for several months before succumbing to infection.

The chemotherapy could not be administered without the attendant nausea and discomfort. In that Joseph's mental capacity did not allow the staff to explain the nature of the illness and why the treatments were necessary, he would probably need to be restrained for the chemotherapy to be delivered. The institution where Joseph was treated appealed to the courts for guidance in the case. Physician consultants were called to testify and spoke against the administration of the chemotherapy. The court ruled that the chemotherapy not be given. The decision was appealed to the Massachusetts Supreme Court which concurred with the lower court ruling. Joseph Saikewicz had died from pneumonia prior to the time the higher court had issued its full opinion. The court ruled that a guardian could be assigned to make the judgment, but that the judgment be based on the best interest of the patient.

Not all legal opinion was sanguine with regard to the Saikewicz decision and in the *In re Storar* (1981) case a New York court, reiterating the comments of an expert witness, stated that asking a guardian to make a choice for an incompetent patient as the patient would have made it had he been competent, was "similar to asking whether if it snowed all summer if it would then be winter?" John Storar was a profoundly retarded 52-year-old man with the mind of an 18-month-old child. When it was discovered that he had cancer in his bladder, physicians requested permission from the state to administer blood transfusions to John, despite the objections of his mother to the contrary. Although the best interest principle has difficulties and inconsistencies, it is still an attempt to honor the constitutional right of the patient to refuse treatment. In the *Storar* case, the court treated the incompetent adult involved as an infant whose parents had decided against treatment. The court therefore concluded that it was in John's best interest to receive the blood transfusion and not bleed to death because "someone as close as a parent or sibling feels that [it] is best for one with an incurable disease."

In the case of Nancy Cruzan, the decision to remove life support was focused on the removal of hydration and nutrition. At 25 years of age, Nancy Cruzan lost control of her car and was thrown into a ditch. She was resuscitated at the scene of the accident but never regained consciousness. Like Karen Ann Quinlan, Nancy was diagnosed as being in PVS and physicians estimated that she could live for another thirty years being supported by feeding tubes. In describing her condition, her father stated that, "Since the accident, she has never had what we felt was a thought-produced response to anything. We feel the most humane and kind thing we can do is to help her escape this limbo between life and death." Faced with this grim prognosis, the family requested that the feeding tube be removed and Nancy be allowed to die. When the Missouri Rehabilitation Center refused the request, the family took the case to the lower courts which ruled in their favor. This affirmation was overturned by the state supreme court on the basis that the state had a greater duty to preserve life than any right that the parents might have to refuse treatment for their daughter (*Cruzan v. Missouri Department of Health*, 1990).

The *Cruzan* case reached the Supreme Court of the United States and gave the Court an opportunity to address this difficult area of law. Recognizing that the right to die is a complex issue, the Court examined whether a state could require that an incompetent's wishes be proved by a standard of **clear and convincing evidence.** The Court explained that the state may decline to make any judgments about an incompetent's "quality" of life and just simply assert an interest in preserving human life. In a five to four decision, the Court explained that:

- The state has a right to assert an unqualified interest in the preservation of human life.

- A choice between life and death is an extremely personal matter.

- Abuse can occur when incompetent patients do not have loved ones available to serve as surrogate decision makers.

- The state has a right to express an unqualified interest in the preservation of human life.

The United States Supreme Court declined to address the issue of whether a state can give effect to decisions made for an incompetent by a surrogate—states are free to legislate in this area. The Court did express, however, a reservation as to lack of assurance it had that a close family member's view would have necessarily been the view of one now in a vegetative state. Following the Supreme Court's decision, three friends of Nancy's came forward claiming that in previous conversations with her, she had indicated a revulsion about being kept alive in a vegetative state. This provided the clear and convincing evidence required by the Court, and the State of Missouri ceased its opposition to the removal of the feeding tube. With this life support removed, Nancy Cruzan died.

Although the Supreme Court held to a narrow focus in Nancy Cruzan's case, several critical aspects were reinforced by the decision. First, the decision upheld the concept that competent individuals could refuse life-sustaining treatment. Second, it made no legal distinction between tube feeding and other life-sustaining measures. Food and water may be withheld when either of the two following conditions are met.

1. The treatment is futile. In cases when all efforts to provide nutrition would be ineffective and cause pain (e.g., those patients whose cardiac status is such that any intravenous fluids would overload the heart), there should be no life-sustaining treatment.

2. There is no possibility of benefit. Although it is most often reasonable practice to provide nutrition and hydration, in those cases when the family and caregivers agree that the practice offers no benefit, such as a PVS case, there should be no barrier to discontinuance.

ADVANCE DIRECTIVES

The call for clear and convincing evidence in regard to these cases has increased interest in **advanced directives.** Following the 1976 California example, a majority of states have passed some form of **living will,** right-to-die, or death-with-dignity statute (Figure 9–4). There is, however, no uniformity in laws on living wills and surrogate decision makers. In some states, the advanced directives go into effect only if a patient is terminally ill, and death is imminent. In others, the physician is given civil and criminal immunity from prosecution when he fails to honor the living will, because in his good faith judgment based on medically valid reason, continued treatment would be of benefit to the patient. In over twenty states such a will is invalidated during pregnancy.

Due to the inconsistencies and limitations found with these statutes many authorities recommend the use of **durable power of attorney** over a living will. This allows you to name someone with authority as proxy to make medical decisions on your behalf should you become incompetent and unable to make the decisions yourself. This form of legal arrangement seems to offer the greatest flexibility in making your wishes known after you have lost competency, as the proxy individual is in the position to react to the unique and specific circumstances of the case. The Society for the Right to Die (1987) suggests the following reasons for establishing a durable power of attorney.

1. To give or withhold consent to specific medical or surgical measures with reference to the principal's condition, prognosis, and known wishes regarding terminal care; to authorize appropriate end-of-life including pain-relieving procedures.

2. To grant releases to health care providers.

3. To employ and discharge health care providers.

4. To have access to and to disclose medical records and other personal information.

5. To resort to court if necessary, to obtain court authorization regarding medical treatment decisions.

6. To expend or withhold funds necessary to carry out medical treatments.

Although both forms of advanced directives promote ethical decision making in these cases and support personal autonomy, it is estimated that less than 20 percent of our citizens have either type in place. Young people and the poor are the least likely to request and implement these forms. As is true for many social issues, the young, the poor, and those poorly informed suffer the consequences of having the least protection. The **Patient Self-Determination Act of 1990 (PSDA)** (Figure 9–5) mandates

I, _____ am of sound mind, and I voluntarily make this declaration.

I direct that life-sustaining procedures should be withheld or withdrawn if I have an illness, disease, or injury, or experience extreme mental deterioration, such that there is no reasonable expectation of recovering or regaining a meaningful life.

These life-sustaining procedures that may be withheld or withdrawn include, but are not limited to:

Cardiac resuscitation, ventilatory support, antibiotics, artificial feeding and hydration.

I further direct that treatment be limited to palliative measures only, even if they shorten my life.

Specific instructions:

A. Specific instructions regarding care I do want:

B. Specific instructions regarding care I do not want:

My family, the medical facility, any physicians, nurses, and other medical personnel involved in my care shall have no civil or criminal liability for following my wishes as expressed in this declaration.

I sign this document after careful consideration.

I understand its meaning and I accept its consequences.

Date:_____ Signed: _____

Address: _____

_____

This Declaration was signed in our presence. The declarant appears to be of sound mind and to be making this declaration voluntarily without duress, fraud, or undue influence.

Signed by witness: _____

Signed by witness: _____

FIGURE 9–4 Living Will Statement

that all certified hospitals, nursing facilities, home health care agencies, hospices, and HMOs receiving federal reimbursement under Medicare and Medicaid comply with the following requirements.

1. Inform every adult, both orally and in writing, of their right under state law to make decisions concerning medical care, including their right to refuse medical or surgical treatment, and their right to make advance medical directives.

Senator John Danforth (R-MO.) drafted the PSDA as part of the Omnibus Reconciliation Act of 1990. PSDA was designed to support the autonomous decision-making authority of patients in regard to accepting or refusing specific medical interventions when admitted to health care facilities receiving federal reimbursements under Medicare or Medicaid. The legislation requires these facilities to:

A. Provide patients at the time of admissions with information concerning their right to accept or refuse medical interventions. The facilities are charged with providing information and assistance in the preparation of advanced directives.

B. The facilities will create and maintain written institutional policies in regard to patient rights. They will provide education for the staff, patients, and community concerning advanced directives.

C. The patient's wishes in regard to refusing or executing an advanced directive will be documented in the medical record.

FIGURE 9–5 Patient Self-Determination Act of 1990 (PSDA)

2. Have and provide written statements of policies of the health care provider concerning the implementation of the patient's rights in the health care decision-making process.

3. Have a written statement affirming that the facility will not condition provision of care or discriminate in any way based on whether the patient has executed an advance directive.

4. Document on the patient's medical record any advanced directives by the patient.

5. Have a written statement ensuring compliance by the facility with the requirements of the state law respecting advanced directives.

6. Conduct programs of education for the facility staff and the community on medical and legal issues concerning advanced directives (Darr, 1991).

ADVANCED DIRECTIVES IN A DIVERSE SOCIETY

An interesting aspect of the implementation of advanced directives is that they not only impact upon the patient, but also upon the family and the surrounding society. We often make the mistake that we are practicing in a void or if not a void, at least in a rather comfortable white, middle-class, Judeo-Christian context. Yet, these issues must be considered in the larger context of a multicultural society.

The patient's race, religion, economic and social class, and ethnic background affect how the information regarding end-of-life decisions will be received and ultimately made.

It is worthwhile to imagine how others might view our desire to provide them with information regarding advanced directives. To the elderly, it may appear as a message that we are setting up a situation where we no longer need to treat them appropriately. To the poor, the language of wills, living or no, may seem like a legal issue for the rich, and may be more associated with the *fact* of dying rather than the *possibility.* To the disadvantaged minority population and elderly, our encouragement of advanced directives may seem like we are trying to persuade them to give up rights to self-determination rather than exercise them. For the Evangelical Christians, the problem may be one of manifesting a lack of faith. If, for instance, they sign the advanced directives are they saying they have given up their faith in a personal miraculous cure?

Because advanced directives and health care in general draw upon and are impacted by the cultural context, they require a special sensitivity to the needs of patients, especially those from other cultures. Even for English-speaking patients, health care providers often are virtually unintelligible given the penchant to technospeak. To be effective in delivering health care, providers must learn to understand why different people respond as they do and communicate with them in an honest and affirming manner. Although they are prohibited from serving as witnesses to durable power of attorney directives that involve the patients they serve, nurses and other health care providers perform a vital service in the education of patients about advanced directives.

INFORMED NON-CONSENT—THE COMPETENT NON-COMPLIANT PATIENT

The case of William Bartling offers a different aspect to the rights of patients in these decisions. Mr. Bartling was a 75-year-old chronic pulmonary disease patient with four other terminal illnesses. There was no question as to his competence when he requested to be removed from his ventilator. The hospital, fearing liability, refused his request due to the fact that if the device was removed it would surely hasten his death. This altered the role of the institution from one of following the directives of a competent patient to one that is forcing treatment on an unwilling patient. The ventilator caused Mr. Bartling severe emotional distress and on several occasions he attempted to remove himself from the respirator. To ensure that Mr. Bartling would not remove the ventilator, the physician ordered restraints. When the hospital refused to accept his living will as a rationale for removing the ventilator, he appealed to the courts. It was felt that there was some ambiguity in his reasoning, for when asked if he wanted to live, he stated in the affirmative, and when asked if he wanted to be removed from the ventilator, he answered in the affirmative. His lawyer stated that this was not ambiguity. Although he preferred to live, he did not prefer to live with his illness and with the necessity of his every breath being sustained by a ventilator.

The lower court judge was not persuaded and affirmed the institution's decision to not remove the ventilator or the restraints. The lower court did so in spite of the fact that Mr. Bartling had a living will and a durable power of attorney for health care, both of which stated his desire to die naturally. Although Mr. Bartling and his wife made repeated requests in regard to his desire to refuse the care, he spent the last six months of his life on the ventilator and died before the appeals court overturned the lower court decision and ruled in his favor. The court reasoned that "if the right of the patient to self-determination as to his own medical treatment is to have any meaning at all, it must be paramount to the interests of the patient's hospital and doctors" (*Bartling,* 1984).

A second case similar to that of Mr. Bartling is that of Elizabeth Bouvia, a 28-year-old quadriplegic suffering from severe cerebral palsy from birth as well as arthritis. Elizabeth had attended college, earned a degree, had married, and divorced. By the time she entered the hospital she was completely dependent upon others for her needs, including feeding, washing, toileting, and placement in bed. Previously, she had depended upon her family for her care; however, due to changes in her family situation, her father informed her that they could no longer provide her care.

During her hospitalizations, she asked that her pain be controlled and she be allowed to starve herself to death. Physicians and hospital authorities refused her request and she was force-fed through a nasogastric tube to maintain body weight. She requested that the feeding be stopped. The hospital refused even though her competency was not questioned. Bouvia went to court several times during the next several years making media headlines and becoming a symbol of the **right-to-die movement.** The lower courts affirmed the hospital's decisions stating that "she could not ask society in the person of the hospital to help her because she was not a terminal patient." The decision allowed the hospital to force-feed the patient.

In June 1986 the California Supreme Court upheld a lower court decision allowing her to end the force-feeding. The court in its ruling, determined that the fact that Ms. Bouvia was young and therefore had a potential for a long life was essentially irrelevant. The court held that Ms. Bouvia's desire to let nature take its course did not amount to a choice of suicide. The court stated that it was not "illegal or immoral to prefer a natural albeit sooner, death than a drugged life attached to a mechanical device." The decision stated that the time allotted for continued life was not the issue, only the perceived quality of that life and that "if a right exists, it matters not what motivates its exercise." Although the *Bouvia* case did not affirm a basic right to die, it did become a landmark decision regarding the right to informed non-consent in a nonterminal patient.

The *Bartling* and *Bouvia* cases seem to indicate a growing consensus with regard to the allowance of personal autonomy and informed non-consent. The legal rights of patients to refuse medical treatment have been upheld in literally hundreds of court decisions. The courts appear to be moving closer to the view that patients are entitled to be allowed to die. Several critical elements have been reinforced by these court decisions.

1. The acuity of the patient is irrelevant to the allowance of treatment refusal. The patient's right to refuse care is not dependent upon having a terminal illness.

2. The patient's own perceived view of the quality of life and the treatment requirements necessary to preserve it are of paramount importance. The fact that Elizabeth Bouvia could potentially live for another four decades and be a productive citizen could not overcome her autonomous choice to refuse care.

3. There is no meaningful legal distinction between mechanical life support and nasogastric feeding; both are invasive.

4. Distinctions between withholding and withdrawing care are legally irrelevant.

5. The surrogate's decision is most trustworthy when it is in keeping with clear and convincing evidence that it is in keeping with the patient's authentic wishes.

6. The state's duty to protect the life of citizens is weakened under the conditions of terminal unconsciousness, intractable pain, or terminal illness (*Bouvia v. Superior Court,* 1986).

With the court's decisions in the *Cruzan* and *Bouvia* cases, nutrition and hydration were elevated to the status of life support and under certain conditions could be defined as extraordinary care, which could be discontinued. Although this position gained public and legal support, others in the ethicist community had grave concerns (Curtin, 1994). Many argued that food and water were not in a real sense medical issues or prerogatives, but rather a subsistence right that we owed to all members of our species. Somehow, the suspension of nutrition seems to not fulfill the humanitarian role that we ascribe to health care providers. Although physicians could order a special diet, provide feedings in a series of ways, or even under certain conditions temporarily suspend nutrition, it was generally not a medical option to suspend nutrition on a permanent basis. Subsistence right is a form of human right that is gained by recognizing a universal human need. Although the right is not in itself defined by the need, it is a just fulfillment of it.

The dilemma that is inherent in the nature of nutrition and hydration and its withdrawal as life support is not lost upon health care professionals. In a carefully worded opinion the Council on Ethical and Judicial Affairs of the American Medical Association (1992) states:

> The social of the physician is to sustain life and relieve suffering. Where the performance of one duty conflicts with the other, the preferences of the patient should prevail. If the patient is incompetent and did not indicate his or her preferences, the family or other surrogate decision maker in concert with the physician, must act in the best interest of the patient.
>
> For humane reasons, with informed consent a physician may do what is medically necessary to alleviate severe pain, or cease or omit treatment to permit a terminally ill patient to die when death is imminent. . .
>
> Life-prolonging medical treatment includes medication and artificially or technologically supplied respiration, nutrition, or hydration. In treating a terminally ill or permanently unconscious patient, the dignity of the patient should be maintained at all times.

From the statement, it is clear that the medical profession is differentiating regular feedings from technically providing nutrition and hydration through invasive means.

It is this invasive technology that seems appropriate to discontinue in cases when the treatment is futile, when there is no possibility of benefit, or when its provision causes a severe disproportionate burden on behalf of the patient.

DO-NOT-RESUSCITATE ORDERS

Cardiopulmonary resuscitation (CPR) and advanced cardiac life support (ACLS) are interventions that could theoretically be offered to all patients within the hospital. Following its rather general application in the mid 1960s, it became obvious that CPR was not in the best interest of all patients and, for some, offered a more violent death rather than salvation. With this recognition, hospitals began to seek appropriate criteria that would allow **do-not-resuscitate (DNR) orders.** What is the purpose of CPR if it offers no meaningful possibility of patient benefit? The late 1970s and 1980s were a period of confusion when health care support staff struggled to find their way through an ambiguous maze of verbal orders, orders for slow codes, show codes, partial codes, purple dots, etc. Figure 9–6 is an example of an article that shows the frustration with the ambiguous state of DNR orders during this time period (Whitacre, 1980).

DNR policies are now required of all hospitals by the Joint Commission on Accreditation of Healthcare Organizations (JCAHO). Figure 9–7 provides general guidelines that one might expect for the establishment of DNR policies within a modern health care facility.

Even given the wide use and acceptance, the selection of patients for DNR orders still raises some concern. In our age of cost containment and stretched resources, do DNR patients belong in the intensive care units? Studies show that these patients in ICU are sicker, have longer stays, have poorer prognoses, consume more resources (both human and fiscal), and have a higher mortality rate than do non-DNR patients. Thirty-nine percent of the ICU patient deaths occur with those who have DNR orders (Edwards, 1990).

In the *Guidelines for the Appropriate Use of Do-Not-Resuscitate Orders,* the Council of Ethical and Judicial Affairs of the American Medical Association (1991) concluded that the intent of DNR orders did not preclude the use of any other treatment modalities, nor admission and treatment in an intensive care unit. When treatment (either curative or palliative) cannot be obtained in other units outside of intensive care, the patient's right to autonomy, beneficence, and nonmaleficence coupled with the requirements of fidelity make the ICU usage a reasonable choice.

The initiation of DNR orders is best performed after an understanding between physicians, patients, family, and staff has been reached. This is an area where value preference will make a great deal of difference. The place where communication often fails between the patient's family and the providers is in the consideration of what is being offered by CPR. Many families see the situation as one where the choice is between life and no life. In this decision they will opt for life. What is missing is the discussion that CPR and life support techniques may in fact preserve a quality of life that would not be valued by the patient. The truth is that these techniques can often only offer a period of life extension that inflicts additional suffering and harm that is grossly out of proportion to any possibility of benefit.

"A month or so ago, a young lady who had two heart surgeries and a couple of (cardiac) arrests during the past two years, which resulted in hypoxic brain damage that had left her feeble-minded and with a convulsive disorder, arrested again at home one evening because of a failed pacemaker. She was resuscitated and brought into the hospital, with no oxygen in the ambulance. There in the medical intensive care unit where everyone knew her from prior admissions, she arrested AGAIN about an hour later. Since she was not **red-tagged** we were obliged to resuscitate her AGAIN, and put her on a ventilator. There she literally rotted away for 3 or 4 weeks (they had promptly fixed her pacemaker so that her heart wouldn't be able to stop again), until in spite of Hell (which included dialysis for renal failure for over a week) she finally managed to "die."

Now if one of the male staff had jumped into her bed and raped her, this would have been regarded as a criminal assault, and everyone would have been outraged, right? But what we did was far more damaging physically, far more protracted, and not one whit less immoral. Just the same, in the eyes of our curious social system, it was OK. Some system!

Another time recently I was privileged to attend a **Code Blue** on a patient who had arrested during cobalt therapy! That was only one of a whole series of resuscitations, done routinely on terminal cancer patients at that hospital.

Why, when such patients have literally nothing going for them, must we be so hell-bent on interfering with this perfectly natural process which would relieve them of their hopeless suffering? Have our physicians taken complete leave of their senses? These are outrageous prostitutions of the art and science of resuscitation.

Resuscitation is the most literally life-saving act the therapist performs. It is the noblest, loftiest, most heroic, and should be the most God-like thing one mortal can do for another. But every time I am called to one of these grossly inappropriate codes, I am sick in my soul at this UN-godly, beastly business. The dictum that we are required to resuscitate ANYbody who arrests if he is untagged, no matter what's wrong with him or how long before we find him the arrest may have occurred, really sticks in my craw. It is just reckless irresponsibility of the most irrational and immoral sort.

What's behind this tragedy? NEGLECT! Nobody talked with the patient or his family about whether he (they) wanted him resuscitated if he should arrest. Doubtless the rule always to do so in the absence of a **No Code** order was put there because of the policy that nobody but a physician should make this decision. This can of course be construed as protecting non-physicians of being accused of not resuscitating a patient who was in their judgment non-salvageable.

But we all know of all too many instances where the doctor has specified NOTHING either way, and where the wishes of the patient or his family have NOT been explored. This situation is, of course, inescapable when there is no time; but usually the subject was just plain avoided because it was too unpleasant.

I think we should complain about this to our medical directors, and try to get them to use their influence on medical staffs to face this responsibility squarely, and then definitely to red tag or No Code all patients who are either (a) not regarded as salvageable, or (b) who have expressed their desire to be allowed to die in peace. Actually, hospitals could relieve doctors of some of this unpleasantry, in case (c), by making this question a part of the admissions interview with either the patient or next of kin.

FIGURE 9–6 Article about Inappropriate Resuscitation

1. DNR orders should be documented in the written medical record.

2. DNR orders should specify the exact nature of the treatment to be withheld.

3. Patients, when able, should participate in DNR decisions. Their involvement and wishes should be documented in the medical record.

4. Decisions to withhold CPR should be discussed with the health care team.

5. DNR status should be reviewed on a regular basis.

6. DNR is not equivalent to medical or psychological abandonment.

FIGURE 9–7 DNR Guidelines

The key to the decision process is communication. Institutional policies must be in place which provide opportunities for the patient and family to be fully informed in regard to these decisions. When disagreement occurs between the providers and the family or in cases when no one represents the patient, the DNR decision should be taken to the institutional ethics committee for review and further consultation in regard to the appropriateness of the order and whether it is within the scope of the institution's policy.

The use of DNR orders seems inappropriate for cases when it is determined that no medical benefit would occur as a result of the procedure, or when a poor quality of life existed prior to CPR. Perhaps it would be more useful to have the order stated in the terms of "care and comfort only" rather than DNR as this would indicate to both patient and staff alike that the order does not indicate a withdrawing of care for the patient.

BABY DOE

Unlike the informed non-consent of autonomous adults or the substituted judgment cases involving those who are irreversibly incompetent to make decisions are those situations involving withholding or withdrawing care from infants. These decisions are filled with anguish for all involved, parents and health care providers alike. In the spring of 1982 an infant known as Baby Doe was born with an esophageal-tracheal fistula and trisomy 21, a form of congenital anomaly known commonly as Down syndrome. The esophageal-tracheal fistula needed immediate surgery if the infant was to be fed. The decision of whether to do the surgery would not have been questioned for a "normal" infant. The physicians split in their recommendations as to whether to provide the surgery in this case and the parents with court concurrence elected to refuse the surgery on behalf of their child, and the infant died. The parents based their decision on their view that it would not be in their son's best interest to survive, because he would always be severely retarded (Rhoden, 1986).

In March 1983, in response to this case and others like it, the United States Department of Health and Human Services issued the *Interim Final Rule*. The rule directed all health care facilities dealing with infants less than 1 year of age, who received federal funding, to prominently display an antidiscrimination notice protecting these infants. The notice provided a handicapped infant hotline for those who might witness cases when infants were receiving less than "customary medical care" (Annas, Rosenblatt, & Wing 1990). Anyone in the nursery could then call and complain about care and the federal government would send representatives to investigate the allegations. The fear of Baby Doe squads descending upon the health care facility and involving themselves in what had previously been a rather private parent-physician arena of decision making had a serious chilling effect upon these private deliberations. The force of the notices was to place a potential conflict between the law and the moral obligations of the health care providers (Moscop & Saldanha, 1986). Legal duties in and of themselves do not establish moral duties or vice versa.

The definition of "customary medical care" is sufficiently vague as to seemingly include the necessity to preserve life regardless of the potential quality or value of that life to the individual. It appeared that medicine was to be forced away from any decision-making role with regard to these issues, even in those instances when the infants were born with complete absences of vital parts of their brains. The national media picked up the Baby Doe issue and began to relate it to the Civil Rights movement and the Holocaust. This feeling that something was basically wrong and that the government had a duty to protect these infants was forcefully stated by the conservative columnist Patrick Buchanan (1983) in the following interesting, although overblown, **slippery slope** or **wedge argument.**

> Once however, we embrace this utilitarian ethic—that man has the sovereign right to decide who is entitled to life and who is not—we have boarded a passenger train on which there are no scheduled stops between here and Birkenau.

> Once we accept that there are certain classes, i.e., unwanted, unborn children, unwanted infants who are retarded or handicapped, etc.—whose lives are unworthy of legal protection, upon what moral high ground do we stand to decry when Dr. Himmler slaps us on the back, and asks us if he can include Gypsies and Jews?

As with most important issues, responsible forces lined up on both sides. Opposing the regulations were groups such as the American Academy of Pediatrics and the American Medical Association. In support were groups such as the American Association of Retarded Citizens, who felt that the decision to provide care should be neutral in respect to handicap. In other words, if a "normal" infant would have received the surgery, then infants with handicaps should also. Of the almost four million infants born each year, approximately 10 percent are born prematurely or with major birth defects. Modern surgery and neonatal care have been rather miraculous; however, many of these still face life severely handicapped. In the investigations of more than 1,500 hotline reports following the Baby Doe case, the government found three cases in which infants were allegedly being denied appropriate care.

In 1984, Congress passed the Child Abuse Amendment which provided guidelines as to when it was appropriate to withhold medically indicated treatment from such infants. The physician is not obliged to provide care beyond palliative care when in the physician's reasonable medical judgment any of the following circumstances apply.

1. The infant is chronically and irreversibly comatose
2. The provision of such treatment would merely

    a. prolong dying
    b. not be effective in ameliorating or correcting all of the infant's life-threatening conditions
    c. be futile in terms of survival

3. The provision of such treatment would be virtually futile in terms of the survival of the infant and the treatment itself under such circumstances would be inhumane (DHHS, 1985)

The Child Abuse Amendment (P.L. 98-457) was also important in that it encouraged the development of infant care review committees (ICRC) within health facilities, especially those with tertiary level neonatal units. These specialized ethics committees have been useful in recommending institutional policies, educating families and practitioners, and offering counsel and review.

In 1986, following the recommendations of the President's Commission on Medical Ethics, the Supreme Court of the United States ruled that the Baby Doe regulations were not authorized under Section 504 of the Rehabilitation Act of 1973. The court emphasized that child protection was a state responsibility and that the primary decision makers for the child should be the parents, provided that such decisions were in the child's best interest. With this ruling, the federal government was out of the Baby Doe business and parents and physicians once again could wrestle with these problems somewhat out of the public eye. Regardless of who the primary decision makers are, the ethical problems remain. Whereas parents have a right to privacy and to be left alone in their decisions with regard to their children, it is not an absolute right and does not extend to child abuse. The standard, and perhaps most appropriate decision-making criteria cited, is that of the "best interest" of the infant.

Many feel that if mental and physical handicaps are overwhelming, then it would be inhumane to provide life-extending care and to salvage infants to lives whose only awareness is pain and suffering. Conversely, to refuse care to a child on the whimsy of being dissatisfied with a particular model is equally distasteful. The right choice for these babies is easy to determine at the extremes, but becomes a true problem when deciding for those infants when it is not clear as to what constitutes their best interest. Perhaps these are cases that are best served by basing the judgments upon the potential for **quality of life** or **personhood.** Some believe that to have value, life must contain some aspects of quality such as awareness and the potential for human relationships. This view is in keeping with the writings of Richard McCormick (1979), a Jesuit priest who defends a quality of life determination. "It is neither inhuman nor unchristian to say that there comes a point where an individual's condition itself represents the negation of any truly human—i.e., relational-potential. When that point is reached, is not the best treatment no treatment?" Translated into the language of personhood, an infant that has no present or future potential for self-awareness and relationships can be said to have no interests at all. It then becomes incomprehensible to provide life-extending care based on the child's best interests, as it makes no difference to the child whether the equipment is maintained for five minutes or five years.

PERSONHOOD

It is clear that the reasoning involved in questions of personhood are of vital importance to the study of biomedical ethics. Most of the focus of ethical thought is on the person, the being who bares personal rights and responsibilities. Judgments in this regard have in the past excluded such groups as women, African-Americans, and Native Americans.

Personhood is a rather controversial line of reasoning that seems appropriate for cases involving patients in a persistent vegetative state or infants with no potential for self-awareness. In Chapter 3 on basic human rights, we examined the concepts of natural and human rights which posit that human beings have certain rights and privileges, and that these rights are not extended to rocks, trees, or animals. In fact, somehow the very recognition of our humanity and our basic needs created an essential difference. The discussion of personhood examines what types of beings can be thought of as bearers of rights. What types of beings can be thought of as persons?

Philosophers such as Mary Ann Warren (1984) and Joseph Fletcher (1972) have attempted to define which characteristics a being must possess to be considered a bearer of rights. Although one is human by virtue of one's genetic code, a "person" is a member of the moral community. One becomes a member of the community by having certain characteristics recognized by the community as grounded in moral status and, in particular, moral and legal rights. Suggested criteria include the following:

1. One who could be said to have interests, a person for whom something can be said to be good for the person's own sake.

2. One who has cognitive awareness, a being of memories, expectations, and beliefs.

3. One who is capable of relationships. Interpersonal relationships seem to be at the very essence of what we idealize in truly being a person.

4. One who has a sense of futurity. How truly human is someone who cannot realize there is a time yet to come as well as a present. The question "What do you want to become." only makes sense in relation to a person.

5. Self-motivated activity.

If these criteria were accepted as being necessary for one to be thought of as a bearer of rights (a person), then patients in PVS do not meet the criteria. Prior to her accident, Karen Ann Quinlan may have had the right to vote, the right to freedom of speech, etc. It becomes incomprehensible to consider her as a possessor of these rights once she irreversibly lost neocortical function. These patients cannot be thought of as being the kinds of beings for whom rights make sense, either the right to live, or the right to die. Because the patient who has become irreversibly comatose is not one who can be thought of as having interests, nothing we do can run counter to the patient's interests. In this sense, what we can or cannot do is rather dependent upon the interests of others—society, family, and health care practitioners—who can be thought of as bearers of rights. The patients themselves can be left out of the equation. Some have suggested that personhood should replace brain death as the legitimate criteria for death. For others, the personhood argument is a rather slippery slope that could allow some monstrous wrong to be perpetrated against a helpless minority in the future. The argument drawn from historical precedence of one group denying others the classification of personhood and then using their lack of this quality to justify slavery or sterilization, rings frighteningly true and appalling.

The problem with this analysis, based on historical events, is that the criteria currently being used for personhood is very basic. So long as the definitions remain at the level of self-awareness, any potential group of targeted and persecuted minorities could be excluded. Denying personhood to those with PVS does not say anything about them or suggest what it is that we might do to or for them, it just excludes them from the community of those who can be thought to bear rights.

EUTHANASIA AND ASSISTED SUICIDE

The moment had come. With a nod from Janet I turned on the ECG and said "Now." Janet hit the Mercitron's switch with the outer edge of her palm. In about ten seconds her eyelids began to flicker and droop. She looked at me and said, "Thank you, thank you." I replied at once as her eyelids closed, "Have a nice trip."

Jack Kevorkian, M.D. (1991)

In June of 1990, Janet Adkins ended her life in a secluded county park with the assistance of the now famous Dr. Jack Kevorkian. By the end of June 1996, Dr. Kevorkian had participated in over thirty similar events using his suicide machine (Thanatron-Mercitron). Among those whom he has assisted with **medicide** have been individuals with emphysema, Alzheimer's, rheumatoid arthritis, multiple sclerosis, as well as those declared terminally ill by their physicians. Janet Adkins, although the first, is also perhaps the most troubling. At the time of her death, Mrs. Adkin's memory loss from Alzheimer's disease was still at the stage of forgetting to take her purse or missing a tennis lesson. The last evening of her life was spent among friends, in cogent conversation regarding the music of Bach. Prior to her death, she had arranged with a therapist to assist her family through the bereavement period. These are not the activities of someone who normally is thought of as the classic candidate for **assisted suicide.** Although common wisdom teaches "It is better too early than too late," it would seem that her death was a bit premature. In Carol Gilligan's (1982) value development writing, she postulates that the highest value for women is responsibility. It is troubling to consider that perhaps Janet Adkins had a double measure of this characteristic and her rush to death was created by wanting her final exit to occur prior to her becoming a burden on the family.

Dr. Kevorkian has become a central figure in the **euthanasia** controversy. For some, he is nothing more than a serial killer with a gimmick. A killer who specializes in exploiting the vulnerable, especially women (Caplan, 1992). The American Medical Association has consistently opposed Kevorkian's actions and the practice of assisted suicide (ERGO, 1996). For others, he is the Che Guevara of the revolution that will usher in the new specialty of medicide, dedicated to bringing death within the realm of human determination. A recent *British Medical Journal* proclaimed "Jack Kevorkian: a medical hero" (Roberts, 1996). Yet, regardless of how one feels personally about assisted suicide and euthanasia, Dr. Kevorkian's actions do appear extreme. In August 1996 he assisted four people in dying. The patients had disease states as varied as multiple sclerosis to chronic fatigue syndrome.

One consideration that seems basic to the discussion is the need for human beings to die a dignified death. Individuals on both sides of the debate can probably agree that humans should not die in isolation away from friends and family, technologically tethered, and in pain. It seems equally true that it cannot be right for someone regardless of intent, to advertise in a newspaper, find a vulnerable individual, take the "patient" to a secluded park, assist her in killing herself, videotape the event, drop the body off at a convenient spot, and hold a press conference.

Etymologically, *euthanasia* means a "good death" or an "easy death," a death free from suffering and pain. Often the term **mercy killing** is used as a synonymous term with euthanasia when the intent of the killing is to bring about the complete end of suffering for an individual. What Dr. Kevorkian is practicing is a form of assisted suicide, as the patient is performing the act with the equipment that the doctor has provided.

Current practice allows for passive euthanasia in which the deadly process is allowed to proceed without intervention when treatment is considered futile and no possibility of patient benefit exists. Every day, in a hundred clinical settings, "DNR" orders are written, respirators are disconnected, IV lines are removed, and proposed surgeries are canceled. Although somewhat controversial, the issue today does not revolve around passive euthanasia.

However, American common law and criminal law regard life as sacred and a health care practitioner who deliberately hastens the death of a patient under the guise of active euthanasia has entered a practice prohibited under the homicide laws. "Consent and humanitarian motive" is never a defense under the law of murder (*Notre Dame Lawyer,* 1973). Although this is true for the letter of the law, in several cases in which a jury has focused on the motivation of a spouse who has taken the life of a mate suffering from illness, the juries have often found the individual not guilty on the basis of temporary insanity or have mandated long periods of probation (DeRamus, 1991).

Holland is the only modern nation to sanction the practice of physician-assisted euthanasia. In 1991 only 590 cases were reported, but recent surveys have reported approximately 5,000 cases annually. Physicians allow at least 3,000 handicapped newborn Dutch babies to die each year. Following a review of the process in 1993, the House of Parliament gave immunity to physicians who followed the official guidelines in their practice but did not strike from the criminal codes penalties for assisted suicide (Humphry, 1993). Yet, there have been some signs that the loosening of barriers regarding **active euthanasia** has led some physicians to move beyond acceptable practice. An article in *National Review* in 1994 described a case when a psychiatrist assisted a physically healthy woman to commit suicide. The woman was depressed over the death of her two children and a broken marriage. In response to the courts allowing the physician to ignore the guidelines, the Dutch Patient's Association, a disability rights group, has begun to distribute a wallet card to its members instructing doctors that "no treatment be administered with the intention of terminating life" (Smith, 1994). Members of this group in a letter to the Parliamentary Committees for Health Care and Justice wrote:

> We feel our lives are threatened. We realize that we cost the community a lot. Many people think we are useless, often we notice that we are being talked into desiring death. We will find it extremely dangerous and frightening if the new medical legislation includes euthanasia.
>
> Fenigsen, 1989

Some opponents to the legalization of active euthanasia oppose the practice on the basis of the principle of beneficence and the fear of beginning a slippery slope. Under this scenario the practice would at first be limited only to voluntary patients. In that those lacking capacity must be provided the same rights as the competent, the practice could then be extended to include the noncompetent patient if the surrogate agreed. Finally the process could be extended to include others based on a perceived need of society such as rationing (Brock, 1995).

Often those opposed to the legalization of euthanasia point to Nazi-style genocide as the final point on the slippery slope. The problem with an analysis that includes Nazi Germany is that this government did not go from mercy killing to the final solution. They began with a flawed system that sought to bring about the ends of the state through the involuntary control of its citizens. A wide chasm exists between the grossness of the actions of certain totalitarian states and the perceived need for voluntary euthanasia in the context of an American medical-moral-legal framework. Yet, the Netherlands experience gives some pause as observers such as Carlos Gomez (1991) see hints of abuse as a result of the lowering of the sanctity of life barriers.

> Throughout my study and analysis of the situation in the Netherlands, I have been plagued with the sense that something other than autonomy was at work. I have had the sense that some (physicians) felt that certain patients were better off dead and that it was a humane act to kill them.

In recent years, polls have indicated that a majority of American citizens favor some form of physician-assisted suicide, and in November 1995 Oregon voters approved a ballot initiative (Measure 16) that would allow terminally ill patients to obtain a physician's prescription for a fatal drug for the expressed purpose of ending their lives (Capron, 1995). This decision was challenged in court with plaintiffs claiming Measure 16 violated the equal protection and due process clauses of the Fourteenth Amendment to the Constitution (*Lee*, 1994). The judge found that the constitutional challenge merited the postponement of the implementation of the legislation until the concerns are fully heard and analyzed.

Two recent appellate court decisions appear to have moved the practice of euthanasia closer to a legal reality. On 6 March 1996 the Ninth U.S. Circuit Court of Appeals overturned a Washington State ban on physician-assisted suicide. This was followed on 2 April 1996 by the Second U.S. Circuit Court of Appeals overturning a State of New York Southern District Court decision forbidding the practice. In both cases the courts argued that if a competent, terminally ill patient could ask for the removal of life support and be allowed to die, then it was unfair that a competent, terminally ill patient not on life support had to wait for death to occur naturally. The courts acknowledged that the state had a legitimate interest in protecting life but that this interest was diminished in light of an expressed wish to die by a terminally ill or permanently comatose patient. The focus of the decisions was on the right of physicians to provide prescriptions to end a life. Questions regarding the role of nursing, pharmacy, and allied health personnel were not addressed by the cases. In the Washington case an appeal has been made to the U.S. Supreme Court (Brodeur, 1996).

The ethical arguments for the practice of euthanasia can be expressed in both utilitarian and duty-oriented terms. The consequence approach is strongly put forward by the noted ethicist and theologian Joseph Fletcher (1974) who believes:

> It is harder to justify letting someone die a slow and ugly death, dehumanized, than it is to justify helping him to escape from such misery. This is a case at least in any code of ethics which is humanistic or personalistic, i.e., in any code of ethics which has a value system that puts humanness and personal integrity above biological life and function.

The duty-oriented defense of the practice of euthanasia is usually centered on an extension of personal autonomy—the right accorded those in Western societies to live their lives according to a personal vision, unrestricted by the views of others. If life can be lived according to a personal vision, why not extend this to the controlling of the time of death?

Those opposed to euthanasia usually do so on the utilitarian basis of the slippery slope. One analogy often drawn is that of the grossness of the German experience under Nazi Germany. The duty-oriented analysis is often drawn from a religious context. If our lives are not ours but a gift from God, then we are bound to hold not only our life but the lives of others inviolate.

It would seem that perhaps the debate involving active euthanasia in the United States is premature. Prior to deciding whether individuals have a right to self-determination regarding this issue, it would be wise to consider why the concept is so popular. When one considers that modern death often involves overwhelming fiscal costs, pain, isolation among strangers, invasion of one's body by technology, and the chance that one will not be allowed to die at all but rather will be continued in an elongated state of unconsciousness, it is no wonder that a now rather than later mentality has infected the population. In the 14 February 1996 *Journal of the American Medical Association,* the Council on Scientific Affairs provided a report on "Good Care of the Dying." Essentially the report stated that sound information regarding how the health care system should serve dying patients does not currently exist. The council found little literature on the epidemiology or symptoms of dying, or the service requirements needed by the ill, or even the decision-making processes that ought to be involved in the treatment of dying patients. The council concluded that at a time when so little is known about the comprehensive care needed by these patients that it was premature to embrace physician-assisted suicide as a definitive answer, even for a small segment of the terminally ill. Perhaps the debate involving active euthanasia should wait until better answers are known or at least until the problems associated with modern death have been ameliorated.

CONCLUSION

Within our culture the concept of death has a variety of meanings and applications. To the religious, death may be nothing more serious than a transition during which the spirit advances from the earthly body to a celestial one. For the philosopher, death may signify the loss of one's position in the moral community, as only those who are alive can be thought of as being bearers of rights and participants in the community. In the area of law, death is a medical definition. Based on this definition, wills are probated, organs are removed, and determinations are made as to whether an action is an assault or a homicide.

Medically, in a less complicated age, death could be defined on the basis of cardiopulmonary function. One died when the heart or lungs ceased to function. This is clearly inadequate today given that patients in the midst of open heart surgery would by this criteria be dead.

Medical science can now save biological life so effectively that we have been forced away from using a cardiopulmonary definition of death to the certification of death by brain function. We have also as a product of our technology and therapeutics moved into a time of being able to fend off brain death, only to expose the patient to continued misery and suffering. Health care providers have reached a quandary where the duty to respect and preserve life comes into direct conflict with the duty to prevent and relieve pain.

In this chapter we have examined several classes of patients where decisions of withdrawing and withholding care have been reasoned. These decisions have gained some cultural, legal, and ethical acceptance. Reasoning for the profoundly handicapped infant, the PVS patient, those who choose informed non-consent, and the mentally retarded each requires a different basis. In some instances, the framework of what is to be done has been postponed and the issue has become instead, who is to decide.

Some instances of nontreatment seem to have gained acceptance and are rather noncontroversial. The 98-year-old with severe dementia and not a relative in the world who contracts pneumonia might be allowed to die quietly. The real questions in regard to health provider duty do not lie in the extremes, such as an infant born with no brain or the terminally ill centenarian, but in the middle ground where the potential for personhood and meaningful life exists.

In the extreme cases when no potential exists, or the best interests of the individual seem best served by withholding or withdrawing treatment, a form of **passive euthanasia** has been allowed. Euthanasia which literally means a gentle or easy death has been divided into two major groupings, passive and active. Active euthanasia has in the last decade become a popular national issue. Whatever the convictions of the health care provider, they should follow closely the current arguments regarding euthanasia. Currently, active euthanasia is considered professionally unethical and illegal. In the near future, this may change, and with the change will come changes in the specialty codes of ethics and legal status of the practice.

Legal Case Study: A Question of Futility—Baby K, 832 F. Supp. 1022 (E.D.Va. 1993).

In this case, the infant girl was born with the congenital malformation anencephaly which left only her brain stem functioning. This limited function allowed for a continuation of respiration but the infant was permanently unconscious; she could not see, or interact with her environment. At birth the physicians and an institutional ethics committee advised the mother that the use of a ventilator that had been put into place awaiting a firm diagnosis was futile and should be withdrawn. The mother resisted these recommendations and, because of the disagreement, the hospital attempted to have the baby transferred to another hospital. When no comprehensive hospital would accept the transfer, the infant was moved to a nursing home.

On several occasions following the transfer, the infant was readmitted to the hospital and given ventilatory support. Although the hospital attempted to resist these admissions, the courts held that they must provide the services. The court determined that to refuse care to the infant would be in violation of the Emergency Medical Treatment and Active Labor Act (EMTALA), a federal statute concerning child abuse, the Americans with Disabilities Act (ADA), the Rehabilitation Act of 1973, and parental decision-making rights as guaranteed by the Fourteenth Amendment to the Constitution.

1. How would you resolve this dilemma?
2. In a time of scarce resources is it reasonable to require the hospital to provide seemingly futile services?
3. How would you define futility?
4. Read over the EMTALA statute to see why the courts have used it to cover this case.

REVIEW EXERCISES

1. Respond to the idea that our current acceptance of a right to die, especially for those who are unconscious and need a proxy decision maker, is a rather slippery slope that may in the future be used not to protect individual autonomy or privacy but rather to serve as a facade to rid us of individuals whose lives we do not value.
2. Respond to the following cases and determine what is the appropriate legal and moral action.
   a. Ms. Jones is brought into the hospital following an overdose of a variety of prescription drugs. It is clear that this is a suicide attempt. While in the emergency room she was intubated and placed on a ventilator and later transferred to the intensive care. The following morning she begins to awaken but is angry with the health care providers for interfering with her decision to end her life.

After she has been in the hospital for forty-eight hours she spikes a temperature and begins to suffer respiratory distress. Diagnostic tests reveal that she has acquired nosocomial pneumonia, which requires a regimen of antibiotics. The morbidity of this condition within the intensive care setting often is as high as 50 percent.

Upon hearing of her diagnosis and prognosis, Ms. Jones smiles and refuses the treatment.

b. In 1987 Michael Martin was injured in a car accident. Following the accident Martin has been unable to walk, feed himself, or talk and requires round-the-clock care by family or caregivers. Martin is aware of those around him and appears to respond through smiles and some hand and head movements. Mr. Martin has been declared incompetent by the courts and prior to his injury he had not executed any form of advanced directive although he had said that he would not want to live in a persistent vegetative state. His current condition is somewhat different than PVS.

His wife has made a request to the Michigan Supreme Court seeking authorization to remove the feeding tube which is keeping her husband alive. She contends that her husband would never have wanted to live in his current state. Is a surrogate bound only to what is written or can a surrogate decision maker move beyond clear and convincing evidence based on an intimate knowledge of the patient's authentic wishes?

3. Differentiate between the various lines of reasoning and arguments needed to decide the following types of cases in regard to withdrawing or withholding care.

   a. Persistent vegetative state cases

   b. Profoundly retarded patient cases

   c. Baby Doe cases

   d. Informed non-consent cases

   e. Which of these case types is best served by proxy judgments, and if so, what form—best interest or substituted judgment?

4. The nurses attending Karen Ann Quinlan were Catholic nuns and based on their personal religious beliefs weaned the patient from the ventilator so that she could continue to live in a persistent vegetative state. One prominent Catholic scholar commented angrily that "some nuns were holier than the church," indicating that the church doctrine did not require extraordinary care to be provided.

This exercise is not intended to defame the motives of the nurses as they were individuals of great integrity. However, did the nurses act appropriately? If not, what would have been appropriate? Must they participate in something that they feel is morally wrong? How is this case an example of one of the basic criticisms of virtue ethics?

5. State why an order for "care and comfort only" might be superior to a DNR order.

6. Assuming that Baby Doe would have grown up to know himself, know those around him, walk, talk, play, and perhaps even go to school, was the decision to not provide the surgery ethical? Regardless of how you answer, justify your decision using ethical criteria. Also note that legal decisions are ethics neutral, and vice versa. Something truly can be legally correct, medically correct, socially correct, and morally reprehensible. An example is the work of Dr. Mengele (Nazi war criminal who performed ghoulish experiments in the death camps), for he surely felt that relative to his society what he was doing was socially, medically, and legally correct.

7. Mr. Joseph was a 75-year-old chronic obstructive disease patient. He was in the hospital because of an upper respiratory tract infection. He and his wife had requested that CPR not be performed should he require it. A DNR order was written in the charts. In his room on the third floor he was being maintained with antibiotics, fluids, and oxygen and seemed to be doing better. His oxygen was inadvertently turned up, and this caused him to go into respiratory failure. When found by the therapist, he was in terrible distress and lay gasping in his bed.

Should Mr. Joseph be transferred to the intensive care where his respiratory failure can be treated by a ventilator, and his oxygen level monitored? Whatever your answer, provide an ethical rationale. Does a patient with a written DNR belong in an intensive care?

8. In a recent nursing journal question-and-answer column the individual asked the question as to what his duty was when a physician wrote DNR orders for all his AIDS patients, even though it was known that the patients wanted everything done that was possible. When questioned the physician just shrugged and said, "I know what is best for my patients." How would you advise the nurse? Is this a case when the legal requirements are lower than ethical practice?

9. The article in regard to inappropriate resuscitation (Figure 9–6) outlines the basic problem encountered by health professions prior to the establishment of reasonable DNR orders. What he wanted was guidelines much like those outlined in Figure 9–7. With these guidelines in mind, first underline the sections within the article that appear inflammatory and devoid of collegiality. Second, rewrite the article so that it is less inflammatory and more persuasive. Third, decide on a plan (who, what, where, why, and when) on how you are going to present your ideas in regard to changing the resuscitation policy so that it coincides with these guidelines.

10. In this chapter, the section on advanced directives stressed the need for sensitivity to issues of cultural diversity. Investigate one of the cultural groupings (outside of your own) found within your geographical area and write a short paper on how that particular cultural reference (religious, ethnic, social class) affects their perception of advanced directives.

REFERENCES

Ad Hoc Committee of the Harvard Medical School to Examine the Definition of Death. (1981, November 13). A definition of irreversible coma. *Journal of the American Medical Association, 246* (19).

Andrew, F. (1994). Overview of legal issues for nurses. *Nursing issues for the nineties and beyond.* New York: Springers Publishers.

Annas, G., Law, S., Rosenblatt, R., Wing, K. (1990) *American Health Law*, Boston MA: Little Brown & Co.

Arras, J. D., & Steinbock B. (1995). *Ethical issues in modern medicine.* Mountain View, CA: Mayfield Publishing Company.

Baby K. 832 F.Supp. 1022 (E.D.Va. 1993).

Bartling v. Superior Court, 209 Cal. Rptr. 221 (Cal. Ct. App. 1984).

Bouvia v. Superior Court, 225 Cal. Rptr. 297 (Cal. Ct. App. 1986).

Brock, D. Voluntary active euthanasia in *Ethical Issues in Modern Medicine* by Arras, J., Steinbock, B. Mayfield Publishing Company, Mt. View, Calif: 1995.

Brodeur, D. (1996a). Ethical issues and legalizing physician-assisted suicide. *Issues, 11*(5). St. Louis: A publication of the SSM Health Care System.

Brodeur, D. (1996b). Physician-assisted suicide: Appellate court rulings. *Issues, 11*(2). St. Louis: A publication of the SSM Health Care System.

Brodeur, D. (1996c). Uncertainty and ethical decision making. *Issues, 11*(3). St. Louis: A publication of the SSM Health Care System.

Buchanan, P. (1983, November 15). The dividing line. *New York Times,* editorial.

Caplan, A. (1992, June 9). Disabled women are victimized by Kevorkian. *Detroit Free Press,* p. 2C.

Capron, A. (1995, January-February). Sledding in Oregon. *Hastings Center Report.*

Council on Ethical and Judicial Affairs of the American Medical Association. *1992 Code of ethics, current opinions,* pp. 14–15.

Council on Ethical and Judicial Affairs of the American Medical Association. (1991). Guidelines for the appropriate use of do-not-resuscitate orders. *Journal of the American Medical Association, 265*(14), pp. 1868–1871.

Cruzan v. Director, Missouri Department of Health, 497 U.S. 261 (1990).

Curtin, L. (1994). Ethical concerns of nutritional life support. *Nursing Management, 25*(1), pp. 14–15.

Darr, K. (1991). *Ethics in health services management.* Baltimore: Health Professions Press.

Department of Health and Human Services, Office of Human Development Services. (1985, April 15). *Final rule; child abuse and neglect prevention and treatment program.* 45 CFR part 1340.

DeRamus, B. (1991, October). Without a clear law, we can't point fingers at assisted suicide. *The Detroit.*

Edwards, B. (1990, September). Does the DNR patient belong in the ICU. *Critical Nursing Clinics of North America* (pp. 473–479). W. B. Saunders.

ERGO News Bulletins. (1996, June 1).

Feinberg, J. (1984). The problem of abortion. Belmont, CA: Wadsworth Books.

Fenigsen, R. (1989). A case against dutch euthanasia. *Hastings Center Report, 19*(1), 17–19.

Fletcher, J. (1972). Indicators of humanhood. *Hastings Center Report, 2*(5), pp. 1–4.

Fletcher, J. (1974). The right to live and the right to die. *The Humanist, 34*(4).

Furlow, T. (1974). Tyranny of technology: a physician looks at euthanasia. *The Humanist, 34*(4), pp. 6–8.

Gilligan, C. (1982). *In a different voice.* Cambridge, MA: Harvard University Press.

Gomez, C. (1991). *Regulating death: Euthanasia and the case of the Netherlands.* New York: The Free Press.

Humphry, D. (1993). *Lawful exit.* Junction City, OR: Norris Lane Press.

In re Quinlan, 355 A.2d 647 (N.J. 1976).

In re Storar, 438 N.Y.S.2d 266 (1981).

Kelly, G. (1957). *Medico-moral problems* (p. 129). St. Louis: Catholic Hospital Association.

Kevorkian, J. (1991). *Prescription: Medicide.* Buffalo: Prometheus Books.

Kübler-Ross. (1969). *On Death & Dying.* New York: Macmillan.

Lee v. Oregon, B69 F. Supp. 1491 (D. Or. 1991).

McCormick, R. (1979). To save or let die: The dilemma of modern medicine. *Journal of the American Medical Association, 229,* pp. 172–176.

Meilaender, G. (1984). On removing food and water: Going against the stream. *Hastings Center Report, 14,* pp. 11–13.

Moscop, J. C., & Saldanha, R. L. (1986, April). The Baby Doe rule: Still a threat. *Hastings Center Report,* pp. 8–12.

New York Times. (1989, April 15). p. A15.

Notre Dame Lawyer, 48(1973), 1202–1260.

Rhoden, M. (1986, August). Treating Baby Doe: The ethics of uncertainty. *Hastings Center Report,* pp. 34–42.

Roberts, J. (1996, June 8). Editorial. *British Medical Journal* as reported in ERGO! New Bulletins.

Sachs, G., Ahnonheim, J., Rhymes, J., Volicer, L., Lynn, J. (1996). Good care of the dying. Chicago: *JAMA* Feb 14 (275)6: 474–476.

Smith, W. J. (1994). Going Dutch? *National Review,* vol 46 Issue 19, pp. 60–65.

Society for the Right to Die. (1987). *Handbook of living will laws.* New York: Society for the Right to Die.

Spritz, J. K. (1991). Speeding the dying. *Hastings Center Report, 21*(4), p. 4.

Superintendent of Belchertown State School v. Saikewicz. (1977). 370 N.E.2d (Mass 1977) 417.

Uniform Determination Death Act (UDDA). (1981). President's Commission for the Study of Ethical Problems in Medicine and Biomedical and Behavioral Research. Washington, D.C.: U.S. Government Printing Office.

Warren, M. (1984). On the moral and legal status of abortion. In Joel Feinberg (Ed.), *The problem of abortion.* Belmont, Calif.: Wadsworth Books.

Whitacre, J. (1980). Ole nincompoop says: Help stamp out inappropriate resuscitation. *Newsletter of the Missouri Society for Respiratory Therapy,* pp. 11–12.

CHAPTER 10

The American Health Care Delivery System

Goal

The major instructional goal is to arrive at an understanding of the current health care fiscal crisis and to evaluate the alternative solutions.

Objectives

At the conclusion of this chapter, the reader should understand and be able to:

1. Differentiate between Medicare and Medicaid as federal and state programs.

2. Define and differentiate between macroallocation and microallocation as they relate to health care.

3. Discuss prospective payment as an attempt by the federal government to gain control of health care costs.

4. Discuss the process of triage and relate it to the microallocation of scarce beds.

5. Define and differentiate between social utility, public utility, and medical utility as forms of microallocation.

6. Identify the forces within the American health care system responsible for the rapid rise in health care costs.

7. Define managed care and identify the market forces being used to curb health care costs.

8. Identify three incentives used in managed care that create a potential for a conflict of interest within the fiduciary relationship that exists between provider and patient.

9. Define the common law "reasonable man" standard.

10. State how the concept of a natural life span would lower the costs of health care.

11. List managed care practices that could create legal difficulties in the area of standard of care.

12. List managed care practices that could create ethical difficulties in the area of the patient-provider relationship.

Key Terms

capitation	laissez-faire	prospective payment
egalitarianism	managed care	public utility
entitlement programs	medical utility	social utility
fiduciary	portability of insurance	standard of care
free market		triage

AMERICAN HEALTH CARE TODAY

Perhaps the most astounding assertion I've heard during the current debate over health care reform is that there is no "health care crisis in America." This statement often comes before arguments that comprehensive health reform is unnecessary or that the current system just needs a few adjustments and fine tuning. Let's not pull any punches: This argument is bogus.

Donna E. Shalala, Secretary of the U.S. Department of Health and Human Services (1-25-94)

One of the major policy requirements for most Western societies today is to eschew the drama for awhile, and examine critically with scientific techniques the dogmas and clichés with which the policy making for medical care has been encumbered.

Gordon McLachlan, British health care expert (1967)

Advances in health technologies and therapeutics during the first half of the twentieth century brought the practice of health care from nostrums to magic bullets. It appeared, for a time, as if all things were possible as one after another of the dreaded plagues were brought under control and, in the case of entities such as small pox, iradicated. Many of these benefits came from doing simple things better: better sanitation, better nutrition, better vaccines. With the advent of antibiotics, for a period of time the society gained control over bacterial infections, and pneumonia ceased to be feared as a killer of children and the aged. Yet to accomplish these ends, Americans spend more on health care per capita and an aggregate basis than any other nation.

Recently, many have come to question the value of the health care victories and even wonder whether the society is not on a wrong path altogether. Although strides were made improving sanitation, improving the quantity and quality of food and water supplies, and improving vaccines and antibiotics, they have all been reasonably inexpensive measures. Once these benefits had been gained, the problems that remained did not seem amenable to mass action or the inexpensive fix. In some areas such as the antinierobial, health care practice seems to be losing ground to an ever increasing number of highly resistant organisms and new plaguelike diseases such as AIDS and its even more frightening cousin the Eboli virus.

The cost of American health care is staggering by any measure. Currently the society spends more than 14 percent of the gross domestic product on health care. This amounts to more than $1 trillion each year. Over the last half of this century, per capita medical costs have increased by over 1,000 percent. The demographics of the future include an aging population who will place an even greater burden upon an already stressed system. Although the use of high technology in medicine has been and continues to be miraculously dazzling, these miracles come with a heavy economic price. In health care, unlike most other industries, technology has not brought about a decrease in personnel needs. In fact, the opposite has occurred. Often when a new technology such as sonography is developed, it initiates the need for a whole new group of technical specialists to provide the necessary services. If present laws and practices regarding health care were to continue, the yearly cost would reach $1.7 trillion by the year 2000. This would equal approximately 18.0 percent of the American domestic product. Unless major cost reduction systems are put into place, by about the year 2030, when the baby boomers reach their seventies and eighties, the estimated costs for health care are expected to grow to $16 trillion and account for over 30 percent of the gross domestic product.

Humanity is of the species Homo sapiens, not Homo medicus (Figure 10–1)! It is difficult to imagine spending over 30 percent of the gross domestic product on health care. Although health is a priority, it is not the *only* priority. Even in the face of clear evidence as to the negative effects on personal health, there are competent adults who drink too much, eat too much, smoke too much, read too much, and exercise too little. If, in fact, health was viewed as the primary value, this would not be the case. Good health, although a universal positive value, is just one of the competing values to which society must attend. Allowing health care costs to spiral out of control will consume money needed for education, rapid transit, roads, bridges, new investments, social welfare, and military defense. The society is reaching a funding crisis in regard to health care that must be faced. As stated by Daniel Callahan (1990), director and cofounder of the Hastings Center,

> We have come to ever more desire what we cannot any longer have in unlimited measure—a healthier, extended life—and cannot even afford to pursue much longer without harm to our personal lives and other social institutions.

Yet for all the money spent, many still believe that more needs to be done. One out of six Americans under the age of 65 lacks basic health care coverage. The United States and South Africa are the only modern industrial nations that do not provide universal health coverage. A job change, a downsizing, an insurance exclusion for a particular medical condition, or the seemingly ever present rise in premiums can lead to a loss of insurance. It is estimated that on any given day in 1993 over thirty-nine million individuals had neither public nor private health care insurance coverage. Even those Americans who are currently covered cannot be sure that a change in fortunes will not place them in the ranks of the uninsured tomorrow. Over half of

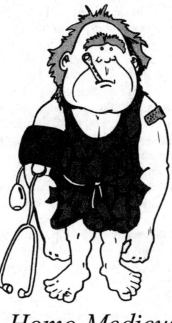

Homo Medicus

FIGURE 10–1 Homo Medicus. Courtesy of Jeff Ek.

all Americans say they worry that they will lose coverage sometime within the next five years. In general, the health care insurance crisis is largely a middle-class problem as the poor are covered by Medicaid. Working adults and their dependents constitute the vast majority—84 percent—of the uninsured (Senate Committee on Labor and Human Resources, 1994).

Being uninsured causes a fiscal problem and also impacts health care outcomes. Children in families without health insurance often do not receive the preventive care or hearing, vision, and developmental screening needed for early intervention. Even children without chronic health problems sometimes miss or delay recommended immunizations which places them at greater risk of acute and chronic illness (Kogan et al., 1995). Adults unable to afford coverage will often ignore ailments and forgo routine care that might detect and cure a problem in an early stage. As a result, uninsured adults often access the health care system late in the process when their conditions have reached an advanced state and the remaining solutions are expensive. As a group, they are twice as likely as insured patients to be at risk of dying prior to reaching the hospital.

Another negative characteristic of the American health care system is maldistribution of access. For the urban poor, the problem is that of poverty, and they face the same problems in gaining access to health care as they do to other goods and services. For rural populations, the problems go beyond just poverty and are complicated by the low physician to population ratio which is much lower than that found in urban areas. In regard to critical incidents, such as heart attacks and cerebral vascular accidents, when early treatment is often vital, a patient in a major urban area can expect to receive emergency care within the first few minutes. In contrast, a patient in some rural sites may wait for hours prior to receiving vital emergency assistance.

An important aspect of the maldistribution problem has been the historical shift of physicians from general practice to specialty practice. Prior to World War II, the typical physician was in a general fee-for-service practice working alone and delivering a variety of services, from pediatrics to geriatrics. As the end of this century nears, we find a shortage of general practitioners, and currently most physicians are specialists confining their attention to a particular branch of medicine or to a particular age group. The earlier individual practices are now outnumbered by physicians who practice in groups, are salaried employees of hospitals, or have joined some other nontraditional delivery mode.

As Americans, we are therefore ending the twentieth century with a feeling of unease regarding our health care system. Although the media is replete with stories such as the discovery of new drugs and therapies which brilliant researchers and clever physicians use to enable the spinal injury patient to walk, to reduce brain damage following stroke, to facilitate conception of infertile couples, and to provide prenatal diagnosis for the high risk fetus, a general feeling of crisis still exists. Too many dollars are being consumed by a health care system that is spiraling out of control, and yet for all our spending, too many citizens lack basic health care coverage and must depend upon emergency rooms as their primary health care access point. Somehow, two seemingly contradictory feats must be accomplished; that is, to cut back on health care costs and widen health care access.

GOVERNMENT INTERVENTION

Throughout most of the nineteenth century the American government took a **laissez-faire** position toward private enterprise, including the practice of health care. This hands-off policy was superimposed upon a religious and philosophical foundation that idealized hard work, thrift, and personal responsibility. The effects of this pro-growth policy were remarkable increases in both material goods and services. However, the invisible hand as described by Adam Smith, an eighteenth century Scottish economist, did not distribute these goods and services equally and the system produced a form of social Darwinism which promoted the strong and perhaps predatory at the expense of the weak and disorganized.

As the nation entered the twentieth century, public sentiment decried the harshness of laissez-faire principles. Government was called upon to curb rampant individualism and to adopt a positive role in providing services to the population. If, in the nineteenth century, people held a general view that the government had no responsibility for the individual, some intellectuals of the twentieth century proclaimed that the individual had no responsibility for resolving personal difficulties and that collective action was required to solve most problems. Many voices resounded, calling for a right to health care, but few voices called for individuals to live their lives in such a way as to make the provision of health care less necessary (*Congressional Digest,* 1994).

A right to health is an interesting concept, as it supposes that somewhere in society there is a supply of health that can be distributed, and if the society could organize itself appropriately, it could deliver this service to its citizens. This becomes even more difficult to imagine when we realize that no unified definition exists of exactly what constitutes health. Certain groups such as the World Health Organization (WHO) define it in the broadest terms: "a state of complete physical, mental, and social well being, and not merely the absence of infirmity" (Constitution of the World Health Organization, 1946). Whereas it is difficult to imagine a right to health or the distribution system that could deliver it, it is less difficult to imagine a right to health care. Within this area of thinking, two questions should be considered. If health care is a right, does it create an obligation for citizens to use it? If it is a right, who has the duty to pay for its usage?

Society is bedeviled by the fact that even in instances when access to preventive care measures such as early childhood vaccinations are available and free, many children remain unprotected. Can a society require changes in personal behavior to use such services? Should parents be punished if they fail to take a child to a free clinic to receive standard vaccinations? Can a liver transplant be denied to someone who has destroyed the original organ through alcohol abuse? Before signing on too quickly to a system that punishes those who actively participate in their own ill health, consider the great number of individuals who eat too much, drink too much, smoke too much, and drive too fast. What is to be done with them? Even if society decided that it would be correct to somehow deny benefits to smokers, drinkers, or overeaters, what about those who eat too much red meat, mountain climb, hunt mushrooms in the wild, or do all sorts of interesting things that may have an unfavorable impact on health?

During the twentieth century the government assumed an increasing role in the provision of health care for the society. The following is a chronology of some of the major events in the national debate over increasing the access of health care through government programming.

1935—Social Security Act included funding for maternal and child health grants and support for the disabled. This act was the first federal acknowledgment of a positive role in the provision of health care to the public. The act was endorsed by President Franklin D. Roosevelt and was passed by Congress.

1945—Senators Wagner and Murray and Representative Dingell introduced the first national health insurance bill with funding to be paid by a payroll tax. This was followed with a call by President Harry S. Truman for a compulsory national health insurance, funded by payroll deductions and providing every citizen with medical and hospital services.

1957—Representatives Roberts and Forand introduced the first Medicare legislation to provide national health insurance for the elderly.

1959—The Federal Employees Health Benefits program was established to provide basic hospital and major medical health insurance to active federal employees and their families. The program provides two basic types of health care insurance: fee for service and prepaid plans.

1960—Senator Kerr and Representative Mills introduced a bill later enacted into law that provided federal support to state medical programs for the elderly poor.

1965—Medicare and Medicaid authorization. President Lyndon B. Johnson signed both into law. The authorization provided health insurance for the elderly, disabled, and the poor. Medicare provides assistance to pay for health services for people 65 and older and for persons receiving

Social Security disability benefits after two years. The system also assists those of any age who have end stage renal disease (ESRD) and need dialysis or kidney transplants. By 1995 Medicare covered more than thirty-eight million people, including approximately four million Social Security disability patients and 257 thousand ESRD patients. Medicare provides two types of coverage: Part A. Hospital Insurance, which assists with inpatient hospital services, skilled nursing facility care, and hospice care for the terminally ill; and Part B. Medical Insurance, which helps pay for physician services, outpatient hospital services, outpatient surgery, diagnostic tests, clinical laboratory services, and medical equipment and supplies.

Medicaid (Title XIX of the Social Security Act) authorizes federal matching funds to assist the states in providing health care for certain low income groups. By 1995, approximately thirty-six million persons were receiving health care under Medicaid. The major groups that the states are required to cover include recipients of Aid to Families with Dependent Children (AFDC), the aged and blind who receive cash assistance from the federal Supplemental Security Income (SSI) program, and pregnant women and children existing at or near the federal poverty line. The total federal expenditures for Medicaid including state administrative costs were approximately $152 billion in 1995. The state paid $66 billion (43%) and the federal government paid $86 billion (57%).

The care provided under Medicaid and Medicare was paid on a cost-basis (for hospitals) and charge-basis (for physicians), whereby providers were reimbursed for most of the costs and charges incurred while providing the care. This payment system was a powerful incentive toward the escalation of health care costs. The patient had virtually no incentive to curtail costs because the insurance program was paying most of the costs. Another factor in the process that tended to create the spiraling costs was that for the most part the patients turned the decisions as to whether to order treatments over to their doctors, because the patients lacked the expertise to make these decisions themselves. This sets up a strange situation where the buyer turned the buying decisions over to the seller. Not only did the physicians make the decision as to what and how much care was being ordered, they also controlled the amount of costs for the services provided determined by a process known by the acronym UCR "usual, customary, and reasonable" fees (Hall & Ellman, 1990). This is not to say that the physicians and hospitals were acting out of pure self-interest. In fact, many ethicists maintain that health care providers have a **fiduciary** duty to their patients. If costs are of no consequence and one is acting on behalf of the patient, then perhaps more is better. The end result was a "spare no expense" mentality that infected the whole system.

Both Medicare and Medicaid are **entitlement programs** and provide benefits automatically to all individuals who qualify. Medicare has an autonomous trust fund that does not require an annual appropriation from Congress. Current expenditure trends threaten the trust fund with insolvency early in the next century. Over the last twenty years the health care expenditures focused on the last year of life have accounted for about 30 percent of the total Medicare budget.

1971—President Richard Nixon proposed expansion of health maintenance organizations (HMOs) and incentives for employers to provide health insurance for their employees.

1974—Employee Retirement Income Security Act became the first comprehensive law regulating employee pensions and health plans under the direction of President Gerald Ford.

1977—President Jimmy Carter proposed hospital cost containment that would place a cap on public and private payments for hospital services.

1983—The Medicare **prospective payment** system was initiated, under which program rates were set in advance for each medical diagnosis. This system moved Medicare from a system of retrospective cost-based payments to a prospective payment system. Prospective payment was introduced to curb the spiraling health care costs as the traditional fee-for-service plans had provided the institutions with an incentive to increase spending. Because payments for a given illness were predetermined and fixed, health care facilities had a powerful incentive to contain costs. Prospective payment in some sense was an attempt to provide the hospitals with a profit-or risk-based incentive to bring about economies within the system. The most common forms of cost containment efforts were centered around reducing services, decreasing staff, and shortening the length of patient stay. The patients were, in effect, being sent home "sicker and quicker."

In that the prospective payment plan was directed at controlling hospital costs, one of the results was that many services were shifted out of the hospital. In some way it was analogous to squeezing a balloon in the middle; while hospital costs were restrained, many of the services that were previously provided there were shifted to outpatient care sites which became lucrative fee-for-service payment sites. It became obvious that the only way the government was going to gain control over the costs was to initiate a **capitation** system.

1988—The Medicare Catastrophic Coverage Act expanded Medicare coverage for catastrophic illness costs and prescription drugs, signed into law by President Ronald Reagan. The 1990 budget reconciliation bill replaced the 1988 Medicare Catastrophic Coverage Act, with a new physician payment system to be phased in from 1992 to 1996 based on the amount of work involved in a treatment, geographical area, and other factors.

1993—President Bill Clinton appointed a Task Force on National Health Care Reform, headed by First Lady Hillary Rodham Clinton, to devise a plan for overhauling the health care system. The efforts of the task force appeared overreaching to most Americans and were defeated in Congress.

1991 to 1994—Representative Stark sponsored legislation known as Stark I and Stark II. Although allowing limited exceptions, the legislation was designed to prevent physicians from referring Medicare and Medicaid patients to health care facilities in which they held a proprietary interest. Stark I applied to clinical laboratory facilities. Stark II added physical therapy, occupational therapy, radiological services, diagnostic services, services related to durable medical equipment, and services related to home health care. The assumption of the legislation was that physician referrals to facilities in which the physicians had a proprietary interest were often made for unnecessary treatment and made primarily to increase the amount of fees charged to Medicare and Medicaid.

In the election of 1996, the crisis within the health care system was not a major election issue and most congressional initiatives regarding health care were taken at the margins of the problem, such as providing **portability of insurance** for citizens between jobs. The crisis in health care, however, is not a problem that will go away just because politicians fail to make it a vital election issue. In fact, a health care crisis exists, and the costs of American health care are at present too high and rising. Ways must be found to maintain quality, increase access, and control costs. Whether these changes occur as a result of government intervention or by market forces is a real issue that must be addressed as Americans enter the twenty-first century. These are frustrating times for health care providers. The current practice dilemma was clearly stated by a practitioner who wrote,

> *We are presently committed to providing the best of care, equally to all, while maintaining provider and receiver choice, though at the same time engaging in cost containment. It should be clear that one cannot pursue all of these four goals at the same time. We confront a conflict of values and goals.*

> Englehardt, 1986

POSITIONS ON MACROALLOCATION OF HEALTH CARE

Although most agree about the health care crisis, no one agrees as to how to allocate the available health care resources. Some call for a free-market approach where health care is treated much like any other service, while others claim that it is a natural right and therefore must be available to all on the basis of need. The three major theoretical positions are **free market,** egalitarian, and utilitarian.

Free-market

Free-market advocates call for a return to the open market, believing that the current government interventions not only do not help but also have created the crisis. These advocates hold that, if the government would cease all efforts to manipulate the market, the price of health care would find its natural level. They point to research groups such as the Rand Corporation, whose studies seem to indicate that persons who have access to free health care use significantly more services than do those who must pay a portion of the costs (Newhouse et al., 1981). Advocates who feel that government intervention is the problem usually adopt a free-market approach to provide solutions. Free-market thinkers usually emphasize personal rights to social and economic liberty. They are not particularly concerned with, nor do they attempt to outline, the requirements of how material goods and services are allocated in a society; only that the choice of allocation system be freely chosen without governmental interference. In the United States, outside of charity, social welfare, and military duty, goods and services have generally been allocated using a free-market approach.

The free-market system operates on the material principle of ability to pay, and usually invokes some form of libertarianism as its justification. Given the national traditions of personal freedom and individualism, it is quite likely that some aspect of the free market will continue to coexist within any national health care plan that evolves in the United States. Figure 10–2 provides one humorous vision of a future free-market world under managed competition.

Recently most health care reform efforts have been in the area of **managed care** systems which attempt to bring free-market restraint to spiraling health care costs. Essentially, managed care is an umbrella term for plans that coordinate health care through primary care generalists. In that this is a dynamic period of health care when change is occurring at a dizzying rate, it is difficult to say exactly what managed care is. Because of the diversity of current systems, one author has described managed care as a modern Jekyll and Hyde, saying the term "managed care" does not necessarily tell you what you are getting (Clancy & Brody, 1995). As Victor Cohn of the *Washington Post* remarked, "If you've seen one managed care system, you've seen one managed care system." As a result, there are many terms and models of managed care to consider.

- Health Maintenance Organization (HMO)—Prepaid health care systems that cover preventive services, checkups, and serious illnesses.

- Group Model—The traditional HMO with salaried doctors who only treat plan members, who in turn are only covered when they use the HMO doctors and hospitals.

- Independent Practice Association—An HMO that contracts with independent networks of independent doctors who are paid an annual fixed sum or a per-visit

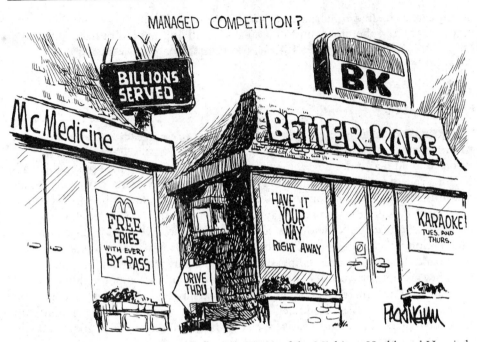

FIGURE 10–2 Managed Competition? Courtesy of the Michigan Health and Hospital Association.

fee for each enrollee. Members are covered only when using HMO doctors and designated hospitals.

- Preferred Provider Organization—A hybrid HMO in which members choose from a roster of doctors who provide care according to a set fee schedule. Members can choose an out-of-plan physician if they are willing to pay a higher co-payment.

- Point of Service—Plans that allow members to use non-HMO health services, again, if they are willing to pay higher premiums and co-payments.

- Fee-for-Service Plan—The traditional "old system" where patients see any physician and choose use of any hospital. They usually pay a deductible and co-payment, and the insurer pays the rest (Rivo et al., 1995).

Figure 10–3 provides an interesting attempt in applying managed care cost containment techniques to an orchestra concert. From the cost containment processes described, it is easy to see why many health care providers at all levels of practice find the trends unsettling. Because physician activities account for 60 to 80 percent of the expenditures within the hospital, the following discussion will focus primarily on managed care as it affects physician practice. Managed care systems use a variety of approaches to alter the practice behaviors of physicians and other health care providers. The use of case managers to coordinate care, financial incentives to conserve resources, and health care protocols to guide the delivery of care all seek to bring about changes in health provider behavior with a lower expenditure of funds.

The President of a large California health insurance company was also the chairman of the board of his community's symphony orchestra. He could not attend one of the concerts and gave his tickets to the company's director of health care cost containment. The next morning he asked the director how he enjoyed the performance. Instead of the usual polite remarks, the director handed him a memorandum which went like this.

"The undersigned submits the following comments and recommendations relative to the performance of Schubert's Unfinished Symphony by the Civic Orchestra as observed under actual working conditions:

- The attendance of the orchestra conductor is unnecessary for public performances. The orchestra has obviously practiced and had the prior authorization from the conductor to play the symphony at a predetermined level of quality. Considerable money could be saved by merely having the conductor critique the orchestra's performance during a retrospective peer review meeting.

- For considerable periods, the four oboe players had nothing to do. Their numbers should be reduced and their work spread over the whole orchestra, thus eliminating peaks and valleys of activity.

- All twelve violins were playing identical notes with identical motions. This is unnecessary duplication; the staff of this section should be drastically cut with consequent savings. If larger volume of sound is required, this could be obtained through electronic amplifications, which has reached very high levels of reproductive quality.

- Much effort was expended playing 16th notes. This seems like an excessive refinement as most of the listeners are unable to distinguish such rapid playing. It is recommended that all notes be rounded up to the nearest 8th. If this were done, it would be possible to use trainees and lower grade operators with no loss of quality.

- No useful purpose would appear to be served by repeating with horns the same passage that has already been handled by the strings. If all such redundant passages were eliminated, as determined by a utilization review committee the concert could have been reduced from two hours to twenty minutes, with still greater savings in salaries and overhead. In fact, if Schubert had attended to these matters on a cost containment basis, he probably would have been able to finish his symphony."

ANONYMOUS

FIGURE 10–3 Musings on Managed Care

High Managed Care Cities
Costs	11.2% Below National Average
Length of Stay	6.3% Below National Average
Mortality Rate	5.3% Below National Average
Complication Rate	0.9% Higher than National Average

Low Managed Care Cities
Costs	7.9% Above National Average
Length of Stay	3.4% Above National Average
Mortality Rate	2.9% Below National Average
Complication Rate	2.0% Below National Average

St. Louis Dispatch, Thursday, February 1, 1996, 8C.

FIGURE 10–4 Managed Care Comparisons

Case managers may review health care records and deny physicians payment for unnecessary health care services, and seemingly ration certain services provided within the plan. The results of managed care activities have been to lower the rising costs of health care. It is difficult to argue with the results, as reported in Figure 10–4 which compares cities with high and low penetration of managed care systems.

The media also carry disquieting stories of conflicting interests between managed care participants. Every HMO organization has at least four different stakeholders who have a vested interest in the success of the enterprise. Figure 10–5 indicates the dimensions of the stakeholders in managed care systems. Each of the four major anchor groups has a right to reasonable expectations but must recognize innumerable points where a conflict of interest may occur. Patients have the right to expect quality care, with reasonable access, delivered in a timely and respectful fashion. Health care providers and staff have a right to fair wages, career advancement, and the maintenance of working conditions that allow for the provision of quality services. Owners have a right to an appropriate return on investment and that providers will, within reason, protect the bottom line. The community has a right to expect that the institution will be a good neighbor, provide stable employment, and provide community services and health care access. How can society be assured that the interests of patients, health care providers, and owners and community remain in appropriate balance? How does it ensure that the legitimate goals of reducing expenditures, increasing efficiency, and eliminating unnecessary treatments do not lead to a system that results in patients receiving less individual attention and poorer care? How can society be assured that pressures upon providers to cut corners to keep jobs does not lead to less access to quality care for the community?

Conflicting goals between stakeholders do not necessarily result in abuses. Yet it is also clear that market forces have at times failed to protect the vulnerable, especially when there was a disparity of power and information. Society has recognized this problem and under law has identified certain groups as fiduciaries. A fiduciary is one who holds a thing in trust, a trustee. A fiduciary relationship occurs when one person has a legal duty to another for which the former is accountable and is required by law

[handwritten margin note: Conflicting rights (?) leaves us with no winners]

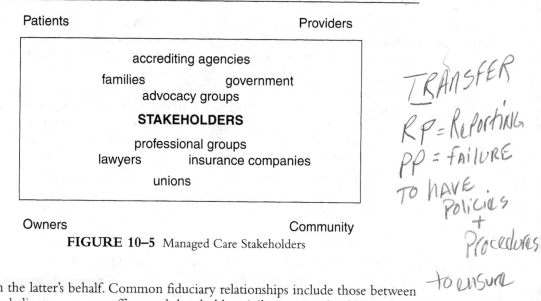

FIGURE 10–5 Managed Care Stakeholders

to act on the latter's behalf. Common fiduciary relationships include those between lawyer and client, corporate officer and shareholder, civil servant and public, partners in business, and in some contexts, physicians, nurses, and health care providers and their patients. The central feature of a fiduciary relationship is some form of duty. In the case of the health care provider and the patient, once the relationship is established, the provider has a duty to offer a proper standard of care. If the health care professional fails to provide an appropriate standard of care, that professional may become subject to liability for violating the fiduciary duty to the patient.

Consider the following three stories recently reported in the news, in light of their potential impact upon the fiduciary relationships between the physicians and the patients.

- Recently a physician signed on with a large east coast HMO system. Following his contractual agreement, the physician gave a slide presentation at the National Managed Care Congress, where among other things he called attention to a portion of the contract that he described as being a "gag clause." The clause in the contract stated:

  Physicians shall agree not to take any action or make any communication which undermines or could undermine the confidence of enrollees, potential enrollees, their employees, their unions, or the public . . .

- Three days following the *Donahue Show* the company terminated the physician's contract, contending that "Given the fact that he has expressed a lack of comfort with us . . . we assumed . . . he would have welcomed the notice we provided him" (Cole, 1996).

- A psychologist reported working with a 10-year-old child, who exhibited the behavior of compulsive hand washing. The managed care policy allowed for only ten sessions with the psychologist. At the end of the ten sessions, the psychologist informed the mother that the child needed continued care and offered to continue treatment at a reduced rate. He directed the mother to the insurance company. The woman then brought the problem to the company asking that treatment be continued beyond the ten-session limit. Within a month of the complaint, the psychologist was dropped from the provider list.

- A young mother who complained of abdominal pain and rectal bleeding was seen by her physician. The members of the woman's family were part of a family practice plan with a local physician group. The physician group contract was with an HMO operated by a major insurance company and the plan was a fixed capitation system.

  After three months of care, the pain and bleeding continued and the family demanded action. The physician ordered a barium enema X ray which was inconclusive. After three additional visits the costs of care provided had risen to a level that the physician group under contract had to assume the next $5000 in charges. The woman died twenty months later of undiagnosed colon cancer.

This third incident although troubling is also one when great caution needs to be taken before conclusions are drawn. In fact, it is difficult if not impossible to know what motivated the level of care provided. Health care provision is both an art and a science and requires individual judgment. Everyone will not make the same decision and not every case will come to the desired conclusion. Although the fiscal incentive raises the question, it may not have played any part in the decisions made or the case outcome.

The three stories describe potential interference with the patient-provider relationship. The contractual constraints that require physicians to refrain from informing patients of information regarding care, and fiscal incentives that promote cost containment at the expense of diagnostic tests, emergency room usage, length of hospital stays, and specialty referral, all may directly affect the **standard of care.** Health care providers are frustrated because managed care has placed others between them and their patients, others who make decisions as to what type of care can be provided. Figure 10–6 points to the potential for having nonhealth care providers deciding access to health care modalities.

The American Medical Association (1995) expressed its concern regarding the potential deleterious effects of managed care upon the physician–patient relationship and have offered the following four guidelines regarding physician practice within the system.

- Efforts at cost containment should not place patient welfare at risk.
- Plan coverage should not affect the practitioner's duty to provide informed consent.
- The practitioner has a duty to serve as patient advocate.
- Patients must assume responsibility for selecting their own health care plan.

Health care providers must assume greater responsibility in determining the nature of managed care systems. As a result of the fiduciary relationship between the patient and provider, the patient has a right to expect that personal interests will be protected. These expectations contain the important elements of professional competence, professional autonomy, respect for persons, continuity of care, beneficence or nonmaleficence, patient advocacy, confidentiality, and perhaps most importantly, no conflicts of interest.

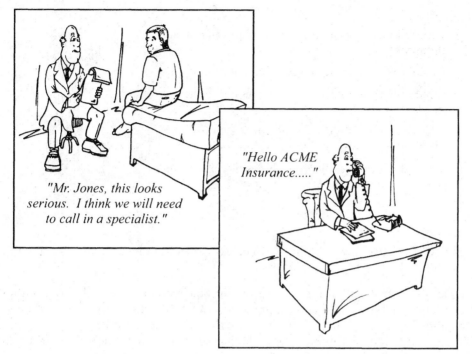

FIGURE 10–6. Courtesy of Jeff Ek.

If health care professionals cannot guarantee these elements, then a new form of informed consent should be adopted where questions such as those listed in Figure 10–7 are answered. The morality of the marketplace is a new arena for health care providers, and if fully adopted, health care professionals have an obligation to inform the patients that care is being provided under the standard caveat aeger—let the patient beware.

Egalitarianism

At the opposite end of the spectrum from the free-market proponents are the advocates of **egalitarianism.** These thinkers believe that an affluent society such as ours must find a way to provide universal health care to all its citizens. It is within the egalitarian end of the spectrum that the advocates of a right to health care are most comfortable. Egalitarian proponents often point to socialistic, universal access health care systems such as those found in Canada and the United Kingdom as being models worth emulation. In its most extreme form, these thinkers hold that any deviation from absolute equality in distribution is unjust. Some take a romantic view to the health care problem and fail to consider the scarcity of resources relative to human wants. They see the barrier to free and available health care to all in unlimited quantities as being caused by human error and organization rather than to basic human choices that must be made between health care and other needed goods and services. When confronted with the inevitable gap of tragedy between available resources and human desires, the romantics often point to human error such as waste,

- Is the doctor's salary affected by patient load and amount of care provided?

- Is there a fiscal incentive provided for limiting care?

- Can the physician tell you about options not covered in the plan?

- What consequences will the physician face for being an advocate for you with the HMO over additional care?

- If the care provided exceeds the physician's annual compensation, does the doctor pay the excess?

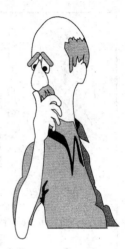

FIGURE 10–7 Morality of the Marketplace—New Informed Consent Questions

fraud, or a stingy political system, claiming that these are the real barriers, thus protecting their illusion that no scarcity exists. Victor Fuchs (1974) likened this romantic view to confusing the real world with the Garden of Eden.

A more rational formulation of egalitarianism can be found in the contractarian writings of John Rawls (1971), which hold that a just society is one whose social arrangement is based on a contract between members to advance the good of all who are in the society. Ethicists such as Beuchamp and Childress (1989) have argued that this collective protection coupled with the fair opportunity rule form the basis of a right to health care. According to this philosophy, members of a society are bound in a social contract, and a need among any of its membership creates a moral obligation on the part of the society as a whole. This then is a collective obligation to provide the needed goods and services to the extent of the society's available resources.

Utilitarianism

A middle system that one finds in the macroallocation discussion is that of utilitarianism. These theorists propose a mixture of criteria so that **public utility** is maximized. Public utility is the key to this strategy, and is captured in the phrase "the greatest good for the greatest number." Utilitarians accept governmental planning and intervention as methods of redistributing goods and services within a society to advance public utility. The public health policies of many Western nations have been based upon utilitarian reasoning. Many authorities in the United States, such as former governor and reform party candidate Richard Lamm of Colorado (1986), see health care as just one of the many goods and services found within the bounds of public utility and see our current policy as one that treats "our illnesses at the expense of our livelihoods. We spend more than a billion dollars a day for health care while our bridges fall down, our teachers are underpaid, and our industrial plants rust." An examination of most small towns in America will show that the local hospital is the building in town with the highest level of technology, whereas the lowest level of technology is found in the elementary schools. Given limited resources and choices that must be made, is the allocation between health care provision and education of children appropriate?

Authorities such as Lamm and Daniel Callahan, director of the Hastings Center, believe that health care must take its place among the whole array of limited resources and must be rationed when there is a shortage and provided only to those who would benefit most and be denied to those who will benefit least. An example of this approach can be seen in the practices of Great Britain where a social, political, and medical consensus exists that allows practitioners to deny frail or demented elderly patients hospitalization or intensive care, even in such treatable cases as pneumonia. Prior to being critical, it should be noted that this same system provides extensive home and geriatric day care; in fact, they are making what they consider to be utilitarian choices (Edge & Groves, 1994).

The Oregon Plan. By the mid-1980s it became clear that Oregon did not have the resources to offer everyone everything and that the "spare no expense" mentality could not be maintained. The decision was to increase the number of potentially eligible citizens to health care access through Medicaid by removing access to some medically important treatments. Citizens attended state meetings throughout Oregon to assess the relative value of the services provided. They ranked each service on three factors—the public's perception of value, the effectiveness or outcome, and the cost. The services considered most valuable were prenatal care, and those least valued involved infertility and cosmetic surgery. The 1988 legislature acted on these initiatives making Oregon the first jurisdiction to explicitly decide on a rationing system for health care in the United States (Coombs, 1990).

Natural Life Span Argument. In Psalm 90:10 the prophet writes "The days of our years are three score and ten." Callahan (1987) argued that a natural life span exists, although at a somewhat higher age span than three score and ten, and that it ends with death, which occurs as a natural component of the life cycle. Figure 10–8 lists the criteria used to establish the end of the natural life cycle. The limits of a natural life span would be reached when the criteria were met, and at that point, Callahan offered the following principles of practice:

1. After a person has lived out a normal life span, medical care should no longer be oriented toward resisting death.

2. Medical care following a natural life span would be limited to the relief of suffering.

3. The existence of technologies capable of extending life beyond a normal life cycle creates no technological imperative for its use.

Adopting these principles would have the result of decreasing overall health care costs as we presently concentrate the largest portion of our health care dollars in the last year of people's lives. One of the benefits of the natural life span view is that it

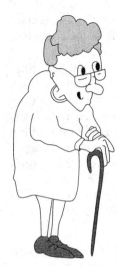

1. One's life work is completed.

2. One's moral obligations to those for whom one has responsibility have been discharged.

3. One's death does not seem to others an offense to sense or sensibility or tempt others to despair and rage at human existence.

4. When the process of dying is not marked by unbearable and degrading pain.

FIGURE 10–8 End of the Natural Life Cycle

would preclude the spending of vast sums to stave off the inevitable death that occurs at the end of the natural life cycle. For all the criticism of the natural life span argument it may be an ethically persuasive model if it operated as a closed system, where all savings gained from limiting technology at the end of life could be used to enhance health during the other phases of a natural life span. Using a closed system model would also assist in the current problem of intergenerational inequity as the federal expenditure for children is about one-sixth of that for the elderly, even though a greater number of our children live in poverty.

Some have called for a mixed system of allocation designed to maintain the free-market access to health care for those who can afford it and yet provide a decent minimum for those who require public assistance. This two-tiered system would guarantee coverage for basic care and the catastrophic health needs for all Americans. The coverage at the basic level would be distributed on the basis of need, with everyone being assured equal access. The other tier would be based on the ability to pay, and would provide expanded and perhaps better care at private expense. This blending of free-market and utilitarian values may have real appeal in the United States as we attempt to increase access and yet curb governmental costs. The basic minimum package if coupled with individual responsibility for personal health (diet, lifestyle, environmental factors) may in fact prove adequate. Many authorities believe that once a basic minimum is achieved, factors outside of medical care have more to do with health and longevity than the provision of more or less health care (Hall, 1990).

STANDARD OF CARE

Many of the health care provision questions regarding which allocation system to select revolve around legal issues involving standard of care requirements. For example, the fiscal incentives within some managed care systems to provide less care, the contractual requirements that specialists not discuss treatment options outside of the plan, ridged treatment protocols that replace professional judgment, and the replacement of nurses and therapists with lesser educated practitioners all raise questions involving a breach of duty to provide a reasonable standard of care.

Essentially what the law requires is that health care providers conform to a specific standard of care to protect others. A provider such as a nurse who assumes the care of a patient, assumes a duty to provide that care with the degree of skill and knowledge ordinarily possessed and exercised by other nurses. Whereas the health care provider is expected to act with professional judgment, this judgment must remain within the bounds of accepted practice for that specialty group. The courts have over the last several decades moved toward a national standard of care rather than allow for a local focus. Continuing education and national conferences are important elements of current health care practice as the national standard requirements for specialties continue to rise (*Dickinson v. Milliard,* 1970).

We are responsible for both our actions and our failure to act. Under common law we are held to the "reasonable man" standard. This standard has evolved as a fairness standard; that is, we may be charged with negligence if someone is injured because we failed to perform an act that a reasonable person in similar circumstances would have done, or if we commit an act that a reasonable person would not commit. As health care professionals, we are held to a higher standard than laypersons. If a patient is injured because a specialist failed to exercise the skill and expertise that under similar circumstances could reasonably be expected of a professional with similar experience and training, then that health care provider may be liable for negligence. Differing levels of education, training, and specialization then give rise to differing standards of care required.

THE PROCESS OF MICROALLOCATION

Macroallocation is usually the province of legislative bodies, insurance companies, foundations, and health organizations as they attempt to determine what types of goods and services will be available. In some sense this is a far easier task than the more personal process of determining who gets what intensive care bed, what organ, or advanced technology. These are the difficult decisions of microallocation. In the past these decisions may have been made on the basis of lifeboat ethics. When the American ship, *William Brown,* struck an iceberg off the coast of Newfoundland, the survivors found themselves in overburdened lifeboats in heavy winds. After twenty-four hours with the boats taking on water, the crew became concerned that all lives would be lost unless they decreased the numbers in the boat. The decision was made on the basis of **social utility,** that families and women should be spared. Under these rules fourteen young men were thrown overboard, and two young women, sisters of men in the water, joined them. Shortly thereafter the survivors were rescued. Upon their return to Philadelphia all the crew with the exception of Seaman Holmes disappeared. Holmes was brought to trial and he was defended on the basis that the decision was made on the grounds of social utility, of keeping families intact and the duty-oriented value of protecting helpless women.

The court, however, ruled against Seaman Holmes, holding that given the sacred nature of each life a random lottery would have been a more ethically preferable method of making the decision. Seaman Holmes was convicted (*United States v. Holmes,* 1842). The concept that justice requires a random selection among equals has been forcefully defended in the works of the ethicist Paul Ramsey (1970):

> [T]he equal right of every human being to live, and not relative personal worth, should be the ruling principle. When not all can be saved and all need not die, this ruling principle can best be applied by random choice among equals.

Another equally unsatisfactory attempt to microallocate vital health services on the basis of social utility was that of an anonymous Seattle committee set up in the early 1960s to determine which patients with kidney failure would be placed on kidney dialysis. This committee was composed of a physician, lawyer, housewife, businessman, labor leader, state governmental official, and minister and became known as the "God Squad." These were life-and-death decisions as those who were not selected had few other alternatives. The committee used factors such as age, sex, marital status, number of dependents, net worth, educational background, future potential, and emotional stability as decision criteria. One member recorded the following from the experiences:

> . . . . I remember voting against a young woman who was a known prostitute . . . . I also voted against a young man who, until he learned he had kidney failure, had been a ne'er-do-well, a real playboy . . . .

Due to the lack of neutrality of the criteria, the committee favored male patients, Caucasians, and those with middle-class status or above. One critical observer as quoted by Ramsey (1970) called the selection "a disturbing picture of the bourgeoisie sparing the bourgeoisie," and held that the "Pacific Northwest is no place for a Henry David Thoreau with bad kidneys." In cases such as the Seattle situation, a random selection or first come first serve seem more suitable than social utility.

A total lack of neutrality also seems inappropriate to making certain decisions. The process in the military known as **triage** is based on a form of **medical utility.** When used in time of war, the system usually is to divide the wounded into three groups. The first group is the walking wounded who have received superficial wounds that require minimal care. These troops are often ignored during the first few minutes or are patched up immediately so that they can return to the battle. The second group includes the fatally wounded who are given available narcotics to ease their pain but are not treated for their injuries. The third group is the severely but not fatally wounded. These troops are treated immediately, as their care will bring about the highest percentage of survivors. A similar process often used to make bed allocations when the intensive care is overcrowded is the criteria of best prognosis or medical utility.

CONCLUSION

In the United States, although we have a high standard of health care, it is clear that the current inflationary spiral and limitations to access for many of our citizens threaten the viability of the system. As a people we do not have a national consensus regarding how to allocate health care resources. There is no real consensus for providing a universal national health care insurance such as that found in Canada and Great Britain and yet there is only minimal faith that the free market will be a sufficient force to deliver appropriate care for all our citizens. Our current attempts to control costs by using the free-market forces of managed care appear to have possibilities and problems in equal portions. Although it is clear that the costs are being restrained by these systems, there are also ethical and perhaps legal problems associated with some of the current managed care practices.

Utilitarian mixtures such as the Oregon plan have both proponents and critics. We at times seem to want to have it both ways—open unlimited access for all but at low cost. This unfortunately is a romantic view that fails to take into account that when one matches unlimited wants with a truly finite resource, a gap must inevitably occur. Whatever system is finally selected, to be ethically sound it must not fall more heavily upon the socially disadvantaged or those incapacitated by illness. Theorists and planners should consider the principle of material justice and the fair opportunity rule when making their final macroallocation or microallocation choices.

Legal Case Study: *Helman v. Sacred Heart Hospital,* 381 P.2d 605 (Wash. 1963).

This case involved a patient who had sustained chest injuries, left hip dislocation, multiple fractures in the area of the left hip socket, and was paralyzed from the waist down. He was placed in a two-patient room following his surgery. The patient in the next bed complained of a boil on his right arm. Over the next week the nursing staff administered to both patients, gave baths, and back rubs, changed dressings, and generally moved from one patient to another without washing their hands. Eight days following the surgery, the boil was cultured and three days later was found to be infected with *Staphylococcus aureous.* The patient with the boil was then transferred to an isolation area. Following the transfer, the surgical site on the hip surgery patient erupted with discharge containing the same organism. The tissue destruction associated with the infection created the need for another surgery of the hip. Following this surgery, the patient's hip was fused and was essentially rendered immobile.

The court affirmed a judgment for the patient holding that there was a sufficiently strong chain of circumstantial evidence from which the jury could deduce that the patients were infected with the same organism because hospital personnel failed to follow sterile techniques while ministering to the two patients. The court concluded that the hospital, via its nurses, was negligent because it failed to follow well-known and widely practiced precautions and procedures to prevent the spread of staphylococcus.

The hospital's standard of care was to make sure its nurses knew of the preventive techniques and that those nurses were implementing and following such procedures.

1. Could the nurses have been found negligent for a failure in their duty to provide an appropriate standard of care separate from the hospital?

2. Can a patient care assistant be held for the standard of care of professional nurses on staff?

3. Would the nurses have a fiduciary trust relationship with the patient?

REVIEW EXERCISES

1. The states of Utah and Nevada lie side by side in the West, and they are similar in climate, levels of income, level of health care delivery, and in many other aspects. Yet, the inhabitants of Utah are among the healthiest in the United States and those of Nevada among the least healthy. This appears to be a function of lifestyle choice. The state of Utah is inhabited primarily by Mormons who by doctrine avoid tobacco, alcohol, and illicit drugs and live in rather large stable families, whereas in Nevada tobacco and alcohol consumption are high and the family structure less stable.

   Assuming you agree that individuals should be more responsible about choices that impact upon the costs of health care which the public must bear, what prohibitions would you consider putting in place to curb alcohol, cigarettes, and drug use? What incentives might be considered to promote stable families which seem to have a positive impact upon health care costs?

   An example of something that might be considered is a risk analysis component to health insurance deductibles. If the person was a heavy smoker, drinker, or divorced adult, that person would pay higher premiums or deductibles much the same way that those with poor driving records pay higher rates.

2. Many health care practitioners see ethical problems associated with some of the business practices dealing with managed care and have offered the following as a new ethic for managed care.

   • Prohibit all schemes for the use of salary incentives or bonuses tied to provider test ordering patterns.

   • Require that all managed care plans have a board of health care providers (physicians, nurses, therapists, technologists) to approve policies regarding length of stay, quality indicators, etc.

   • Create an independent review board to assess the reliability and validity of all quality indicators before they are approved or required.

   • Require that all managed care plans have clear procedures allowing health care professionals to advocate for treatments for individual patients.

   • Require all managed care plans to have clear procedures under which patients, surrogates, and health professionals may challenge a denial for services.

   Others see these rules simply as attempts by health care providers to return to the good old days of spend, spend, spend. How do you view this issue? Would you want to add additional rules to the new ethic for managed care?

3. Robert Frost (1874–1963) the great American poet wrote the following lines.

   I shall be telling this with a sigh
   Somewhere ages and ages hence;
   Two roads diverged in a wood, and I
   I took the one less traveled by.
   And that has made all the difference.

   Within the traditions of ancient Greece are two cults (options)—Aesculapius and Hygeia—which dealt with health care delivery. Aesculapius was a strict patient and health care provider model that was aggressively patient centered, whereas Hygeia was a public health model that focused on prevention in the context of public interest. It is clear that American medical care is built on a Aesculapian model. When one considers our concerns regarding the allocation of health care, is it possible that some of our problems are associated with this choice made over 1,000 years ago? Consider how the debate would be altered had we taken the Hygeia model (option) as the standard for health care provision.

4. In our society we have distributed goods and services by many systems.
   * To each person an equal share (elementary and secondary education)
   * To each person according to need (aid to dependent children)
   * To each according to merit (promotions)
   * To each according to contribution (retirement benefits)
   * To each according to ability to pay (most goods and services)
   * To each according to social worth (positions on a traditional Mardi Gras float)

   Which of these systems do you consider the best method of distributing health care in the United States? Defend your selection.

5. The following is a limited listing of health care services that a society may desire.

   Prenatal care
   Well baby care
   Neonatal intensive care
   Transplants
   Rehabilitation services
   Burn units
   Pulmonary disease care
   AIDS
   Cardiovascular surgery
   Genetic therapy
   Cosmetic surgery
   Alternative medicine
   Fertility care
   Trauma centers
   Geriatrics
   Home care
   Hospice care
   Sports medicine

   Imagine yourself in the position of the Oregon citizens and must make decisions based on perception of value, outcomes, and costs. In this case you may fund up to fifteen areas and allocate $120 million. No funded area may receive less than $8 million but may receive more.

6. The "Musings on Managed Care" (Figure 10–3) came as an anonymous evaluation of managed care. Is it a fair criticism? In what ways does it capture true problems with managed care practice that are being experienced by nursing and the allied health professions? Defend or criticize the "Musings on Managed Care."

7. Assume that a nurse in a physician's office improperly dressed a wound and as a result further injuries occurred. In defense, the nurse stated and was able to demonstrate that although the wound was dressed improperly, the dressing and techniques used were in accordance with the dressing standard of care used by medical assistants in the community. Do you think that this defense will work? If not, why?

8. The great American baseball hero Mickey Mantle died in 1996. By his own account his lifestyle had been self-destructive and he had a history of alcoholism. It is estimated that the medical costs of keeping Mantle alive during the last three months of his life, including his liver transplant, exceeded $300,000. Respond to the following two ideas.
   a. Should someone with a history of alcoholism be provided with a scarce resource such as a liver for transplantation?

b. Mark Siegler, a highly respected ethicist, said that providing the liver to Mickey Mantle was acceptable even with his history of alcoholism because Mantle was an American hero. This is an example of what form of utility?

REFERENCES

American Medical Association, Council on Ethical and Judicial Affairs. (1995). Ethical issues in managed care. *JAMA, 273* (4), pp. 330–335.

Beuchamp, T., & Childress, J. (1989). *Principles of biomedical ethics.* New York: Oxford University Press.

Callahan, D. (1990). *What kind of life?* New York: Simon and Schuster.

Callahan, D. (1987). Setting limits. *Medical goals in an aging society.* New York: Simon and Schuster.

Clancy, C. M., & Brody, H. (1995). Managed care—Jekyll or Hyde? *Journal of the American Medical Association, 274* (4).

Cohn, V. A map of the health care maze, *Washington Post.* 12:2 May 30, 1995.

Cole, W. (1996). Gagging the doctors. *Time Magazine, 147* (2).

Congressional Digest. (1994, October), pp. 226–232.

Constitution of the World Health Organization (1946). Preamble.

Coombs, B. (1990, September). Two ethics compete in debate on health care rationing. *Journal of American Academy of Physician Assistants.*

Dickinson v. Milliard, 175 N.W. 2d 588 (Iowa 1970).

Edge, R., & Groves, R. (1994). *The ethics of health care* (chap. 11). Albany: Delmar Publishers, Inc.

Englehardt, H.T. (1986). The importance of values in shaping professional direction and behavior. In *Occupational therapy education: Target 2000.* American Occupational Therapy Association.

Fuchs, V. (1974). Who shall live? *Health, economics, and social choice* (pp. 63–64). New York: Basic Books, Inc.

Hall, M. A., & Ellman, I. M. (1990). *Health care law and ethics.* St. Paul, MN: West Publishing Company.

Helman v. Sacred Heart, 381 P.2d 605 (1963).

Kogan, M., Alexander, G., Teitelbaum, M., Jack, B., Kotelchuck, M., & Pappas, G. (1995). The ...effect of gaps in health insurance on continuity of a regular source of care among preschool-aged children in the United States. *JAMA, 274* (18), pp. 1429–1435.

Lamm, R. (1986). Rationing of health care: The inevitable meets the unthinkable. *Nurse Practitioner, 11* (5), pp. 581–583.

McLachlan, G. (1967). From medical science to medical care. *Lancet, 7491,* p. 630.

Newhouse, J. P., Corris, C. N. et al. (1981). Some interim results from a controlled trial of cost-sharing in health insurance. *New England Journal of Medicine, 305,* pp. 1501–1507.

Ramsey, P. (1970). *The patient as a person: Exploration in medical ethics.* New Haven: Yale University Press.

Rawls, J. (1971). *A theory of justice.* Cambridge: Harvard University Press.

Rivo, M. L., Mayes, H. L., Katzoff, J., & Kindig, D. A. (1995). Managed health care. *Journal of the American Medical Association, 274* (9).

Senate Committee on Labor and Human Resources. (1994). Report 103–317.

Shalala, D. (1994). "Let's Face Facts, There Is a Health Care Crisis," reprinted from *Washington Post* Article. 94012501.txt at www.05.dhhs.gov.

Smith, A. (1991). *The Wealth of Nations.* Westminster Maryland, Everymans Library.

United States v. Holmes, 26 Cas. 360 (E.D. Pa. 1842).

List of Cases Used in Text

CITATIONS

Matter of Baby K, 832 F. Supp. 1022 (E.D. Va. 1993).   p. 183

Bartling v. Superior Court, 209 Cal. Rptr. 221 (Cal. Ct. App. 1984).   p. 169–170

Bouvia v. Superior Court, 225 Cal. Rptr. 297 (Cal. Ct. App. 1986).   p. 170–171

Estate of Behringer v. Medical Center at Princeton, 592 A.2d 1251
  (N.J. Super. Ct. Law Div. 1991).   p. 128, 134, 178

Bradley v. University of Texas M.D. Anderson Cancer Center,
  3 F.3d 922 (5th Cir. 1993).   p. 125

Canterbury v. Spence, 464 F.2d 772 (D.C. Cir. 1972).   p. 63, 128, 178

Clayman v. Bernstein, 38 Pa. D. & C. 543 (1940).   p. 89

Cohn v. Mark, 211 P.2d 320 (Cal. Dist. Ct. App. 1950).   p. 93

Cobb v. Grant, 502 P.2d 1 (Cal. 1972).   p. 75

Cruzan v. Director, Missouri Department of Health, 497 U.S. 261
  (1990).   p. 164–165, 171

Danforth v. Planned Parenthood of Central Missouri, 428 U.S. 52
  (1976).   p. 50, 53, 141

De May v. Roberts, 9 N.W. 146 (Mich. 1881).   p. 90

Dickinson v. Milliard, 175 N.W.2d 588 (Iowa 1970).   p. 205

Doe v. Centinela Hospital, No. CV87-2514, 1988 WL 81776
  (C.D. Cal. June 30, 1988).   p. 124–125

Elliot v. Board of Weld County Commissioners, 796 P.2d 71
  (Colo. Ct. App. 1990).   p. 53–54

Faya v. Almaraz, 620 A.2d 327 (Md. 1993).   p. 129

Geddes v. Daughters of Charity of St. Vincent DePaul, Inc., 348 F.2d 144
  (5th Cir. 1965).   p. 77

Gilson v. Knickerbocker Hospital, 116 N.Y.S.2d 745 (N.Y. App. Div. 1952).   p. 88

Glover v. Eastern Nebraska Community Office of Retardation, 867 F.2d 461
  (8th Cir. 1989).   p. 128

Griswold v. Connecticut, 381 U.S. 479 (1965).   p. 88–89

Harris v. McRae, 448 U.S. 297 (1980).   p. 142

The Lawsuit

It is often confusing to laypersons, as well as to many law students, as to how a case proceeds through the American legal system. This appendix is an attempt to help you sort out what occurs should you ever become involved with a lawsuit as a plaintiff or as a defendant.

Initiating the Suit—the Complaint and the Answer

A plaintiff in any action has a duty to establish a prima facie case. To initiate a suit, the plaintiff files a complaint with the court which addresses the elements of the prima facie case and the number of offenses (counts) of which the plaintiff alleges the defendant is guilty of violating (in federal court it is called a complaint, in state court it is usually called a petition). The complaint must also be "served" on the defendant to give notification that a suit is being initiated against the individual. (Here the old adage is usually true: you can run but you cannot hide—a process server will usually find you.) If you are a defendant in a case, being "served with process" may anger you but should really only give cause for disturbance for what it really is—notice of a lawsuit and nothing more. After being served, the defendant usually has a statutorily required period in which a complaint must be answered. (Defendants should not answer a complaint without the assistance of an attorney because it will become part of the court's record and the defendant will be held to anything stated therein.)

After the answer has been filed, a defendant may file a motion for summary judgment or a motion to dismiss. The motion for summary judgment may be directed at all or part of a claim. It asks a judge to make a ruling on a dispute of law; therefore, it requires that there be no dispute of fact between the parties. If there is a dispute as to the facts of the case, then a motion for summary judgment will not stand. Alternatively, the defendant may bring a motion to dismiss which in essence claims that the plaintiff has not established a prima facie case in the complaint or that the complaint does not state a remedy for which the law provides. Either of these motions may be brought anytime before the trial begins.

The Interim—Discovery

This is the longest part of a suit and is usually the place where most lawsuits end. Discovery may be engaged in by either party once the defendant has been notified and certain statutory procedures have been complied with by both parties (e.g., scheduling conference to set deadlines for discovery and the trial). Even though the federal system, and most states, have deadlines by when certain discovery orders must be completed (an effort by the legislature to expedite cases more quickly), extraneous circumstances usually require attorneys to file motions to continue which grant them more time in which to complete their discovery.

Discovery is basically the fact-finding phase when each party has the opportunity to find out relevant, if any, information from the other side. Most often, information that is normally private may be brought to light (e.g., patient records, bank account information, personal histories). Because discovery is the only opportunity both sides have to discover information that will help their case, great latitude is given to the parties in their discovery efforts. Hence, information that may never be brought to light in court may be discovered in this phase of a lawsuit.

The major elements in discovery usually involve interrogatories, document requests, and depositions. Each of these elements should be posed or answered with the help of an attorney because they will all become a permanent part of the court record. An interrogatory is a series of questions sent by one side to the other. Some jurisdictions limit the number of interrogatories a party may ask (e.g., federal courts limit the number of interrogatories to twenty). Document requests are just that—a request for documents. Documents must be requested separately from an interrogatory. Also, depositions are an opportunity for each side to depose witnesses and parties to a suit in order to elicit information that will be helpful to the case. Each party from which a deposition is requested may only be deposed once by the party requesting the deposition. Overall, with the exception of depositions, each of these items may be requested several times before trial.

As stated earlier, discovery is when most suits end because, sooner or later, information is discovered that is detrimental to one party. The resulting information may be in the form of a "smoking gun" (e.g., an e-mail from a hospital administrator stating that a particular person was fired because he was homosexual and that he hates homosexuals), or merely a realization that the plaintiff has in fact not been able to establish a prima facie case. Whatever the reason, either the suit is dropped or the parties proceed to arbitration. Arbitration is recognized in a majority of states and involves a neutral third party of whom both sides have agreed will have the power to decide the outcome and render a binding decision.

The Trial

More often than not, a trial will be a jury trial. (Trials heard by only a judge usually involve a dispute of law and not a dispute of fact; one of the few exceptions to this rule is the small-claims court.) The jury is impaneled through a process called voir dire. If you have ever been called for jury duty, you have an understanding of this stage of the trial. In voir dire, the judge and the attorneys for both sides are allowed an opportunity to ask questions from potential jurors to discover information about their lives and attitudes. The information elicited ranges from the mundane (Where do you live?) to the more personal (What is your opinion about capital punishment?). Following the questioning, the judge and the attorneys, in private, will make a decision as to who will be asked to be on the jury. In federal court, the jury is composed of twelve people; some state courts only require six people.

Once the jury is impaneled, the trial may begin. With the plaintiff leading, both sides are allowed an opening statement to present what they intend to prove at trial. The plaintiff, who has the burden of proving the prima facie case to the jury, begins by putting on evidence and witnesses. If, at this stage, a plaintiff has hopelessly been unable to prove a prima facie case, the defense can request a motion for a directed verdict. This request asks the judge to render a verdict without allowing the jury to consider any of the case before them. Basically, it is the same as a motion to dismiss but at the trial level. If the motion is denied, then the trial continues and the defendant is allowed to put forth evidence and witnesses to rebut the plaintiff's claims and argue available defenses. Sometimes, depending upon the issue being litigated, if the plaintiff successfully proves a prima facie case, the burden of proof shifts to the defendant to prove particular elements of a defense. Remember, the party who does not have the burden of proof has to prove nothing and could, technically, remain silent. When each side has had a chance to present its case and cross-examine witnesses, then each side is allowed time for a closing argument. After the closing argument, the jury is instructed by the court on any applicable law and any presumptions which the jury should consider in the deliberations, and then the jury is dismissed to deliberate.

The trial usually ends with the verdict. A federal jury trial requires that the decisions of the jury be unanimous; some states only require a majority. Regardless, unless the requisite number of jurors is reached to form a consensus, the jury is hung and a mistrial is declared, thereby requiring another trial. If a verdict is rendered by a jury which one side believes to be totally unfounded in law and when no substantial evidence supports the jury's conclusion, then the losing side may make a motion for judgment notwithstanding the verdict (JNOV). A JNOV allows a judge to basically overturn the decision of the jury and enter a judgment for the losing party. If the evidence was insufficient, or there was jury misconduct, or other errors on other grounds, then the losing party may make a motion for a new trial. If neither of these motions are granted or applied, then the trial court will enter a judgment in accordance with the jury's decision; such a judgment becomes a final judgment.

The Appeal

The losing party may appeal a trial court decision to a higher court in that particular jurisdiction, but only a final judgment may be appealed. The higher court will accept appellate arguments from both parties, but an appellate court will not entertain any new issues. Essentially, an appellate court is a trier of law, reviewing the processes of the lower court and the applicable decisions of law rendered by the lower court. The appellate court is not a trier of fact; that responsibility belongs solely to the lower court. Consequently, if the appellate court finds that a particular factual issue was never brought before the lower court that has bearing on the outcome of a case, the appellate court will remand the case back to the lower court to try that factual issue. The appellate court has the power to affirm, reverse, and/or remand a case back to the lower court. It is due to this particular procedural aspect that cases can drag on for years. For example, if a motion for summary judgment is granted at the pretrial stage, such a judgment is final and may be appealed. If the appellate court finds that the lower court abused its discretion in rendering a judgment on the motion, then it remands the case back to the lower court so that a trial may proceed.

Doing Legal Research

When one enters a law library for the first time, the frustration of where to begin becomes quite intense. You will soon realize, however, that legal research is easier than it appears. Most libraries have many search mechanisms you can use to locate the information you seek. This appendix is meant to help you get started in locating that information, but you will find that the law librarian will become your greatest source of information and will be able to direct you to avenues of research of which you are unaware.

An understanding of court authority

All ABA-accredited law schools have a law library. If there is not a law school in your area, or if access to it is restricted, then you should be able to go to your local courthouse. Most courthouses hold at least a limited number of volumes; most federal courthouses have fairly extensive holdings.

Before you can begin researching, you need to understand how the court system works. Our legal system works off the principle of stare decisis, which dictates that lower courts must follow the decisions of a higher court in the same jurisdiction. To understand whether a case is binding on a court, you must understand the difference between mandatory and persuasive authority. A decision by a court that is directly above another court in the same jurisdiction (e.g., a court of appeals) provides mandatory authority for that particular lower court—the lower court must follow the decision of the higher court on any directly applicable issue related to the case it is deciding. Persuasive authority is authority that a court may follow, but is not binding on the court because it usually comes from a court outside of the jurisdiction (e.g., a New York Court of Appeals decision vis-a-vis The Colorado Supreme Court).

The Supreme Court of the United States is the ultimate authority for all issues related to federal law and the Constitution. The federal system is divided into thirteen circuits. Each circuit has a trial court (the district court) and a court of appeals (the circuit court). The federal system also has several specialty courts which hear only certain types of cases such as tax and bankruptcy courts. Nevertheless, the power of authority of each court depends upon its location. There are several district courts in a circuit and each district court's decision is only persuasive authority for the other district courts in the circuit. However, all district courts in a circuit are bound by the mandatory authority of the circuit court. Yet, each circuit court is only persuasive authority for another circuit court. For example, if the Southern District of Illinois has a case before it, any similar issues decided by the Northern District of Illinois will be persuasive authority. However, the Court of Appeals for the Seventh Circuit is mandatory authority, as opposed to any decisions by the Ninth Circuit which would only be persuasive authority on both the Southern District of Illinois and the Seventh Circuit. Furthermore, federal law is mandatory authority on all federal courts, and all state law is mandatory authority on courts within the state.

Most state courts are divided in a similar fashion to that of the federal system. There are trial courts (usually a county circuit court), courts of appeal, and a state supreme court. State courts hear cases related to state law. More often than not, the state supreme court is the highest authority to which most state court cases rise. Nevertheless, depending upon the issues at stake (usually ones involving rights guaranteed by the Constitution), the Supreme Court of the United States may grant a **writ of certiorari** and hear the case on appeal. Unless a case is granted a writ of certiorari, the decision of the state supreme court will stand.

Locating cases

Germane to any legal research is an understanding of where cases are recorded. Cases are published in books called **reporters**. Reporters publish cases chronologically according to the date the decision was issued. Every level of court has at least one reporter for its decisions. Supreme Court decisions are located in the *U.S. Reporters* (U.S.) or the *Supreme Court Reporter* (S.Ct.). The federal circuit court decisions are located in the *Federal Reporter* (F.,F.2d,F.3d). Federal district court decisions are located in the *Federal Supplement* (F. Supp.). State court decisions are found in regional case reporters which are divided geographically (e.g., California cases are located in the *Pacific Reporter* (P.,P.2d), whereas Missouri cases are located in the *South Western Reporter* (S.W.,S.W.2d)).

Using the citations

Legal citations seem ominous at first glance, but, in all reality, are extremely easy to understand. For example:

115 S. Ct. 2724 (1993) 889 F.2d 56 (4th Cir. 1986) 58 S.W.2d 347 (Mo. Ct.App. 1950)

The first number in a citation is the volume number of the reporter. The letters identify which reporter is being cited. In the examples above, "S. Ct." identifies the Supreme Court Reporter; the "F.2d" identifies the Federal Reporter Second; the "S.W.2d" identifies the South Western Reporter Second. The last number is the first page on which the case is found. Any information that follows in parentheses tells you which court decided the case and when, helping you, the researcher, to quickly distinguish between mandatory and persuasive authority. Once you have a citation, you go to the shelves, locate the area in which the particular reporter you need is shelved, and then find the volume which will be organized in ascending numeric order.

Using the descriptive word approach

The most common situation that attorneys and paralegals face is not knowing the citation of a particular case. It is a situation that can quickly become tedious and frustrating. Hence, most practitioners turn to an electronic database (LEXIS or WESTLAW) to do a quick subject search. However, electronic research is expensive and requires an account-access number before you can begin any research. If you do not have access to an electronic database, never fear, the old fashioned way of doing research is still rather efficient and can sometimes be more rewarding.

To begin, identify the issue you want to research and write down key descriptive words that relate to the issue. For example, if your issue was whether a doctor could be held liable for an inadvertent disclosure by his nursing staff about the HIV status of a patient, your key word list may include *doctor, nursing staff, HIV, disclosure,* and *patient.* However, because your mind and the mind of an editor will most likely never be in synchrony, it is best if you also include related key words, such as *physician, employee, AIDS,* or *consent.*

Next, locate the set of reporters that apply to the jurisdiction you wish to search. Because most doctor-patient relationships are governed by state law, you will most likely find yourself in the applicable regional reporter (unless a federal law applies, then you could turn to the applicable federal reporters). Each set of reporters has a case digest complete with an index. First, locate the index and begin looking to find your key descriptive words. You will find that some of your descriptive words will not be in the index, so you should look for related terms. The index will direct you to subject headings and key notes in the digest. As you will find, the subject headings in the digest may organize subjects differently than you would by placing cases under the headings of *physicians and surgeons* or *hospitals,* rather than under *doctors.* The next step is to locate the volume of the digest (usually arranged alphabetically according to subject) and turn to the relevant key note number. There you will find a one-paragraph summary of a case as well as its citation. Then, follow the previous steps above for when you know the citation. You will find that once you begin researching, the process quickly becomes rote and you will be more efficient each time.

Finally, after doing all the research and finding a case right "on point," you need to make sure that the case you found is still good law. As stated earlier, the American court system is based on the principle of stare decisis, meaning that once a case is overturned by a higher court, it is no longer good law. The tool for locating whether your case is still good law is in the *Shepard's Citations.* An explanation of the use of these books would be too confusing at this point. It will be easier if you approach the law librarian for assistance in "shepardizing" your case. The *Shepard's Citations* are organized chronologically, but each volume is not cumulative and requires some extra searching into other volumes; hence, turn to the librarian for assistance to ensure that your case is current.

Regional Centers for Ethical Study

The Hastings Center
255 Elm Rd.
Briarcliff Manor, NY 10510
(914) 762-8500
Dr. Strachan Donnelley, President

Boston University School of Health
80 E. Concord
Room A-509
Boston, MA 02218
(617) 638-4626
George J. Annas, Director of Health Law
Michael Grodin, Director of Law, Medicine, and Ethics

C. Everett Koop Institute
at Dartmouth College
7025 Strasenburg
Hanover, NH 03755
(603) 650-1450
Michael Caputo, Director, Telemedicine Program

Ethics Institute of Dartmouth College
6031 Parker House
Hanover, NH 03755
(603) 646-1110
Prof. Ronald Green, Director of Ethics Institute

Center for the Study of Society and Medicine
Columbia College of Physicians
630 West 168th St.
New York, NY 10032
(212) 305-4096
David J. Rothman, Ph.D., Director

Department of Epidemiology and Social Medicine
Albert Einstein College of Medicine of Yeshiva University
1300 Morris Park Ave.
Bronx, NY 10461
(718) 430-3574
Dr. Michael H. Alderman, Chairman

Department of Religious Studies
University of Virginia, Cocke Hall
Charlottesville, VA 22903
(804) 924-6709
Harry Gamble, Ph.D., Chair

Edinboro University of Pennsylvania
Russell B. Roth, Professor of Clinical Bioethics
Edinboro, PA 16444
(814) 732-2604
James F. Drane, Ph.D., Director

Department of Medicine
University of Illinois at Chicago
Section of General Internal Medicine
840 South Wood St.
Chicago, IL 60612
(312) 996-1599
Lawrence Frohman, M.D., Director

University of Wisconsin Center for Health Science
Program in Medical Ethics
1300 University Ave.
Medical Science Center
Room 1420
Madison, WI 53706
(608) 263-3414
Norman Fost, M.D., Director
Fax # (608) 262-2327
E-mail: mdethics@macc.wisc.edu

Division of Medical Ethics and Humanities
University of South Florida
Department of Internal Medicine
12901 Bruce B. Downs Blvd.
MDC Box 19
Tampa, FL 33612
(813) 974-2918
Fax # (813) 974-5460
E-mail: rowalker @com1.med.usf.edu
Robert Walker, M.D., Director

Program on Human Values and Ethics
University of Tennessee
College of Medicine
956 Court Street, Box 11
Memphis, TN 38163
(901) 448-5686
Fax # (901) 448-4103
E-mail: dstallings@utmem1.utmem.edu
Terrence F. Ackerman, Ph.D., Chair

Medical College of Wisconsin, Bioethics
8701 Watertown Plank Rd.
Milwaukee, WI 53226
(414) 456-8498
Fax # (414) 266-8654
Robyn Shapiro, Director

Medical Humanities Program
Southern Illinois University
School of Medicine
P.O. Box 19230
Springfield, IL 62794-1113
(217) 782-4261
Fax # (217) 782-9132
Theodore LeBlang, Chair

Center for Health Care Ethics
St. Louis University Medical Center
1402 S. Grand
St. Louis, MO 63104
(314) 577-8195
Fax # (314) 268-5150
E-mail: troyd@wpogate.slu.edu
Kevin O'Rourke, O.P.J.C.D., Director

Michigan State University
Center for Ethics
C-208 East Fee Hall
East Lansing, MI 48824
(517) 355-7550
Fax # (517) 353-3289
E-mail: brody@pilot.msu.edu
Howard Brody, M.D., Director

Midwest Bioethics Center
1021-25 Jefferson
Kansas City, MO 64105
(816) 221-1100
Fax # (816) 221-2002
E-mail: midbio@qni.com
Web site: HTTP://www.midbio.com
Myra Christopher, President and CEO

Institute for Medical Humanities
U.T.M.B.
2210 Ashvel Smith Bldg.
301 University Blvd.
Galveston, TX 77555-1311
(409) 772-2376
Fax # (409) 772-5640
E-mail: racarson@utmb.edu
Ronald A. Carson, Ph.D., Director

University of Arizona College of Medicine
1501 North Campbell Ave.
Tucson, AZ 85724
(520) 626-6214
Fax # (520) 626-4884
Shirley N. Fahey, Ph.D., Director,
Social Perspectives in Medicine

Center for Bioethics
St. Joseph Health System
440 South Batavia Street
Orange, CA 92668
(714) 997-7690
Fax # (714) 997-7907
E-mail: ethics@corp.stjoe.org
Jack Glaser, Director

East Caroline University
School of Medicine
2 S. 17 Brody Medical Sciences Bldg.
Greenville, NC 27858-4354
(919) 816-2618
Fax # (919) 816-2319
E-mail: kopelman@brody.med.ecu.edu
Loretta M. Kopelman, Chair

University of Michigan
School of Public Health
109 Observatory
Ann Arbor, MI 48109-2029
(313) 764-5464
Fax # (313) 763-5455
E-mail: nmclark@umich.edu
Noreen Clark, Dean

Codes of Professional Ethics: Selected Health Professions

AMERICAN DENTAL ASSOCIATION PRINCIPLES OF ETHICS AND CODE OF PROFESSIONAL CONDUCT

With official advisory opinions revised to October 1996 © **ADA**
ADA Principles of Ethics and Code of Professional Conduct

CONTENTS

I. INTRODUCTION

The dental profession holds a special position of trust within society. As a consequence, society affords the profession certain privileges that are not available to members of the public-at-large. In return, the profession makes a commitment to society that its members will adhere to high ethical standards of conduct. These standards are embodied in the *ADA Principles of Ethics and Code of Professional Conduct (ADA Code).* The *ADA Code* is, in effect, a written expression of the obligations arising from the implied contract between the dental profession and society.

Members of the ADA voluntarily agree to abide by the *ADA Code* as a condition of membership in the Association. They recognize that continued public trust in the dental profession is based on the commitment of individual dentists to high ethical standards of conduct.

The *ADA Code* has three main components: The **Principles of Ethics,** the **Code of Professional Conduct,** and the **Advisory Opinions.**

The **Principles of Ethics** are the aspirational goals of the profession. They provide guidance and offer justification for the *Code of Professional Conduct* and the *Advisory Opinions.* There are five fundamental principles that form the foundation of the *ADA Code:* patient autonomy, nonmaleficence, beneficence, justice, and veracity. Principles can overlap each other as well as compete with each other for priority. More than one principle can justify a given element of the *Code of Professional Conduct.* Principles may at times need to be balanced against each other, but, otherwise, they are the profession's firm guideposts.

The **Code of Professional Conduct** is an expression of specific types of conduct that are either required or prohibited. The *Code of Professional Conduct* is a product of the ADA's legislative system. All elements of the *Code of Professional Conduct* result from resolutions that are adopted by the ADA's House of Delegates. The *Code of Professional Conduct* is binding on members of the ADA, and violations may result in disciplinary action.

The **Advisory Opinions** are interpretations that apply the *Code of Professional Conduct* to specific fact situations. They are adopted by the ADA's Council on Ethics, Bylaws, and Judicial Affairs to provide guidance to the membership on how the Council might interpret the *Code of Professional Conduct* in a disciplinary proceeding.

The *ADA Code* is an evolving document and by its very nature cannot be a complete articulation of all ethical obligations. The *ADA Code* is the result of an ongoing dialogue between the dental profession and society, and as such, is subject to continuous review.

Although ethics and the law are closely related, they are not the same. Ethical obligations may—and often do—exceed legal duties. In resolving any ethical problem not explicitly covered by the *ADA Code,* dentists should consider the ethical principles, the patient's needs and interests, and any applicable laws.

II. PREAMBLE

The American Dental Association calls upon dentists to follow high ethical standards which have the benefit of the patient as their primary goal. Recognition of this goal, and of the education and training of a dentist, has resulted in society affording to the profession the privilege and obligation of self-government.

The Association believes that dentists should possess not only knowledge, skill, and technical competence but also those traits of character that foster adherence to ethical principles. Qualities of compassion, kindness, integrity, fairness, and charity complement the ethical practice of dentistry and help to define the true professional.

The ethical dentist strives to do that which is right and good. The *ADA Code* is an instrument to help the dentist in this quest.

III. PRINCIPLES, CODE OF PROFESSIONAL CONDUCT, AND ADVISORY OPINIONS

Section 1—PRINCIPLE: PATIENT AUTONOMY ("self-governance"). The dentist has a duty to respect the patient's rights to self-determination and confidentiality.

This principle expresses the concept that professionals have a duty to treat the patient according to the patient's desires, within the bounds of accepted treatment, and to protect the patient's confidentiality. Under this principle, the dentist's primary obligations include involving patients in treatment decisions in a meaningful way, with due consideration being given to the patient's needs, desires, and abilities, and safeguarding the patient's privacy.

CODE OF PROFESSIONAL CONDUCT

1.A. PATIENT INVOLVEMENT.

The dentist should inform the patient of the proposed treatment, and any reasonable alternatives, in a manner that allows the patient to become involved in treatment decisions.

1.B. PATIENT RECORDS.

Dentists are obliged to safeguard the confidentiality of patient records. Dentists shall maintain patient records in a manner consistent with the protection of the welfare of the patient. Upon request of a patient or another dental practitioner, dentists shall provide any information that will be beneficial for the future treatment of that patient.

ADVISORY OPINIONS

1.B.1. FURNISHING COPIES OF RECORDS. A dentist has the ethical obligation on request of either the patient or the patient's new dentist to furnish, either gratuitously or for nominal cost, such dental records or copies or summaries of them, including dental X-rays or copies of them, as will be beneficial for the future treatment of that patient. This obligation exists whether or not the patient's account is paid in full.

1.B.2. CONFIDENTIALITY OF PATIENT RECORDS. The dominant theme in Code Section 1.B. is the protection of the confidentiality of a patient's records. The statement in this section that relevant information in the records should be released to another dental practitioner assumes that the dentist requesting the information is the patient's present dentist. The former dentist should be free to provide the present dentist with relevant information from the patient's records. This may often be required for the protection of both the patient and the present dentist. There may be circumstances where the former dentist has an ethical obligation to inform the present dentist of certain facts. Dentists should be aware, however, that the laws of the various jurisdictions in the United States are not uniform, and some confidentiality laws appear to prohibit the transfer of pertinent information, such as HIV seropositivity. Absent certain knowledge that the laws of the dentist's jurisdiction permit the forwarding of this information, a dentist should obtain the patient's written permission before forwarding health records which contain information of a sensitive nature, such as HIV seropositivity, chemical dependency, or sexual preference. If it is necessary for a treating dentist to consult with another dentist or physician with respect to the patient, and the circumstances do not permit the patient to remain anonymous, the treating dentist should seek the permission of the patient prior to the release of data from the patient's records to the consulting practitioner. If the patient refuses, the treating dentist should then contemplate obtaining legal advice regarding the termination of the dentist/patient relationship.

Section 2—PRINCIPLE: NONMALEFICENCE ("do no harm"). The dentist has a duty to refrain from harming the patient.

This principle expresses the concept that professionals have a duty to protect the patient from harm. Under this principle, the dentist's primary obligations include keeping knowledge and skills current, knowing one's own limitations and when to refer to a specialist or other professional, and knowing when and under what circumstances delegation of patient care to auxiliaries is appropriate.

CODE OF PROFESSIONAL CONDUCT

2.A. EDUCATION.

The privilege of dentists to be accorded professional status rests primarily in the knowledge, skill, and experience with which they serve their patients and society. All dentists, therefore, have the obligation of keeping their knowledge and skill current.

2.B. CONSULTATION AND REFERRAL.

Dentists shall be obliged to seek consultation, if possible, whenever the welfare of patients will be safeguarded or advanced by utilizing those who have special skills, knowledge, and experience. When patients visit or are referred to specialists or consulting dentists for consultation:

1. The specialists or consulting dentists upon completion of their care shall return the patient, unless the patient expressly reveals a different preference, to the referring dentist, or, if none, to the dentist of record for future care.

2. The specialists shall be obliged when there is no referring dentist and upon a completion of their treatment to inform patients when there is a need for further dental care.

ADVISORY OPINION

2.B.1. SECOND OPINIONS. A dentist who has a patient referred by a third party for a "second opinion" regarding a diagnosis or treatment plan recommended by the patient's treating dentist should render the requested second opinion in accordance with this Code of Ethics. In the interest of the patient being afforded quality care, the dentist rendering the second opinion should not have a vested interest in the ensuing recommendation.

2.C. USE OF AUXILIARY PERSONNEL.

Dentists shall be obliged to protect the health of their patients by only assigning to qualified auxiliaries those duties which can be legally delegated. Dentists shall be further obliged to prescribe and supervise the patient care provided by all auxiliary personnel working under their direction.

2.D. PERSONAL IMPAIRMENT.

It is unethical for a dentist to practice while abusing controlled substances, alcohol, or other chemical agents which impair the ability to practice. All dentists have an ethical obligation to urge chemically impaired colleagues to seek treatment. Dentists with first-hand knowledge that a colleague is practicing dentistry when so impaired have an ethical responsibility to report such evidence to the professional assistance committee of a dental society.

ADVISORY OPINION

2.D.1. ABILITY TO PRACTICE. A dentist who becomes ill from any disease or impaired in any way shall, with consultation and advice from a qualified physician or other authority, limit the activities of practice to those areas that do not endanger the patients or members of the dental staff.

Section 3—PRINCIPLE: BENEFICENCE ("do good"). The dentist has a duty to promote the patient's welfare.

This principle expresses the concept that professionals have a duty to act for the benefit of others. Under this principle, the dentist's primary obligation is service to the patient and the public-at-large. The most important aspect of this obligation is the competent and timely delivery of dental care within the bounds of clinical circumstances presented by the patient, with due consideration being given to the needs, desires, and values of the patient. The same ethical considerations apply whether the dentist engages in fee-for-service, managed care, or some other practice arrangement. Dentists may choose to enter into contracts governing the provision of care to a group of patients; however, contract obligations do not excuse dentists from their ethical duty to put the patient's welfare first.

CODE OF PROFESSIONAL CONDUCT

3.A. COMMUNITY SERVICE.

Since dentists have an obligation to use their skills, knowledge, and experience for the improvement of the dental health of the public and are encouraged to be leaders in their community, dentists in such service shall conduct themselves in such a manner as to maintain or elevate the esteem of the profession.

3.B. GOVERNMENT OF A PROFESSION.

Every profession owes society the responsibility to regulate itself. Such regulation is achieved largely through the influence of the professional societies. All dentists, therefore, have the dual obligation of making themselves a part of a professional society and of observing its rules of ethics.

3.C. RESEARCH AND DEVELOPMENT.

Dentists have the obligation of making the results and benefits of their investigative efforts available to all when they are useful in safeguarding or promoting the health of the public.

3.D. PATENTS AND COPYRIGHTS.

Patents and copyrights may be secured by dentists provided that such patents and copyrights shall not be used to restrict research or practice.

3.E. CHILD ABUSE.

Dentists shall be obliged to become familiar with the perioral signs of child abuse and to report suspected cases to the proper authorities consistent with state laws.

Section 4—PRINCIPLE: JUSTICE ("fairness"). The dentist has a duty to treat people fairly.

This principle expresses the concept that professionals have a duty to be fair in their dealings with patients, colleagues, and society. Under this principle, the dentist's primary obligations include dealing with people justly and delivering dental care without prejudice. In its broadest sense, this principle expresses the concept that the dental profession should actively seek allies throughout society on specific activities that will help improve access to care for all.

CODE OF PROFESSIONAL CONDUCT

4.A. PATIENT SELECTION.

While dentists, in serving the public, may exercise reasonable discretion in selecting patients for their practices, dentists shall not refuse to accept patients into their practice or deny dental service to patients because of the patient's race, creed, color, sex, or national origin.

ADVISORY OPINION

4.A.1. HIV-POSITIVE PATIENTS. A dentist has the general obligation to provide care to those in need. A decision not to provide treatment to an individual because the individual has AIDS or is HIV seropositive, based solely on that fact, is unethical. Decisions with regard to the type of dental treatment provided or referrals made or suggested, in such instances should be made on the same basis as they are made with other patients, that is, whether the individual dentist believes he or she has need of another's skills, knowledge, equipment, or experience and whether the dentist believes, after consultation with the patient's physician if appropriate, the patient's health status would be significantly compromised by the provision of dental treatment.

4.B. EMERGENCY SERVICE.

Dentists shall be obliged to make reasonable arrangements for the emergency care of their patients of record. Dentists shall be obliged when consulted in an emergency by patients not of record to make reasonable arrangements for emergency care. If treatment is provided, the dentist, upon completion of treatment, is obliged to return the patient to his or her regular dentist unless the patient expressly reveals a different preference.

4.C. JUSTIFIABLE CRITICISM.

Dentists shall be obliged to report to the appropriate reviewing agency as determined by the local component or constituent society instances of gross or continual faulty treatment by other dentists. Patients should be informed of their present oral health status without disparaging comment about prior services. Dentists issuing a public statement with respect to the profession shall have a reasonable basis to believe that the comments made are true.

ADVISORY OPINION

4.C.1. MEANING OF "JUSTIFIABLE." A dentist's duty to the public imposes a responsibility to report instances of gross or continual faulty treatment. However, the heading of this section is "Justifiable Criticism." Therefore, when informing a patient of the status of his or her oral health, the dentist should exercise care that the contents made are justifiable. For example, a difference of opinion as to preferred treatment should not be communicated to the patient in a manner which would imply mistreatment. There will necessarily be cases where it will be difficult to determine whether the comments made are justifiable. Therefore, this section is phrased to address the discretion of dentists and advises against disparaging statements against another dentist. However, it should be noted that, where contents are made which are obviously not supportable and therefore unjustified, such comments can be the basis for the institution of a disciplinary proceeding against the dentist making such statements.

4.D. EXPERT TESTIMONY.

Dentists may provide expert testimony when that testimony is essential to a just and fair disposition of a judicial or administrative action.

ADVISORY OPINION

4.D.1. CONTINGENT FEES. It is unethical for a dentist to agree to a fee contingent upon the favorable outcome of the litigation in exchange for testifying as a dental expert.

4.E. REBATES AND SPLIT FEES.

Dentists shall not accept or tender "rebates" or "split fees."

Section 5—PRINCIPLE: VERACITY ("truthfulness"). The dentist has a duty to communicate truthfully.

This principle expresses the concept that professionals have a duty to be honest and trustworthy in their dealings with people. Under this principle, the dentist's primary obligations include respecting the position of trust inherent in the dentist-patient relationship, communicating truthfully and without deception, and maintaining intellectual integrity.

CODE OF PROFESSIONAL CONDUCT

5.A. REPRESENTATION OF CARE.

Dentists shall not represent the care being rendered to their patients in a false or misleading manner.

ADVISORY OPINIONS

5.A.1. DENTAL AMALGAM. Based on available scientific data the ADA has determined through the adoption of Resolution 42H-1986 (Trans.1986:536) that the removal of amalgam restorations from the non-allergic patient for the alleged purpose of removing toxic substances from the body, when such treatment is performed solely at the recommendation or suggestion of the dentist, is improper and unethical.

5.A.2. UNSUBSTANTIATED REPRESENTATIONS. A dentist who represents that dental treatment recommended or performed by the dentist has the capacity to cure or alleviate diseases, infections, or other conditions, when such representations are not based upon accepted scientific knowledge or research, is acting unethically.

5.B. REPRESENTATION OF FEES.
Dentists shall not represent the fees being charged for providing care in a false or misleading manner.

ADVISORY OPINIONS

5.B.1. WAIVER OF COPAYMENT. A dentist who accepts a third party* payment under a copayment plan as payment in full without disclosing to the third party* that the patient's payment portion will not be collected, is engaged in overbilling. The essence of this ethical impropriety is deception and misrepresentation; an overbilling dentist makes it appear to the third party* that the charge to the patient for services rendered is higher than it actually is.

5.B.2. OVERBILLING. It is unethical for a dentist to increase a fee to a patient solely because the patient has insurance.

5.B.3. FEE DIFFERENTIAL. Payments accepted by a dentist under a governmentally funded program, a component or constituent dental society sponsored access program, or a participating agreement entered into under a program of a third party* shall not be considered as evidence of overbilling in determining whether a charge to a patient, or to another third party* in behalf of a patient not covered under any of the aforecited programs constitutes overbilling under this section of the Code.

5.B.4. TREATMENT DATES. A dentist who submits a claim form to a third party* reporting incorrect treatment dates for the purpose of assisting a patient in obtaining benefits under a dental plan, which benefits would otherwise be disallowed, is engaged in making an unethical, false, or misleading representation to such third party.*

5.B.5. DENTAL PROCEDURES. A dentist who incorrectly describes on a third party* claim form a dental procedure in order to receive a greater payment or reimbursement or incorrectly makes a non-covered procedure appear to be a covered procedure on such a claim form is engaged in making an unethical, false, or misleading representation to such third party.*

5.B.6. UNNECESSARY SERVICES. A dentist who recommends and performs unnecessary dental services or procedures is engaged in unethical conduct.

*A third party is any party to a dental prepayment contract that may collect premiums, assume financial risks, pay claims, and/or provide administrative services.

5.C. DISCLOSURE OF CONFLICT OF INTEREST.

A dentist who presents educational or scientific information in an article, seminar, or other program shall disclose to the readers or participants any monetary or other special interest the dentist may have with a company whose products are promoted or endorsed in the presentation. Disclosure shall be made in any promotional material and in the presentation itself.

5.D. DEVICES AND THERAPEUTIC METHODS.

Except for formal investigative studies, dentists shall be obliged to prescribe, dispense, or promote only those devices, drugs, and other agents whose complete formulae are available to the dental profession. Dentists shall have the further obligation of not holding out as exclusive any device, agent, method, or technique if that representation would be false or misleading in any material respect.

ADVISORY OPINIONS

5.D.1. REPORTING ADVERSE REACTIONS. A dentist who suspects the occurrence of an adverse reaction to a drug or dental device has an obligation to communicate that information to the broader medical and dental community, including, in the case of a serious adverse event, the Food and Drug Administration (FDA).

5.D.2. SALE OF PRODUCTS. Dentists who engage in the sale of dental products to their patients must take care not to exploit the trust inherent in the dentist-patient relationship for their own financial gain. Dentists should not induce their patients to buy a dental product by misrepresenting the product's therapeutic value. It is not enough for the dentist to rely on the manufacturer's representations about a product's safety and efficacy. The dentist has an independent obligation to enquire into the truth and accuracy of the manufacturer's claims and verify that they are founded on accepted scientific knowledge or research. Dentists should disclose to their patients all relevant information the patient needs to make an informed purchase decision, including whether the product is available elsewhere.

5.E. PROFESSIONAL ANNOUNCEMENT.

In order to properly serve the public, dentists should represent themselves in a manner that contributes to the esteem of the profession. Dentists should not misrepresent their training and competence in any way that would be false or misleading in any material respect.*

5.F. ADVERTISING.

Although any dentist may advertise, no dentist shall advertise or solicit patients in any form of communication in a manner that is false or misleading in any material respect.*

ADVISORY OPINIONS

5.F.1. ARTICLES AND NEWSLETTERS. If a dental health article, message, or newsletter is published under a dentist's byline to the public without making truthful disclosure of the source and authorship or is designed to give rise to questionable expectations for the purpose of inducing the public to utilize the services of the sponsoring dentist, the dentist is engaged in making a false or misleading representation to the public in a material respect.

5.F.2. EXAMPLES OF "FALSE OR MISLEADING." The following examples are set forth to provide insight into the meaning of the term "false or misleading in a material respect." These examples are not meant to be all-inclusive. Rather, by restating the concept in alternative language and giving general examples, it is hoped that the membership will gain a better understanding of the term. With this in mind, statements shall be avoided which would: a) contain a material misrepresentation of fact, b) omit a fact necessary to make the statement considered as a whole not materially misleading, c) be intended or be likely to create an unjustified expectation about results the dentist can achieve, and d) contain a material, objective representation, whether express or implied, that the advertised services are superior in quality to those of other dentists, if that representation is not subject to reasonable substantiation.

Subjective statements about the quality of dental services can also raise ethical concerns. In particular, statements of opinion may be misleading if they are not honestly held, if they misrepresent the qualifications of the holder or the basis of the opinion, or if the patient reasonably interprets them as implied statements of fact. Such statements will be evaluated on a case by case basis, considering how patients are likely to respond to the impression made by the advertisement as a whole. The fundamental issue is whether the advertisement, taken as a whole, is false or misleading in a material respect.

5.F.3. UNEARNED, NONHEALTH DEGREES. The use of an unearned or nonhealth degree in any general announcements to the public by a dentist may be a representation to the public which is false or misleading in a material respect. A dentist may use the title Doctor, Dentist, DDS, or DMD, or any additional earned advanced degrees in health service areas. The use of unearned or nonhealth degrees could be misleading because of the likelihood that it will indicate to the public the attainment of a specialty or diplomats status.

For purposes of this advisory opinion, an unearned academic degree is one which is awarded by an educational institution not accredited by a generally recognized accrediting body or is an honorary degree. Generally, the use of honorary degrees or nonhealth degrees should be limited to scientific papers and curriculum vitae. In all instances state law should be consulted. In any review by the council of the use of nonhealth degrees or honorary degrees the council will apply the standard of whether the use of such is false or misleading in a material respect.

5.F.4. FELLOWSHIPS. A dentist using the attainment of a fellowship in a direct advertisement to the general public may be making a representation to the public which is false or misleading in a material respect. Such use of a fellowship status may be misleading because of the likelihood that it will indicate to the dental consumer the attainment of a specialty status. However, when such use does not conflict with state law, the attainment of fellowship status may be indicated in scientific papers, curriculum vitae, third party payment forms, and letterhead and stationery which is not used for the direct solicitation of patients. In any review by the council of the use of the attainment of fellowship status, the council will apply the standard of whether the use of such is false or misleading in a material respect.

5.F.5. REFERRAL SERVICES. There are two basic types of referral services for dental care: not-for-profit and the commercial. The not-for-profit is commonly organized by dental societies or community services. It is open to all qualified practitioners in the area served. A fee is sometimes charged the practitioner to be listed with the service. A fee for such referral services is for the purpose of covering the expenses of the service and has no relation to the number of patients referred. In contrast, some commercial referral services restrict access to the referral service to a limited number of dentists in a particular geographic area. Prospective patients calling the service may be referred to a single subscribing dentist in the geographic area and the respective dentist billed for each patient referred. Commercial referral services often advertise to the public stressing that there is no charge for use of the service and the patient may not be informed of the referral fee paid by the dentist. There is a connotation to such advertisements that the referral that is being made is in the nature of a public service. A dentist is allowed to pay for any advertising permitted by the Code, but is generally not permitted to make payments to another person or entity for the referral of a patient for professional services. While the particular facts and circumstances relating to an individual commercial referral service will vary, the council believes that the aspects outlined above for commercial referral services violate the Code in that it constitutes advertising which is false or misleading in a material respect and violates the prohibitions in the Code against fee splitting.

5.F.6. HIV TEST RESULTS. An advertisement or other communication intended to solicit patients which omits a material fact or facts necessary to put the information conveyed in the advertisement in a proper context can be misleading in a material respect. An advertisement to the public of HIV negative test results, without conveying additional information that will clarify the scientific significance of this fact, is an example of a misleading omission. A dental practice should not seek to attract patients on the basis of partial truths which create a false impression.

5.G. NAME OF PRACTICE.

Since the name under which a dentist conducts his or her practice may be a factor in the selection process of the patient, the use of a trade name or an assumed name that is false or misleading in any material respect is unethical. Use of the name of a dentist no longer actively associated with the practice may be continued for a period not to exceed one year. *

ADVISORY OPINION

5.G.1. DENTIST LEAVING PRACTICE. Dentists leaving a practice who authorize continued use of their names should receive competent advice on the legal implications of this action. With permission of a departing dentist, his or her name may be used for more than one year, if, after the one year grace period has expired, prominent notice is provided to the public through such mediums as a sign at the office and a short statement on stationery and business cards that the departing dentist has retired from the practice.

5.H. ANNOUNCEMENT OF SPECIALIZATION AND LIMITATION OF PRACTICE. This section and Section 5-I are designed to help the public make an informed selection between the practitioner who has completed an accredited program beyond the dental degree and a practitioner who has not completed such a program. The special areas of dental practice approved by the American Dental Association and the designation for ethical specialty announcement and limitation of practice are: dental public health, endodontics, oral and maxillofacial pathology, oral and maxillofacial surgery, orthodontics and dentofacial orthopedics, pediatric dentistry, periodontics, and prosthodontics. Dentists who choose to announce specialization should use "specialist in" or "practice limited to" and shall limit their practice exclusively to the announced special area(s) of dental practice, provided at the time of the announcement such dentists have met in each approved specialty for which they announce the existing educational requirements and standards set forth by the American Dental Association. Dentists who use their eligibility to announce as specialists to make the public believe that specialty services rendered in the dental office are being rendered by qualified specialists when such is not the case are engaged in unethical conduct. The burden of responsibility is on specialists to avoid any inference that general practitioners who are associated with specialists are qualified to announce themselves as specialists.

GENERAL STANDARDS.

The following are included within the standards of the American Dental Association for determining the education, experience, and other appropriate requirements for announcing specialization and limitation of practice:

1. The special area(s) of dental practice and an appropriate certifying board must be approved by the American Dental Association.

2. Dentists who announce as specialists must have successfully completed an educational program accredited by the Commission on Dental Accreditation, two or more years in length, as specified by the Council on Dental Education, or be diplomates of an American Dental Association recognized certifying board. The scope of the individual specialist's practice shall be governed by the educational standards for the specialty in which the specialist is announcing.

3. The practice carried on by dentists who announce as specialists shall be limited exclusively to the special area(s) of dental practices announced by the dentist.

STANDARDS FOR MULTIPLE-SPECIALTY ANNOUNCEMENTS.

Educational criteria for announcement by dentists in additional recognized specialty areas are the successful completion of an educational program accredited by the Commission on Dental Accreditation in each area for which the dentist wishes to announce. Dentists who completed their advanced education in programs listed by the Council on Dental Education prior to the initiation of the accreditation process in 1967 and who are currently ethically announcing as specialists in a recognized area may announce in additional areas provided they are educationally qualified or are certified diplomates in each area for which they wish to announce. Documentation of successful completion of the educational program(s) must be submitted to the appropriate constituent society. The documentation must assure that the duration of the program(s) is a minimum of two years except for oral and maxillofacial surgery which must have been a minimum of three years in duration.*

ADVISORY OPINIONS

5.H.1. DIPLOMATE STATUS. A dentist who announces in any means of communication with patients or the general public that he or she is certified or a diplomate in an area not recognized by the American Dental Association or the law of the jurisdiction where the dentist practices as a specialty area of dentistry is engaged in making a false representation to the public in a material respect.

5.H.2. DUAL DEGREED DENTISTS. Nothing in Section 5.H. shall be interpreted to prohibit a dual degreed dentist who practices medicine or osteopathy under a valid state license from announcing to the public as dental specialist provided the dentist meets the educational, experience, and other standards set forth in the Code for specialty announcement and further providing that the announcement is truthful and not materially misleading.

5.I. GENERAL PRACTITIONER ANNOUNCEMENT OF SERVICES.

General dentists who wish to announce the services available in their practices are permitted to announce the availability of those services so long as they avoid any communications that express or imply specialization. General dentists shall also state that the services are being provided by general dentists. No dentist shall announce available services in any way that would be false or misleading in any material respect.*

*Advertising, solicitation of patients or business, or other promotional activities by dentists or dental care delivery organizations shall not be considered unethical or improper, except for those promotional activities which are false or misleading in any material respect. Notwithstanding any *ADA Principles of Ethics and Code of Professional Conduct* or other standards of dentist conduct which may be differently worded, this shall be the sole standard for determining the ethical propriety of such promotional activities. Any provision of an ADA constituent or component society's code of ethics or other standard of dentist conduct relating to dentists' or dental care delivery organizations' advertising, solicitation, or other promotional activities which is worded differently from the above standard shall be deemed to be in conflict with the *ADA Principles of Ethics and Code of Professional Conduct*.

IV. INTERPRETATION AND APPLICATION OF PRINCIPLES OF ETHICS AND CODE OF PROFESSIONAL CONDUCT.

The foregoing *ADA Principles of Ethics and Code of Professional Conduct* set forth the ethical duties that are binding on members of the American Dental Association. The component and constituent societies may adopt additional requirements or interpretations not in conflict with the *ADA Code*.

Anyone who believes that a member-dentist has acted unethically may bring the matter to the attention of the appropriate constituent (state) or component (local) dental society. Whenever possible, problems involving questions of ethics should be resolved at the state or local level. If a satisfactory resolution cannot be reached, the dental society may decide, after proper investigation, that the matter warrants issuing formal charges and conducting a disciplinary hearing pursuant to the procedures set forth in the ADA Bylaws, Chapter XII. *Principles of Ethics and Code of Professional Conduct and Judicial Procedure*. The Council on Ethics, Bylaws, and Judicial Affairs reminds constituent and component societies that before a dentist can be found to have breached any ethical obligation the dentist is entitled to a fair hearing.

A member who is found guilty of unethical conduct proscribed by the *ADA Code* or code of ethics of the constituent or component society, may be placed under a sentence of censure or suspension or may be expelled from membership in the Association. A member under a sentence of censure, suspension, or expulsion has the right to appeal the decision to his or her constituent society and the ADA Council on Ethics, Bylaws, and Judicial Affairs, as provided in Chapter XII of the ADA Bylaws.

American Dental Association Council on Ethics, Bylaws, and Judicial Affairs
211 East Chicago Avenue
Chicago, Illinois 60611

With official advisory opinions revised to October 1996.

(Reprinted with permission from the American Dental Association.)

AMERICAN OCCUPATIONAL THERAPY ASSOCIATION CODE OF ETHICS

The American Occupational Therapy Association's Code of Ethics is a public statement of the values and principles used in promoting and maintaining high standards of behavior in occupational therapy. The American Occupational Therapy Association and its members are committed to furthering people's ability to function within their total environment. To this end, occupational therapy personnel provide services for individuals in any stage of health and illness, to institutions, to other professionals and colleagues, to students, and to the general public.

The Occupational Therapy Code of Ethics is a set of principles that applies to occupational therapy personnel at all levels. The roles of practitioner (registered occupational therapist and certified occupational therapy assistant), educator, fieldwork educator, supervisor, administrator, consultant, fieldwork coordinator, faculty program director, researcher/scholar, entrepreneur, student, support staff, and occupational therapy aide are assumed.

Any action that is in violation of the spirit and purpose of this Code shall be considered unethical. To ensure compliance with the Code, enforcement procedures are established and maintained by the Commission on Standards and Ethics. Acceptance of membership in the American Occupational Therapy Association commits members to adherence to the Code of Ethics and its enforcement procedures.

Principle 1 (Beneficence)

Occupational therapy personnel shall demonstrate a concern for the well-being of the recipients of their services.

    A. Occupational therapy personnel shall provide services in an equitable manner for all individuals.

    B. Occupational therapy personnel shall maintain relationships that do not exploit the recipient of services sexually, physically, emotionally, financially, socially, or in any other manner. Occupational therapy personnel shall avoid those relationships or activities that interfere with professional judgment and objectivity.

    C. Occupational therapy personnel shall take all reasonable precautions to avoid harm to the recipient of services or to his or her property.

    D. Occupational therapy personnel shall strive to ensure that fees are fair, reasonable, and commensurate with the service performed and are set with due regard for the service recipient's ability to pay.

Principle 2 (Autonomy, Privacy, Confidentiality)

Occupational therapy personnel shall respect the rights of the recipients of their services.

    A. Occupational therapy personnel shall collaborate with service recipients or their surrogate(s) in determining goals and priorities throughout the intervention process.

    B. Occupational therapy personnel shall fully inform the service recipients of the nature, risks, and potential outcomes of any interventions.

    C. Occupational therapy personnel shall obtain informed consent from subjects involved in research activities indicating they have been fully advised of the potential risks and outcomes.

    D. Occupational therapy personnel shall respect the individual's right to refuse professional services or involvement in research or educational activities.

    E. Occupational therapy personnel shall protect the confidential nature of information gained from educational, practice, research, and investigational activities.

Principle 3 (Duties)

Occupational therapy personnel shall achieve and continually maintain high standards of competence.

    A. Occupational therapy personnel shall hold the appropriate national and state credentials for providing services.

    B. Occupational therapy personnel shall use procedures that conform to the Standards of Practice of the American Occupational Therapy Association.

   C. Occupational therapy personnel shall take responsibility for maintaining competence by participating in professional development and educational activities.

   D. Occupational therapy personnel shall perform their duties on the basis of accurate and current information.

   E. Occupational therapy personnel shall protect service recipients by ensuring that duties assumed by or assigned to other occupational therapy personnel are commensurate with their qualifications and experience.

   F. Occupational therapy personnel shall provide appropriate supervision to individuals for whom the practitioners have supervisory responsibility.

   G. Occupational therapists shall refer recipients to other service providers or consult with other service providers when additional knowledge and expertise are required.

Principle 4 (Justice)

Occupational therapy personnel shall comply with laws and Association policies guiding the profession of occupational therapy.

   A. Occupational therapy personnel shall understand and abide by applicable Association policies; local, state, and federal laws; and institutional rules.

   B. Occupational therapy personnel shall inform employers, employees, and colleagues about those laws and Association policies that apply to the profession of occupational therapy.

   C. Occupational therapy practitioners shall require those they supervise in occupational therapy related activities to adhere to the Code of Ethics.

   D. Occupational therapy personnel shall accurately record and report all information related to professional activities.

Principle 5 (Veracity)

Occupational therapy personnel shall provide accurate information about occupational therapy services.

   A. Occupational therapy personnel shall accurately represent their qualifications, education, experience, training, and competence.

   B. Occupational therapy personnel shall disclose any affiliations that may pose a conflict of interest.

   C. Occupational therapy personnel shall refrain from using or participating in the use of any form of communication that contains false, fraudulent, deceptive, or unfair statements or claims.

Principle 6 (Fidelity, Veracity)

Occupational therapy personnel shall treat colleagues and other professionals with fairness, discretion, and integrity.

   A. Occupational therapy personnel shall safeguard confidential information about colleagues and staff.

   B. Occupational therapy personnel shall accurately represent the qualifications, views, contributions, and findings of colleagues.

   C. Occupational therapy personnel shall report any breaches of the Code of Ethics to the appropriate authority.

(Reprinted with permission from the American Occupational Therapy Association, Inc., copyright AOTA.)

A PATIENT'S BILL OF RIGHTS
AMERICAN HOSPITAL ASSOCIATION

Patient and Community Relations

Introduction:

Effective health care requires collaboration between patients and physicians and other health care professionals. Open and honest communication, respect for personal and professional values, and sensitivity to differences are integral to optimal patient care. As the setting for the provision of health services, hospitals must provide a foundation for understanding and respecting the rights and responsibilities of patients, their families, physicians, and other caregivers. Hospitals must ensure a health care ethic that respects the role of patients in decision making about treatment choices and other aspects of their care. Hospitals must be sensitive to cultural, racial, linguistic, religious, age, gender, and other differences as well as the needs of persons with disabilities.

The American Hospital Association presents *A Patient's Bill of Rights* with the expectation that it will contribute to more effective patient care and be supported by the hospital on behalf of the institution, its medical staff, employees, and patients. The American Hospital Association encourages health care institutions to tailor this bill of rights to their patient community by translating and/or simplifying the language of this bill of rights as may be necessary to ensure that patients and their families understand their rights and responsibilities.

Bill of Rights:

1. The patient has the right to considerate and respectful care.

2. The patient has the right and is encouraged to obtain from physicians and other direct caregivers relevant, current, and understandable information concerning diagnosis, treatment, and prognosis.
   Except in emergencies when the patient lacks decision-making capacity and the need for treatment is urgent, the patient is entitled to the opportunity to discuss and request information related to the specific procedures and/or treatments, the risks involved, the possible length of recuperation, and the medically reasonable alternatives and their accompanying risks and benefits.
   Patients have the right to know the identity of physicians, nurses, and others involved in their care, as well as when those involved are students, residents, or other trainees. The patient also has the right to know the immediate and long-term financial implications of treatment choices, insofar as they are known.

3. The patient has the right to make decisions about the plan of care prior to and during the course of treatment and to refuse a recommended treatment or plan of care to the extent permitted by law and hospital policy and to be informed of the medical consequences of this action. In case of such refusal, the patient is entitled to other appropriate care and services that the hospital provides or transfer to another hospital. The hospital should notify patients of any policy that might affect patient choice within the institution.

4. The patient has the right to have an advance directive (such as a living will, health care proxy, or durable power of attorney for health care) concerning treatment or designating a surrogate decision maker with the expectation that the hospital will honor the intent of that directive to the extent permitted by law and hospital policy. Health care institutions must advise patients of their rights under state law and hospital policy to make informed medical choices, ask if the patient has an advance directive, and include that information in patient records. The patient has the right to timely information about hospital policy that may limit its ability to implement fully a legally valid advance directive.

5. The patient has the right to every consideration of privacy. Case discussion, consultation, examination, and treatment should be conducted so as to protect each patient's privacy.

6. The patient has the right to expect that all communications and records pertaining to her or his care will be treated as confidential by the hospital, except in cases such as suspected abuse and public health hazards when reporting is permitted or required by law. The patient has the right to expect that the hospital will emphasize the confidentiality of this information when it releases it to any other parties entitled to review information in these records.

7. The patient has the right to review the records pertaining to her or his medical care and to have the information explained or interpreted as necessary, except when restricted by law.

8. The patient has the right to expect that, within its capacity and policies, a hospital will make reasonable response to the request of a patient for appropriate and medically indicated care and services. The hospital must provide evaluation, service, and/or referral as indicated by the urgency of the case. When medically appropriate and legally permissible, or when a patient has so requested, a patient may be transferred to another facility. The institution to which the patient is to be transferred must first have accepted the patient for transfer. The patient must also have the benefit of complete information and explanation concerning the need for risks, benefits, and alternatives to such a transfer.

9. The patient has the right to ask and be informed of the existence of business relationships among the hospital, educational institutions, other health care providers, or payers that may influence the patient's treatment and care.

10. The patient has the right to consent to or decline to participate in proposed research studies or human experimentation affecting care and treatment or requiring direct patient involvement, and to have those studies fully explained prior to consent. A patient who declines to participate in research or experimentation is entitled to the most effective care that the hospital can otherwise provide.

11. The patient has the right to expect reasonable continuity of care when appropriate and to be informed by physicians and other caregivers of available and realistic patient care options when hospital care is no longer appropriate.

12. The patient has the right to be informed of hospital policies and practices that relate to patient care, treatment, and responsibilities. The patient has the right to be informed of available resources for resolving disputes, grievances, and conflicts, such as ethics committees, patient representatives, or other mechanisms available in the

institution. The patient has the right to be informed of the hospital's charges for services and available payment methods.

The collaborative nature of health care requires that patients, or their families or surrogates, participate in their care. The effectiveness of care and patient satisfaction with the course of treatment depend, in part, on the patient fulfilling certain responsibilities. Patients are responsible for providing information about past illnesses, hospitalizations, medications, and other matters related to health status. To participate effectively in decision making, patients must be encouraged to take responsibility for requesting additional information or clarification about their health status or treatment when they do not fully understand information and instructions. Patients are also responsible for ensuring that the health care institution has a copy of their written advance directive if they have one. Patients are responsible for informing their physicians and other caregivers if they anticipate problems in following prescribed treatment.

Patients should also be aware of the hospital's obligation to be reasonably efficient and equitable in providing care to other patients and the community. The hospital's rules and regulations are designed to help the hospital meet this obligation. Patients and their families are responsible for making reasonable accommodations to the needs of the hospital, other patients, medical staff, and hospital employees. Patients are responsible for providing necessary information for insurance claims and for working with the hospital to make payment arrangements, when necessary.

A person's health depends on much more than health care services. Patients are responsible for recognizing the impact of their lifestyle on their personal health.

CONCLUSION

Hospitals have many functions to perform, including the enhancement of health status, health promotion, and the prevention and treatment of injury and disease; the immediate and ongoing care and rehabilitation of patients; the education of health professionals, patients, and the community; and research. All these activities must be conducted with an overriding concern for the values and dignity of patients.

(*Reprinted with permission of the American Hospital Association, copyright 1992.*)

THE HIPPOCRATIC OATH

I swear by Apollo, the Physician, by Asclepius, by Hygieia, Panacea, and all the gods and goddesses, making them my witnesses, that I will fulfil according to my ability and judgement this oath and covenant.

To hold him who has taught me this art as equal to my parents and to live my life in partnership with him, and if he is in need of money to give him a share of mine, and to regard his offspring as equal to my brothers in male lineage and to teach them this art—if they desire to learn it—without fee and covenant; to give a share of precepts and oral instruction and all the learning to my sons and to the sons of him who has instructed me and to pupils who have signed the covenant and have taken an oath according to the medical law, but to no one else.

I will apply dietetic measures for the benefit of the sick according to my ability and judgement; I will keep them from harm and injustice.

I will neither give a deadly drug to anybody if asked for it, nor will I make a suggestion to this effect. Similarly I will not give to a woman an abortive remedy. In purity and holiness I will guard my life and my art.

I will not use the knife, not even on sufferers from stone, but will withdraw in favor of such men as are engaged in this work.

Whatever houses I may visit, I will come for the benefit of the sick, remaining free of all intentional injustices, of all mischief and in particular of sexual relations with both male and female persons, be they free or slaves.

What I may see or hear in the course of the treatment or even outside of the treatment in regard to the life of men, which on no account one must noise abroad, I will keep to myself holding such things shameful to be spoken about.

If I fulfill this oath and do not violate it, may it be granted to me to enjoy life and art, being honored with fame among all men for all time to come; if I transgress it and swear falsely, may the opposite of all this be my lot.

AMERICAN PHYSICAL THERAPY ASSOCIATION CODE OF ETHICS

Preamble

This Code of Ethics sets forth ethical principles for the physical therapy profession. Members of this profession are responsible for maintaining and promoting ethical practice. The Code of Ethics, adopted by the American Physical Therapy Association, shall be binding on physical therapists who are members of the Association.

Principle 1.	Physical therapists respect the rights and dignity of all individuals.
Principle 2.	Physical therapists comply with the laws and regulations governing the practice of physical therapy.
Principle 3.	Physical therapists accept responsibility for the exercise of sound judgment.
Principle 4.	Physical therapists maintain and promote high standards for physical therapy practice, education, and research.
Principle 5.	Physical therapists seek remuneration for their services that is deserved and reasonable.
Principle 6.	Physical therapists provide accurate information to the consumer about the profession and about those services they provide.
Principle 7.	Physical therapists accept responsibility to protect the public and the profession from unethical, incompetent, or illegal acts.
Principle 8.	Physical therapists participate in efforts to address the health needs of the public.

(Reprinted with permission from the American Physical Therapy Association.)

AMERICAN MEDICAL ASSOCIATION PRINCIPLES OF MEDICAL ETHICS

Preamble

The medical profession has long subscribed to a body of ethical statements developed primarily for the benefit of the patient. As a member of this profession, a physician must recognize responsibility not only to patients, but also to society, to other health professionals, and to self. The following principles adopted by the American Medical Association are not laws, but standards of conduct which define the essentials of honorable behavior for the physician.

1. A physician shall be dedicated to providing competent medical service with compassion and respect for human dignity.

2. A physician shall deal honestly with patients and colleagues, and strive to expose those physicians deficient in character or competence, or who engage in fraud or deception.

3. A physician shall respect the law and also recognize a responsibility to seek changes in those requirements which are contrary to the best interests of the patient.

4. A physician shall respect the rights of patients, of colleagues, and of other health professionals, and shall safeguard patient confidences within the constraints of the law.

5. A physician shall continue to study, apply and advance scientific knowledge, make relevant information available to patients, colleagues, and the public, obtain consultation, and use the talents of other health professionals when indicated.

6. A physician shall, in the provision of appropriate care, except in emergencies be free to choose whom to serve, with whom to associate, and the environment in which to provide medical services.

7. A physician shall recognize a responsibility to participate in activities contributing to an improved community.

(Reprinted with permission from the American Medical Association.)

AMERICAN ASSOCIATION FOR RESPIRATORY CARE CODE OF ETHICS

The principles set forth in this document define the basic ethical and moral standards to which each member of the American Association for Respiratory Care should conform.

1. Respiratory care practitioners shall practice medically acceptable methods of treatment and shall not endeavor to extend this practice beyond the competence and the authority invested in them by the physician.

2. Respiratory care practitioners shall continually strive to increase and improve their knowledge and skill and render to each patient the full measure of their ability. All services shall be provided with respect for the dignity of the patient, unrestricted by considerations of social or economic status, personal attributes, or the nature of the health problem.

3. Respiratory care practitioners shall be responsible for the competent and efficient performance of their assigned duties and shall expose incompetence and illegal or unethical conduct of members of the profession.

4. Respiratory care practitioners shall hold in strict confidence all privileged information concerning the patient and refer all inquiries to the physician in charge of the patient's care.

5. Respiratory care practitioners shall not accept gratuities for preferential consideration of the patient. They shall not solicit patients for personal gain and shall guard against conflicts of interest.

6. Respiratory care practitioners shall uphold the dignity and honor of the profession and abide by its ethical principles. They should be familiar with existing state and federal laws governing the practice of respiratory therapy and comply with those laws.

7. Respiratory care practitioners shall cooperate with other health care professionals to promote community and national efforts to meet the health needs of the public.

(Reprinted with permission from the American Association for Respiratory Care.)

AMERICAN NURSES ASSOCIATION CODE OF ETHICS

1. The nurse provides services with respect for human dignity and the uniqueness of the client, unrestricted by considerations of social or economic status, personal attributes, or the nature of health problems.

2. The nurse safeguards the client's right to privacy by judiciously protecting information of a confidential nature.

3. The nurse acts to safeguard the client and the public when health care and safety are affected by the incompetent, or illegal practice of any person.

4. The nurse assumes responsibility and accountability for individual nursing judgments and actions.

5. The nurse maintains competence in nursing.

6. The nurse exercises informed judgment and uses individual competence and qualifications as criteria in seeking consultation, accepting responsibilities, and delegating nursing activities to others.

7. The nurse participates in activities that contribute to the ongoing development of the profession's body of knowledge.

8. The nurse participates in the profession's efforts to implement and improve standards of nursing.

9. The nurse participates in the profession's efforts to establish and maintain conditions of employment conducive to high-quality nursing care.

10. The nurse participates in the profession's efforts to protect the public from misinformation and misrepresentation and to maintain the integrity of nursing.

11. The nurse collaborates with members of the health professions and other citizens in promoting community and national efforts to meet the health needs of the public.

(Reprinted with permission from the American Nurses Association.)

CODE OF ETHICS OF THE PHYSICIAN ASSISTANT PROFESSION

The American Academy of Physician Assistants recognizes its responsibility to aid the profession in maintaining high standards in the provision of quality and accessible health care services. The following principles delineate the standards governing the conduct of physician assistants in their professional interactions with patients, colleagues, other health professionals, and the general public. Realizing that no code can encompass all ethical responsibilities of the physician assistant, this enumeration of obligations in the Code of Ethics is not comprehensive and does not constitute a denial of the existence of other obligations, equally imperative, though not specifically mentioned.

Physician Assistants shall be committed to providing competent medical care, assuming as their primary responsibility the health, safety, welfare, and dignity of all humans.

Physician Assistants shall extend to each patient the full measure of their ability as dedicated, empathetic health care providers and shall assume responsibility for the skillful and proficient transactions of their professional duties.

Physician Assistants shall deliver needed health care services to health consumers without regard to sex, age, race, creed, socioeconomic and political status.

Physician Assistants shall adhere to all state and federal laws governing informed consent concerning the patient's health care.

Physician Assistants shall seek consultation with their supervising physician, other health providers, or qualified professionals having special skills, knowledge, or experience whenever the welfare of the patient will be safeguarded or advanced by such consultation. Supervision should include ongoing communication between the physician and the physician assistant regarding the care of all patients.

Physician Assistants shall take personal responsibility for being familiar with and adhering to all federal/state laws applicable to the practice of their profession.

Physician Assistants shall provide only those services for which they are qualified via education and/or experiences and by pertinent legal regulatory process.

Physician Assistants shall not misrepresent in any manner, either directly or indirectly, their skills, training, professional credentials, identity, or services.

Physician Assistants shall uphold the doctrine of confidentiality regarding privileged patient information, unless required to release such information by law or such information becomes necessary to protect the welfare of the patient or the community.

Physician Assistants shall strive to maintain and increase the quality of individual health care service through individual study and continuing education.

Physician Assistants shall have the duty to respect the law, to uphold the dignity of the physician assistant profession, and to accept its ethical principles. The physician assistant shall not participate in or conceal any activity that will bring discredit or dishonor to the physician assistant profession and shall expose, without fear or favor, any illegal or unethical conduct in the medical profession.

Physician Assistants ever cognizant of the needs of the community, shall use the knowledge and experience acquired as professionals to contribute to an improved community.

Physician Assistants shall place service before material gain and must carefully guard against conflicts of professional interest.

Physician Assistants shall strive to maintain a spirit of cooperation with their professional organizations and the general public.

(Reprinted with permission from the American Academy of Physician Assistants.)

Glossary

abandoned: Once a patient-practitioner relationship is established, the health care services must continue or the practitioner may face legal action; that is, abandonment. The relationship may be discontinued only under specific circumstances.

abortifacient: A substance or device used to induce abortion.

abortion: Induced termination of pregnancy before the fetus is capable of survival as an individual.

abortionist: One who performs abortions.

acquittal: A release, absolution, or discharge from obligation, liability, or engagement.

action: In its usual legal sense, a suit to resolve a question of fact or a question of law.

actionable: That for which a legal action will lie, furnishing legal grounds for an action.

active euthanasia: See *euthanasia*.

act utilitarianism: The doctrine that skips any reference to principles and rules, and judges the right action as the one that provides the highest utility such as providing the greatest happiness to the greatest number. Happiness in utilitarian terms is defined in certain types of higher order pleasures such as intellectual aestheticism and social enjoyment, and in terms of minimal suffering.

ad litem: For purposes of litigation; for example, a guardian ad litem is a person given the power and duty to act in behalf of another person, legally incapacitated, for purposes of a lawsuit.

advanced directives: Documents expressing an individual's health care wishes in the event the person loses the ability to relate these matters independently.

agape: Love for humanity, love that is spiritual, not sexual in its nature.

agency: Relation in which one person acts for or represents another by latter's authority.

AIDS: Acquired immunodeficiency syndrome is generally accepted as a collection of specific, life-threatening opportunistic infections that result from an underlying immune deficiency caused by the HIV virus.

alegal: To be neither legal nor illegal. This usually pertains to new areas such as genetic research when the body of law is not complete.

alleged: Stated; recited; claimed; asserted; charged.

altruism: Concern for the welfare of others, selflessness.

251

amicus curiae: Friend of the court. A person with a strong interest in, or views on, the subject matter of an action may petition the court for permission to file a brief ostensibly on behalf of a party, but actually to suggest a rationale consistent with personal views. Such amicus curiae briefs are commonly filed in appeals concerning matters of a broad public interest.

amoral: To be without morals, neither moral nor immoral.

assault: A willful attempt or threat to inflict injury on another, coupled with an apparent present ability to inflict such injury.

assisted suicide: See *euthanasia*.

authentic: An authentic decision is one that is in keeping with the individual's past choices and known preferences.

autonomous: Independent, self-governing, self-determining.

battery: An intentional touching of another person without that person's consent.

beneficence: The principle that imposes upon the practitioner a duty to seek the good for any patient under all circumstances.

best interest standard: A proxy decision-making standard in which the guardian is directed to make the decision in the best interest of the individual. This is often used in cases when the individual was never in a position to make an autonomous decision.

biographical life: Life described by events, relationships, memories, desires, and wishes. Life that is uniquely individual and human.

biological life: That life that separates living from nonliving; for example, that which separates plants from

rocks. Life in this sense is not uniquely human but is that which we share with all other living things.

brain death: Irreversible cessation of all functions of the entire brain, including the brain stem. This is a totally unresponsive, irreversible state beyond coma.

capitation: Numeration by head or individuals. The system creates a fixed payment per patient.

categorical imperative: Under Kantan ethics, persons have duties to one another as moral agents and these duties take precedence over the consequences of any actions. Certain of the duties were considered universal truths which applied to all people for all times, in all situations. These maxims were tested as being "categorical imperatives" meaning they were found to have three elements: (1) universal application, (2) uncondionality, (3) demanding an action.

caveat aeger: Let the patient beware.

civil law: A body of law concerned with civil or private rights and remedies, as contrasted with criminal laws.

classism: The doctrine that holds that one particular social class of persons is superior to another.

clear and convincing evidence standard: A burden of proof which requires more than a preponderance of the evidence but less than a reasonable doubt. The burden requires that the truth of any facts asserted be highly probable. This has created a new emphasis on the need for advanced directives.

cognitive sapient state: A condition in which the individual has the ability to reason.

common law: As distinguished from law created by the enactment of legislatures, the common law comprises the body of those principles and rules of action relating to the government and security of persons and property. Common law derives its authority solely from usages and customs of immemorial antiquity, or from the judgments and decrees of the courts recognizing, affirming, and enforcing such usages and customs.

compensatory justice: The principle in which one is provided compensation for harm done. It is different from retribution, which calls for equal suffering.

competency: Having the ability to make sound, authentic judgments for oneself. Usually, it means that the patient is able to understand the nature of the condition, the options available, and the risks involved.

confidentiality: The principle that binds the practitioner to hold in strict confidence those things learned about a patient in the course of the provision of health care.

consequence-oriented system: An ethical system that believes the right action is one that maximizes some good. The right thing to do in the end is based on what is the good thing to do. One cannot know what is right without an examination of the consequences.

contract: An agreement between two or more persons that creates, modifies, or destroys an obligation to do something.

contractarian theory: A theory of morality that grounds all claims to rights in the principle of justice founded on collective choice. An individual's rights flow from the social contract with others in the society.

correlative obligations: In that rights are justified claims, they create obligations that are correlative to the claim; for example, the patient's right to autonomy creates the correlative obligation of disclosure (informed consent).

criminal law: That law which for the purposes of preventing harm to society (a) declares what conduct is criminal, and (b) prescribes the punishment to be imposed for such conduct. It includes the definition of specific offenses and general principles of liability.

defamation: Injury to a person's reputation or character caused by the false statements of another made to a third party. Defamation includes both libel and slander.

defendant: The person defending or denying; the party against whom relief or recovery is sought in an action; or the accused in a criminal case.

discovery: The ascertainment of that which was previously unknown through a practical investigation; it includes testimony documents that may be under the exclusive control of the other party.

disparagement: To belittle or criticize the skill, knowledge, or qualifications of another professional.

distributive justice: The principle that requires the fair distribution of scarce goods and services.

do-not-resuscitate (DNR) orders: Those orders issued when a determination is made that the level of life that could be sustained following a resuscitative effort would be such that it would not be in the patient's best interest to perform resuscitation.

double effect: A doctrine used to determine whether an action is morally defensible when the action selected has more than one consequence, usually both favorable and ill.

durable power of attorney: A legal instrument enabling an individual to act on another's behalf. This individual is empowered to make decisions for another should that person become unable to make decisions independently or at all. The durable power of attorney is one of the main forms of advanced directives.

duty-oriented systems: An ethical system in which the right action is one that is based on ethical principles that are known to be right, independent of whether they serve good ends.

egalitarianism: A system of allocation that seeks to provide all things equally.

egoism: An exaggerated love of self; refers all knowledge to the phenomena of personal existence.

egoist: One devoted to self-interest and self-advancement.

embryo: In humans, the prefetal product of conception up to the beginning of the third month of pregnancy.

"emergency exception": Hospitals have the right to refuse to extend services under most conditions, the major exception being if the patient is in an emergency situation.

entitlement programs: Government programs that provide benefits automatically to all individuals who qualify unless a change occurs in the underlying law. These programs may require an annual appropriation by Congress. Social Security and Medicare, for example, have autonomous trust funds that possess the authority to pay benefits without an annual appropriation.

equal consideration of interest: The rule that the interests of all individuals must be considered equally. This rule, if adopted, reduces the harm and scapegoatism possible in ethical systems such as utilitarianism.

ethics: Critical reflections about morality and the rational analysis of it. In some sense ethics is a generic term for the study of how we make judgments regarding right and wrong.

euthanasia: An act conducted for the purpose of causing the merciful death of another, usually of an individual suffering from an incurable condition or intractable pain. Over the last decade the following terms concerning euthanasia and assisted suicide have come into general usage.

voluntary euthanasia: To end personal suffering, the individual chooses to stop living. This can be with or without the assistance of others, but the choice is voluntary. Essentially this is the same as suicide.

involuntary euthanasia: In these cases individuals are put to death against their will. The individual bringing about the death does so to relieve the victims of suffering. Clearly, little difference exists between involuntary euthanasia and murder, and the individual involved would be prosecuted for murder.

nonvoluntary euthanasia: In these cases the individual is put to death without having given informed consent or indicating a decision either way in the matter. The intent is to relieve the deceased individual of suffering.

rational suicide: Refers to the suicide of a rational and competent adult who has decided that future prospects do not justify living.

irrational suicide: Refers to suicide by an individual whose depression, anger, fear, or emotional disorder do not allow for competent decision making.

assisted suicide: Suicide when the individual has assistance from others.

passive euthanasia: Ceasing therapies that prolong life so that death can occur.

active euthanasia: Actively assisting the process of death.

indirect euthanasia: Refers to the administration of some process or medications designed to relieve suffering with the incidental consequence of causing sufficient respiratory depression as to result in the patient's death. The primary intent is not the death of the patient.

mercy killing: The act of killing someone for reasons considered to be merciful.

fair opportunity rule: The rule states that "No person shall receive goods and services on the basis of an undeserved advantage nor be denied goods and services on the basis of an undeserved disadvantage."

false claims act: It is a criminal offense to make or present a fictitious or fraudulent claim against the federal government. 18 U.S.C.A. § 287; 31 U.S.C.A. § 231 et seq.

false imprisonment: The unlawful detention of a person without warrant or by illegal warrant in a prison or a place used temporarily for that purpose, or by force and constraint without confinement.

felony: A crime of a graver nature than those designated as misdemeanors; for example, aggravated assault (felony) as contrasted with simple assault (misdemeanor).

fetus: The term used from the time when brain waves can be monitored (beginning at eight weeks' gestation) until birth.

fiduciary: A relationship in which one person has a legal duty to another for which the former is accountable and is required by law to act on the latter's behalf. Common fiduciary relationships include those between lawyer and client, corporate officer and shareholder, civil servant and public, partners in business, and in some contexts, physicians, nurses, and health care providers and their patients. Also, to hold in trust, having the nature of a trust.

fraud: An intentional perversion of the truth in an attempt to induce another in reliance upon it to part with some valuable personal belonging or to surrender a legal right.

free market: A system of allocation that is generally based on the free exchange of goods and services.

gatekeeping: A generic term used for a whole series of activities needed to protect the profession from those who would misuse the appropriate functions of that specialty. An example of the gatekeeping function is the requirement that a professional report the misconduct of another.

Golden Rule: A statement of the idea that one is to "do unto others as one wishes to be done unto."

Good samaritan laws: Laws designed to protect individuals who stop to render aid in an emergency. The laws are designed to provide immunity for specified persons from civil suit arising out of care rendered during an emergency, provided that the one rendering assistance has not done so in a grossly negligent fashion.

harm principle: When the practitioner can foresee a danger to an individual outside of the patient-provider relationship, potentially caused by the patient; the harm principle provides the rationale for breaching confidentiality to warn the vulnerable individual.

hedonic calculus: A system devised by Jeremy Bentham for measuring the pleasure and pain generated from a given situation. The system evaluated seven criteria: intensity, duration, nearness, certainty, fruitfulness, purity, and extent.

hedonism: The doctrine that the chief good of man lies in the pursuit of pleasure.

high risk behaviors: A series of behaviors that are associated with the spread of HIV.

HIV: Human immunodeficiency virus is a retrovirus that is the precursor to AIDS.

homicide: The killing of one human being by the act, procurement, or omission of another.

Homo sapiens: Modern man is the only extant species of the genus *Homo; sapien* is taken from a Latin term meaning "to be wise."

imperfect obligations: Claims that do not create obligations. An example is the duty to be compassionate or charitable. We can sense these as obligations, but their time and place of performance is left to autonomous choice.

indirect euthanasia: See *euthanasia.*

informed consent: A patient's agreement to allow something to happen based on a full disclosure of the facts necessary to make an intelligent decision. Appropriate disclosure requires the physician to make sure the patient understands the nature of the condition, the treatment options, and the risks involved.

institutional ethics committee (IEC): Can be defined as an interdisciplinary body of health care providers, community representatives, and nonmedical professionals who address ethical questions within the health care institutions, especially on the care of patients.

institutional review board (IRB): Boards that examine protocol design for research to ensure that the research conforms to appropriate standards.

interogatories: A list of questions sent from one party in a lawsuit to the other party to be answered under oath.

invasion of privacy: The unwarranted appropriation or exploitation of someone else's personality; publicizing another's private affairs with which the public has no legitimate concern; wrongful intrusion into another's private activities in such a manner as to cause mental suffering, shame, or humiliation to a person of ordinary sensibilities.

involuntary euthanasia: See *euthanasia.*

irrational suicide: See *euthanasia.*

joint venturing: In common usage, the situation in which a health professional has an investment in a health care facility.

justice: The principle that deals with fairness, and entitlements in the distribution of goods and services.

laws: Rules promulgated by government as a means to an ordered society. In common usage it refers to legislative statutes, court made law, as well as administrative rules, regulations, and ordinances.

legal: Conforming to the law; according to the law; required or permitted by the law.

legal right: See *right.*

liability: The state of being bound or obliged by law or justice to do or pay, or make reparations for something.

liability insurance: That type of insurance protection which indemnifies one from liability to third persons as contrasted with insurance coverage for losses sustained by the insured.

libel: A method of defamation expressed through print, writing, pictures, or signs.

litigious: Fond of litigation; prone to engage in suits.

living will: A document where in an individual identifies a preference for withholding life support in the event that individual becomes incapacitated and no longer able to make decisions regarding self.

managed care: A health care plan such as an HMO that manages costs by monitoring health professionals, requiring preauthorization for hospitalization and other services, and limiting referrals to specialists.

materiality test: The test of whether the risk or hazard is of great enough significance to be included within the informed disclosure by the physician. The decision of materiality is made on the basis of whether it would be significant enough to influence the patient's decision.

mean: The moderate position; the position between two extremes.

medical utility: A form of allocation of health care goods and services based on best prognosis.

medicide: The termination of life by a medical specialist; also the title of a book by Dr. Kevorkian.

mercy killing: See *euthanasia*.

misdemeanor: Offenses lower than felonies and generally those punishable by fines rather than time served in a penitentiary.

moral: Of or concerned with the judgment principles of right and wrong in relation to human actions and character.

moral duty: An act or course of action that is required by one on the basis of moral position.

morality: The doctrine of moral duties; quality of an action in regard to right and wrong.

moral option: The power or right to choose among several alternatives on the basis of a moral question.

moral right: See *right*.

natural right: See *right*.

negative right: A form of right that binds others to noninterference, but does not create an obligation on the part of others to supply us goods or services. Most of our unalienable rights (life, liberty, pursuit of happiness) are negative rights. Also, see *right*.

negligence: The failure to do something that a reasonable person would do when guided by those considerations that regulate human affairs; the doing of something that a reasonable and prudent person would not do; the failure to exercise ordinary care; the failure to do something that results in an injury; carelessness, thoughtlessness, disregard, inattention, and oversight.

neocortical death: Irreversible loss of high brain function. Often patients who have lost neocortical function have lost the potential for all uniquely human aspects of life, but still maintain vegetative function.

nonmaleficence: The principle that imposes the duty to avoid or refrain from harming the patient. The practitioner who cannot bring about good for the patient is admonished to at least do no harm.

nonvoluntary euthanasia: See *euthanasia.*

ordinance: A rule established by authority; a permanent rule of action; a law or statute.

ordinary and extraordinary care: A differentiation used to determine what level of care is required and that which might be considered optional due to its high costs, low effectiveness, or other criteria.

original position: An imagined state where individuals make choices under a veil of ignorance, as to natural attributes and social status of the individuals involved. In this situation no one making the choice would know what place they would play in the society—they could be a prince or a pauper. Under these conditions, all choices are made so that even the individual who is in the most disadvantaged position would be willing to accept the decision.

parens patria: Originates from English common law in which the king had the authority to act as guardian for persons with legal disabilities. In the United States, the parens patria function belongs to the individual states.

passive euthanasia: See *euthanasia.*

paternalism: A policy or practice of treating or governing people in a fatherly manner, especially by providing for their needs without giving them responsibility. In these cases one interferes with a person's freedom of action or information with the alleged justification being the good of the person being interfered with.

patient-centered standard: A standard which holds that the patient must have the necessary information to make a rational judgment. This would be a subjective standard given that some patients may not meet the criteria of a hypothetical reasonable person.

Patient Self-Determination Act of 1990: Mandates that all health care providers who receive federal reimbursements for services provide information to each patient and offer the option of initiating an advanced directive.

perfect obligations: Claims that justify and create correlative obligations. The right to informed consent is a perfect obligation in that it creates the correlative obligations of providing appropriate information.

persistent vegetative state (PVS): A state characterized by a permanent eyes-open level of unconsciousness.

person: A living entity with moral standing, possibly a right to life (not necessarily equivalent to human).

personhood: The individual state in which one is accepted as having the criteria of humanity. Discussions of personhood have been important in dealing with issues such as withholding and withdrawing treatment, and abortion.

placebo: Substances thought to be biologically inert which are given to patients so as to make them believe they are receiving medications. Although useful as a research practice, the clinical use of placebos creates real problems in the areas of patient autonomy and the duty of truth-telling.

plaintiff: A person who brings an action; the party who complains or sues in civil action.

portability of insurance: Allowing individuals to continue the same insurance coverage between positions, regardless of employment status.

positive right: See *right.*

potential life: A phrase used in the *Roe v. Wade* case to indicate the status of the fetus.

prima facie case: The elements of a case, as established by case law or statute, which a plaintiff must sufficiently prove before a defendant is required to proceed with the case.

primum non nocere: First do no harm. A restatement of the admonition to abide by the principle of nonmaleficence.

principle of utility: The principle in which the right action is that which leads to satisfaction of those desires that the individual prefers to have satisfied.

procedural justice: The principle of justice that calls for due process.

pro-choice: Favoring or supporting legalized abortion.

professional autonomy: Once a patient-practitioner relationship is established, the practitioner has a duty to provide care; however, they are not obliged to perform services believed morally repugnant. Health care providers may, under such circumstances, withdraw from their obligations to provide services.

professional community standard: A standard in which holds the amount of care or amount of disclosure provided is equal to that which practitioners provide in the local community.

pro-life: Advocating full legal protection of human embryos or fetuses, especially by opposing legalized abortion.

prospective payment: A system by which Medicaid and Medicare payments to hospitals are predetermined by diagnosis. The government is willing to pay only this predetermined fixed amount regardless of other extenuating circumstances.

public utility: A system of allocation that attempts to provide the greatest good for the greatest number.

quality of life issue: Determines whether the potential quality of an individual's life should be considered when making decisions in regard to resuscitation or other extraordinary measures.

quickening: The point usually within the second trimester at which the mother feels the fetus move.

qui tam: Who as well for the King for himself sues in the matter. These suits are often associated with the incentive provided for whistle-blowing by the federal government in the passage of the False Claims Act.

randomized clinical trials: An applied research study when members or a population of patients are assigned to either a "study" group or a "control" group in a random manner.

rational suicide: See *euthanasia*.

reasonable man test: A legal standard of care for negligence that requires the defendant to act as would a reasonably prudent person under similar circumstances, accounting for age, education, physical impairment, and the emergency situation.

reasonable patient standard: A standard in which the physician must provide enough information to the patient, so that a hypothetical reasonable person could understand and make autonomous decisions.

recipient right: See *right*.

relativist: An individual who believes that truth is not an absolute, but is relative to the individual or group that holds the belief.

res ipsa loquitor: The thing speaks for itself. In regular cases of negligence the plaintiff must prove injury.

However, in certain circumstances, such as a surgical instrument being left in a patient, it becomes obvious that an injury has occurred regardless of who directly caused it. In these certain circumstances it is said res ipsa loquitur, the thing speaks for itself.

respect for persons: A basic health care principle that includes these sub-principles: patient autonomy, confidentiality, and veracity.

respondiat superior: The legal principle that the employer is responsible for those acts of his or her employees that are performed within the scope of employment.

right: A justified claim that demands respect. The following list includes different types of rights.

> **human right:** Rights shared by humans as a condition of their humanity. An example would be a right to food and shelter.

> **legal right:** A claim or entitlement, justified by legal principles and rules.

> **moral right:** A claim or entitlement, validated by moral principles or rules.

> **natural right:** One that preexists society and is a component of our existence.

> **negative right:** Justified claims that obligate others to refrain from interfering. One example is the right of personal liberty.

> **positive right:** Justified claims that obligate others to provide something. One example is a veteran's right to health care under the law.

> **recipient right:** A form of positive rights when a justified claim to goods or services exists. Recipient rights are positive rights.

unalienable right: One that cannot be taken away; it exists as a function of human existence. All natural rights are unalienable.

right–to–die movement: A group of individuals who subscribe to the concept that, with the protected rights of life, liberty, and the pursuit of happiness, individuals have the right to decide when life should be ended.

right to privacy: The right to be left alone; the right of a person to be free from unwarranted publicity.

risk management department: A department in a clinical setting that is charged with assessing the legal liability in situations and advising personnel in ways to lower the risk.

role fidelity: The faithful execution of duties required by each practice within the health care system. Role fidelity forms the basis for the ethical system known as virtue ethics.

RU 486: A controversial abortion pill that would allow most abortions to take place without the use of surgical procedures and in a far more private manner.

rule utilitarianism: The doctrine that certain rules have been found to have a high utility; that is, have brought about the greatest happiness for the greatest number. These rules can then be used in similar situations without attempting to measure the exact amounts of happiness gained or pain avoided. An example of such a rule is that one should never yell "fire" (when there is no fire) in a dark and crowded theater.

safe sex: A series of practices designed to allow for sexual contact that minimizes spread of HIV. The most important aspect of these practices is the use of condoms.

scope of practice: The tasks included within the practice of the specialty. Quite often the scope of practice is set forth in the legal regulations that allow the practice within a state.

self-referral: A term used to describe a health care provider's referral of patients to an outside facility in which the provider has a financial interest but no professional responsibility.

slander: The speaking of defamatory words tending to prejudice another in reputation, office, trade, business, or means of livelihood.

Slippery Slope Argument: The argument posits that if a certain act is allowed it will cause or tend to allow other less positive acts to occur. The allusion is to a slippery slope.

social utility: A system that allocates goods and services on the basis of social merit. If the president of the United States needed a heart transplant, he might be given priority based on his position in our society.

standard of care: The degree of care and skill associated with a particular profession, as a whole, in rendering examinations or treatment for a particular condition.

standard precautions: In 1996 the CDC released an update of the universal precautions that protected health care providers from bloodborne pathogens such as HIV and hepatitis B. These new standard precautions include new information from both the universal precautions and body substance isolation, as well as new terminology to avoid confusion with existing systems.

stare decisis: Let the decision stand. A doctrine that requires courts to follow or adhere to previously decided cases.

statutory law: Introduced or governed by statute, as opposed to common law.

substituted judgment standard: A proxy decision-making standard in which the guardian is directed to make the decision compatible with the previous wishes of the individual.

sufficing solution: For every problem there is the best answer and other options that might not be the best but will still suffice. Sometimes one may not choose the absolute best answer due to cost or other factors and will adopt a sufficing solution. A solution that meets present needs.

teleological: The philosophical study of design or purpose in natural phenomena.

therapeutic abortion: An abortion induced for medical reasons, as when pregnancy poses a danger to the woman's health.

third-party payers: Agencies such as insurance companies or governmental programs that are called upon to pay for health care services; also known as fiscal intermediaries.

tort: A legal wrong committed upon a person or property independent of contract; the violation of some private duty by which damages accrue to the individual; a private or civil wrong as opposed to criminal wrong.

triage: A system that divides patient cases into categories so that care can be allocated effectively.

unalienable right: See *right*.

utilitarianism: The doctrine in which utility is the sole standard of moral conduct; often expressed as the greatest happiness for the greatest number. To save the doctrine from becoming a pig-philosophy, happiness is defined in terms of higher order pleasures such as social enjoyments, intellectualism, and aesthetics.

utilization review: A review of the appropriateness of care and the various types of patient care provided within an institution; usually designed to ensure appropriate and cost-effective care.

writ: A written order that is issued to a person, requiring the performance of some specified act or giving authority to have it done.

veracity: To tell the truth. The practice of health care is best served in a relationship of trust when practitioner and patient are bound to the truth.

viability: The stage at which the fetus can live independent of the mother's womb.

voluntary euthanasia: See *euthanasia.*

wedge argument: An argument that posits that if one act is allowed it opens the way for other less positive acts to occur.

world view: An individual's set of subjective values that are received from religious backgrounds, cultural heritage, and personal experiences.

zygote: Comes into being in the first twenty-four hours after conception with the splitting of the conceptus and continues until it becomes implanted into the uterine wall.

Index